Spiritual Care in Nursing Practice

Kristen L. Mauk, PhD, RN, CRRN-A, APRN, BC
Associate Professor of Nursing
Valparaiso University
Valparaiso, Indiana

Nola A. Schmidt, PhD, RN
Assistant Professor of Nursing
Director, Congregational Health Project
Valparaiso University
Valparaiso, Indiana

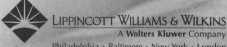

LIPPINCOTT WILLIAMS & WILKINS
A **Wolters Kluwer** Company
Philadelphia • Baltimore • New York • London
Buenos Aires • Hong Kong • Sydney • Tokyo

Senior Acquisitions Editor: Margaret Zuccarini
Senior Developmental Editor: Renee A. Gagliardi
Editorial Assistant: Carol DeVault
Senior Production Editor: Rosanne Hallowell
Director of Nursing Production: Helen Ewan
Managing Editor / Production: Erika Kors
Art Director: Carolyn O'Brien

Design: BJ Crim
Cover: Vasiliky Kiethas
Senior Manufacturing Coordinator: Michael Carcel
Manufacturing Manager: William Alberti
Indexer: Victoria Boyle
Compositor: Lippincott Williams & Wilkins
Printer: R.R. Donnelley/Crawfordsville

9 8 7 6 5 4 3 2 1

ISBN 0-7817-4096-7

Library of Congress Cataloging-in-Publication Data available upon request.

Care has been taken to confirm the accuracy of the information presented and to describe generally accepted practices. However, the authors, editors, and publisher are not responsible for errors or omissions or for any consequences from application of the information in this book and make no warranty, express or implied, with respect to the content of the publication.

The authors, editors, and publisher have exerted every effort to ensure that drug selection and dosage set forth in this text are in accordance with the current recommendations and practice at the time of publication. However, in view of ongoing research, changes in government regulations, and the constant flow of information relating to drug therapy and drug reactions, the reader is urged to check the package insert for each drug for any change in indications and dosage and for added warnings and precautions This is particularly important when the recommended agent is a new or infrequently employed drug.

Some drugs and medical devices presented in this publication have Food and Drug Administration (FDA) clearance for limited use in restricted research settings. It is the responsibility of the health care provider to ascertain the FDA status of each drug or device planned for use in his or her clinical practice.
LWW.com

We dedicate this to God, for His abundant blessings,
and
to all nurses who bless others with their spiritual care.

Contributors

Susan Weber Buchholz, RNC, PhD
Adult Nurse Practitioner
Purdue University Calumet
Hammond, Indiana

Marie T. Cahn, DNS, RN
Associate Professor of Nursing
Purdue University Calumet
Hammond, Indiana

George Fitchett, DMin
Associate Professor and Director of
 Research
Department of Religion, Health and
 Human Values
Rush-Presbyterian-St. Luke's Medical
 Center
Chicago, Illinois

**Christoffer H. Grundmann, M.th:
 Dr. theol.: Dr. habil**
John R. Eckrich Professor of
 Religion and the Healing Arts,
 University Professor
Valparaiso University
Valparaiso, Indiana

Nancy Habermeier, RN, BSN
Lay Minister—Parish Nurse
Pastoral Assistant—Caring Service
 Ministry
Trinity Lutheran Church
Roselle, Illinois

Theodore M. Ludwig, PhD, ThD
Surjit Patheja Professor of World
 Religion and Ethics
Department of Theology
Valparaiso University
Valparaiso, Indiana

Rev. Kevin Massey, MDiv, BCC
Staff Chaplain
Department of Mission and Spiritual
 Care
Advocate Illinois Masonic Medical
 Center
Chicago, Ilinois

Rev. Patricia A. Roberts, DMin
Pastor
Maple Grove United Methodist Church
New Carlisle, Indiana

Cynthia A. Russell, DNSc, RN, CS
Dean and Professor
Samaritan College of Nursing
Grand Canyon University
Phoenix, Arizona

Freda Scales, RN, MDiv, PhD
Associate Pastor
Trinity Lutheran Church
Valparaiso, Indiana

Karon Schwartz, PhD, RN
Nursing Consultant
Bereavement Counselor
Centerville, Michigan

David G. Truemper, PhD
Professor and Chair, Theology
Valparaiso University
Valparaiso, Indiana

LaVerna VanDan, RN, MSN
Advocate and Consultant
Valparaiso, Indiana
Former Parish Nurse Program
 Coordinator
Franciscan Communities
Crown Point, Indiana

Reviewers

Helen E. Ahearn, MS, APRN, BC
Assistant Professor, Coordinator,
 Woburn Program
Department of Nursing
Emmanuel College
Boston, Massachusetts

Katrina Barnes, MS, RN
Assistant Professor of Nursing
Clayton College and State University
Morrow, Georgia

Suzanne H. Carpenter, MSN, RN
Associate Professor of Nursing
Our Lady of the Lake College
Baton Rouge, Louisiana

Janet Dahm, PsyD, RN-C
Associate Professor of Nursing
Saint Xavier University
Chicago, Illinois

Ruth Dankanich Daumer, MSN,
 ARNP, CS
Chairperson and Associate Professor of
 Nursing
Briar Cliff University
Sioux City, Iowa

Cheryl Anne Fenton, RN, BHSc
Professor of Nursing
Mohawk College
Hamilton, Ontario, Canada

Janice C. Ford, RN, MS
Adjunct Faculty
Department of Nursing
Anna Maria College
Paxton, Massachusetts

Katherine S. Gallia, PhD, RN,
 AOCN
Associate Professor of Nursing
University of the Incarnate Word
San Antonio, Texas

Rebecca Gesler, RN, MSN
Associate Professor of Nursing
St. Catharine College
St. Catharine, Kentucky

Barbara Schnell Hansmeier, RN,
 MS
Associate Professor of Nursing
College of Saint Benedict
Saint John's University
St. Joseph, Minnesota

Bryan K. Houser, BS, MS, PhD
Assistant Professor of Nursing
Nursing and Allied Health Professions
 Department
College of Health and Human Services
Indiana University of Pennsylvania
Indiana, Pennsylvania

Mary Leetun, MSN, GNP
Associate Professor, Coordinator FNP
 Program
University of Mary
Bismarck, North Dakota

Linda C. Londo, BSN, MS
Assistant Professor of Nursing
Alverno College
Milwaukee, Wisconsin

Nancy G. McAfee, MSN, RN
Program Director, Upward Mobility
 Program (AND)
Lamar State College, Orange
Orange, Texas

Brenda H. Owens, RN, BSN, MSN,
 PhD, CFNP
Coordinator, Family Nurse Practitioner
 Program
Loyola University New Orleans
New Orleans, Louisiana

Pat Prechter, RN, MSN, PNP, EdD
Associate Professor of Nursing
Our Lady of Holy Cross College
New Orleans, Louisiana

Charlotte Stephenson, RN, DSN
Professor, Academic Coordinator
Department of Nursing
Mississippi College School of Nursing
Clinton, Mississippi

Carol R. Taylor, CSFN, RN, PhD
Director, Center for Clinical Bioethics
Georgetown University
Washington, DC

Golden Tradwell, PhD, RN
Associate Professor of Nursing
McNeese State University
Lake Charles, Louisiana

Preface

Nursing practice has focused increasingly on treating the whole person, including biopsychosocial, cultural, and spiritual needs. The growing body of scientific knowledge about the connectedness of spirituality and health attests to the idea that attention to the spiritual aspects of patients or clients is vital to providing quality nursing care.

One unique feature of *Spiritual Care in Nursing Practice* is the emphasis on interdisciplinary authorship. Nurse educators, theologians, chaplains, ministers, and parish nurses contributed to chapters, providing a comprehensive, collaborative flavor to the work. Use of the nursing process to organize the content is another distinctive feature.

Objectives and key terms appear at the beginning of each chapter. Each chapter has one or more case studies with critical thinking questions and personal reflection questions. References are up-to-date, with additional recommended readings or resources listed. In addition, web sites listed in tables help today's computer-savvy learners link to other information on the World Wide Web. Throughout the text, readers will find symbols, representing the major religions, to help identify content related to the different faiths. A key to these symbols follows this preface.

Chapter 1, Spirituality as a Life Journey, provides a basic introduction to major concepts and philosophies of spiritual care. It examines definitions of spirituality, religion, faith, and spiritual health. It also discusses concepts central to spirituality such as suffering, hope, compassion, grace, and forgiveness. While exploring the relationships between spirituality and health, the unit discusses spiritual care. These concepts are foundational to the case studies in subsequent chapters.

Chapter 2, Spiritual Development Across the Lifespan, presents Fowler's theory of spiritual development in light of the developmental theories of Piaget, Erikson, and Kohlberg. It examines these theories for similarities and differences to show how physical, cognitive, emotional, social, and spiritual developments are related, contributing to the whole person. It also discusses cognitive and affective domains, as well as the generations associated with stages of faith.

Chapter 3, Development of Spiritual Care, presents an overview of the role of nurses through the history of spiritual care nursing. It discusses the events and people who have created a system of caring for the body, mind, and spirit, especially as related to nursing.

Unit 2, The Uniqueness of the Spiritual Journey: Understanding Religious and Cultural Influences on Health and Nursing (Chapters 4 through 12) provides specific information about a wide variety of religions (Judaism, Christianity, Islam, modern religions, Voodoo and indigenous American traditions, South Asian religions, Buddhism, and East Asian religions) and explains how religion and culture are intertwined. The information in this unit will help nurses and other health care providers understand how religious beliefs and practices influence health care and lifestyles, which will enable them to provide more competent care to those who practice these religions. The unit also addresses health care methods related to Eastern philosophies, such as acupuncture, herbs, and touch therapy.

Using the nursing process as a framework, the chapters in *Unit 3, Spiritual Care and the Nursing Process,* provide further insight into the spiritual care of patients. Each chapter describes parts of the nursing process, building on the concepts introduced in Unit 1. *Chapter 13, The Role of the Nurse in the Spiritual Journey,* discusses the role components of the professional nurse and the advanced practice nurse in relation to providing spiritual care. It also presents the four metaparadigm concepts of nursing using a curricular conceptual model from Valparaiso University. It addresses the processes of critical thinking, communication, lifelong learning, and change in relationship to spirituality and nursing practice. *Chapter 14, Assessment and Diagnosis in Spiritual Care,* describes spiritual screening, spiritual history taking, and spiritual assessment, which nurses can use to initiate spiritual care. It also identifies nursing diagnoses, including NANDA terms commonly used when providing spiritual care. *Chapter 15, Planning, Implementing, and Evaluating Spiritual Care,* discusses various interventions based on the Nursing Interventions Classification (NIC) that nurses use to provide spiritually competent care. These include prayer, hope instillation, acupuncture, herbal and vitamin therapy, massage, meditation, yoga, and tai chi, as well as a variety of therapeutic arts, such as drama, music, art, humor, and animal assistance. Using the Nursing-Sensitive Outcome Classification (NOC), this chapter also focuses on ways to evaluate the success of spiritual care, including the importance of documentation. The chapters in this unit conclude with case studies that emphasize the part of the nursing process discussed, featuring patients/clients with a variety of spiritual needs and using primary, secondary, and tertiary levels of prevention.

Unit IV, Nursing Issues in Spiritual Care, provides insight into issues integral to spiritual care. *Chapter 16, Collaboration in Spiritual Care,* explores the importance of teamwork when caring for the spiritual needs of others. It examines the roles of different team members for their contribution to competent spiritual care. With an emphasis on collaboration, it discusses spiritual care both in health care settings and in congregations. *Chapter 17, Ethical Issues in Spiritual Care,* discusses the confusion, complexity, and controversy surrounding the relationships of spirituality and ethics. It examines the two most commonly used frameworks, Deontology and Teleology, in light of spiritual care and the ANA Code of Ethics for Nursing. *Chapter 18, Nursing Research About Spirituality and Health,* explores the role of research in spiritual care and research instruments used to study spirituality, while presenting a cross-section of current nursing studies about spirituality and health. Finally, *Chapter 19, The Nurse's Spiritual Health,* includes strategies to help nurses stay in touch with their spiritual selves and avoid compassion fatigue.

The target audience for this text is broad in scope. The book is appropriate for undergraduate nursing students and their instructors, either in a basic nursing course or an elective course. Graduate nursing students may find this a helpful reference. Clinical cases also assist in making this a useful text for a wide range of staff nurses working in a variety of settings that emphasize spiritual care, such as hospices, oncology units, and religiously affiliated hospitals and facilities. Parish nurses working in the community would likely consider it a key manual for practice. Because of the interdisciplinary authorship of the text, other students, health care providers, and clergy also may find the content helpful.

Nurses often have the unique task of walking with people on portions of their life journey. Using a holistic perspective means to view individuals as biopsychosocial beings with a spiritual core, each component of the self integral to and influencing the others. Nurses must address the spirit to provide holistic and competent care. Through provision of spiritual care, nurses can make both subtle and significant enrichments to the life journeys of their patients.

Kristen L. Mauk, PhD, RN, CRRN-A, APRN, BC
Nola A. Schmidt, PhD, RN

Key

Key for Religious Symbols Used Throughout Text

WORLD RELIGIONS

Hinduism

Buddhism

East Asian

Judaism

Christianity

Islam

NATIVE AMERICAN RELIGIONS

MODERN RELIGIOUS MOVEMENTS OF THE 19TH AND 20TH CENTURIES

Christian
Science

Jehovah
Witnesses

Mormonism

Voodoo

Acknowledgments

We acknowledge our colleagues at the College of Nursing at Valparaiso University for supporting us in this endeavor, as well as allowing publication of their original conceptual model. We are especially indebted to Renee Gagliardi, Senior Developmental Editor at Lippincott Williams and Wilkins, for her guidance and expertise. Thanks to Margaret Zuccarini, Senior Acquisitions Editor at Lippincott Williams and Wilkins, for her assistance during preparation of the proposal, and Rosanne Hallowell, Senior Production Editor, for her assistance during final editing. All chapter authors provided invaluable assistance in the completion of this book. Additionally, we thank Gregg Hertzlieb, Director/Curator of the Brauer Museum of Art at Valparaiso University, for his talented contribution of religious symbols. Lastly, thanks to the reviewers for their critical insights and suggestions.

Contents

1

Spirituality as a Life Journey

Nola A. Schmidt and Kristen L. Mauk

LEARNING OBJECTIVES

At the end of this chapter, the reader will be able to:
- Define common terms related to spirituality.
- Explain the relationship between spirituality and faith.
- Discuss how spiritual health is interrelated with physical, mental, and social components.
- Identify the role of culture in spirituality.
- Distinguish the concepts of suffering, hope, compassion, grace, and forgiveness.
- Recognize the importance of providing spiritual care.
- Discuss common research findings in the area of spiritual care.
- List at least one new strategy to implement when providing spiritual care.

compassion   hope
culture   religion
faith   spiritual care
forgiveness   spiritual health
grace   spirituality
holistic   suffering

The road of life often is filled with twists and turns, ups and downs, and precipitous waysides. People who are facing potentially long-term or debilitating illnesses, confronting acute health crises, or suffering from loss and grief may find themselves re-examining the foundational beliefs they have held since childhood. Usually, at no other time in a person's life is he or she so focused on evaluating the spiritual self than during such crises. Yet the times when patients are most vulnerable also can be opportunities for personal and spiritual growth.

Nurses have the unique task of working with patients at various and multiple points throughout their life journeys. Often, nurses encounter patients during the "rough parts of the trail." The **holistic** nursing perspective requires nurses to view each person as a biopsychosocial being with a spiritual core. Each component of the self (physical, mental, social, and spiritual) is integral to and influences the others. Thus, nurses must be sure to address the spirit along with the other dimensions to provide holistic care (Figure 1-1).

Spirituality is an abstract concept involving many facets. To appreciate its many aspects, one must first understand several related definitions and concepts. This chapter begins by providing a basic overview of spirituality and how it differs from religion. It introduces the reader to how spiritual health is connected with physical, psychological, and social health. It discusses key concepts, such as suffering, hope, compassion, grace, and forgiveness. The chapter concludes with a preliminary discussion of spiritual care in nursing.

OVERVIEW OF SPIRITUALITY

Spirituality and Religion

The term *spirituality* often is used loosely, interchangeably, and mistakenly in place of the term religion. However, these two terms are distinct and not equivalent.

Spirituality is the core of a person's being and usually is conceptualized as a "higher" experience or a transcendence of oneself. Often, such an experience involves a perception of a personal relationship with a supreme being (such as God). However, many who consider themselves spiritual deny such identification with a higher power. Spirituality, then, also encompasses feelings and thoughts that bring meaning and purpose to human existence or to one's life journey.

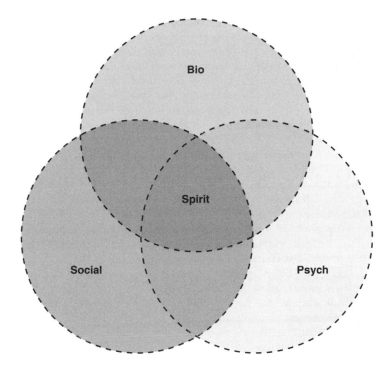

FIGURE 1-1 Holistic person model.

Religion means the organized beliefs, rituals, and practices with which a person identifies and wishes to be associated. It generally involves worshipping a deity or supreme being and gathering with those of like faith or similar beliefs. When comparing these definitions of spirituality and religion, one may observe that a person may claim to be highly spiritual, yet not religious. A common denominator among those who claim to be spiritual yet not religious would be the notion of transcending the commonplace and searching their souls for deeper meaning. Conversely, some people who are religious generally express their spirituality through identification and involvement with an organized religion.

"Spirituality is known and experienced in relationships" (Burkhardt & Jacobson, 2000, p. 95). Relationships with others have been described as a horizontal dimension of spirituality that intersects with a vertical relationship with God (Stoll, 1989). Thus, it is not surprising that people of most religions come together to worship, communing in the presence of God and one another. The nature of a person's connectedness with God can mirror his or her relationships with others. For instance, a person who senses God's love expresses love and compassion for and with others frequently. Conversely, people who harbor anger at God often seem irritated with others. Lack of connection with others can lead to isolation, causing people to become disconnected from themselves as well as others. Isolation erodes the spirit, diminishing one's sense of spiritual well-being and possibly contributing to spiritual distress. It is through relationships based on sharing (both giving and receiving) that people can come to know themselves in life's journey.

🖊 Connectedness with nature also is associated with spirituality. Who has never been inspired by the magnificence of the universe or the wonders of the human body? People can experience a sense of the awesome through connections with nature. Being in nature frequently allows people to reconnect with themselves; thus, it is not surprising that "retreats" frequently occur in places of natural tranquility, rather than in the bustle of the city. For many people, such as Native Americans, spirituality is grounded in their relationship with the earth. People also may find meaning in their relationships with pets. Studies have indicated that interactions with animals can be healing (Johnson & Meadows, 2002; Kaiser, Spence, McGavin, Struble, & Keilman, 2002; Spence & Kaiser, 2002). Our relationship with nature can also be viewed as a horizontal relationship, and these are relationships are depicted in Figure 1-2.

Thus, spirituality is a melding of connectedness—with a higher power, with others, and with the surrounding world—as a person seeks meaning to life's journey. Maddox (2002) states, "Spirituality is a belief system based on intangible elements that impart vitality and add meaning to life events." Walter (2002) suggests that spirituality needs to be individualized "as a particular kind of discourse" (p. 133) and cannot be placed into a restricted mold. Dunne (2001) posits that spirituality is related to the search for "ultimate meaning" (p. 23) beyond ourselves. This idea becomes particularly important at the end of life.

Faith is a multidimensional concept that is significant in discussions of spirituality because it links spirituality to health (Droege, 1991; Wylie & Solari-Twadell, 1999). Faith allows people to hold beliefs that cannot be directly observed. For example, some people have faith that God will heal them or that their friend will keep a promise. Faith can be deeply moving and personal, fostering people as they find meaning in life's journey and view themselves in relation to God and others (Fowler, 1981). For more details about the development of faith, the reader is referred to Chapter 2.

Spiritual and Physical Health

Health generally is defined as the presence or feeling of wellness. However, the term is highly subjective and takes on different meanings for different people. For example, an elderly woman with chronic arthritis may appear frail and worn, yet that woman may report her health as good. Another person may seem to be in wonderful physical condition, yet report his health to be only average or poor.

Some have placed health on a continuum with diametrically opposing ends, saying that each person moves back and forth along this spectrum. When a person re-

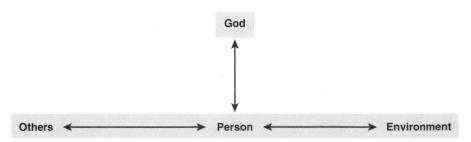

FIGURE 1.2   Vertical and horizontal dimensions of spiritual relationships.

ports feeling healthy, he or she generally is considered to have positive feelings of well-being. When a person feels unhealthy or ill, he or she lacks such feelings of well-being or experiences negative feelings.

Health certainly encompasses the spiritual dimension, and many in the general public, as well as many health care professionals, believe that spiritual and physical health are connected. In a survey conducted in 1996, 99% of 296 family physicians believed that religious beliefs could heal; 75% believed that the prayers of others could promote healing and that "spiritual well-being is an important factor in health" (Larimore, 2001, p. 36). Findings from surveys of the United States public reveal that most believe in the healing power of prayer (Maddox, 2002). Much of this connection between the spiritual and the physical remains a mystery to modern medicine.

Most nurses have encountered or will encounter people whose bodies have been ravaged by disease yet whose spirits remain strong and inspirational. What enables a person to transcend tragedy and illness in this way? How can a person whose life has been forever changed by inexplicable personal loss say that everything is well? Box 1.1 relates the story behind a well-known hymn that illustrates this point.

Likewise, can a person be spiritually ill yet physically healthy? This question is more difficult to answer. Many nurses have observed or will encounter people with relatively minor physical problems who fail to thrive because they have been emotionally and spiritually wounded. Often, the physical body heals faster than does the spiritual self.

Spiritual and Mental Health

When an injury occurs that includes a psychological or emotional component, recovery may take much longer than if the injury had been confined only to the physical dimension. Children who come from homes where they were abused usually carry scars into adulthood that can affect all their mature relationships. Similarly, some women who have been victims of violence at the hands of a father or husband figure often have difficulty relating to God or any other supreme being as loving, caring, and nurturing. Mental and emotional trauma intentionally inflicted by others often leads to distrust and skepticism. Other people suffer mental anguish resulting from their own poor choices or decisions, which later leads to self-blame and guilt. Unchecked, these feelings and emotions can become catastrophic, causing some to turn to negative coping strategies, such as alcoholism, drug abuse, and sexual promiscuity.

Such past experiences, however harmful, also can act as catalysts for true spiritual growth. The spirit can blossom even as a person faces the challenges inherent in working through a painful past. The benefits of health-promoting practices, such as meditating, talking to others, praying, seeking spiritual support, and attending counseling, cannot be overemphasized.

An example of a way that many people achieve spiritual growth by working through psychological and emotional problems is participation in support groups, such as Alcoholics Anonymous (AA). AA and similar organizations were founded to help those with negative habits begin a planned step-by-step program to overcome addictions. Members begin by acknowledging the existence of a power greater than them. People can gain tremendous mental and spiritual support from involvement in such groups, usually resulting in improved physical health as well.

BOX 1.1   "It is Well With My Soul"

The story behind this hymn provides an example of how a person can struggle with enormous personal suffering and loss, yet still experience spiritual wellness. Horatio Spafford lost his only son in 1871 and also lost his fortune in the great Chicago fire. Later, his only four daughters perished at sea when their ship collided with another. Only his wife was rescued. Mr. Spafford penned the words to this famous Christian hymn shortly thereafter when passing the site of his daughters' grave at sea. Read the words and consider how someone experiencing such tragedy can still feel "it is well with my soul." Note the themes of hope and faith in the midst of suffering.

When peace like a river attendeth my way,
When sorrows like sea billows roll;
Whatever my lot, Thou has taught me to say,
It is well, it is well, with my soul.
Chorus:
It is well, with my soul,
It is well, with my soul,
It is well, it is well, with my soul.

Though Satan should buffet, though trials should come,
Let this blest assurance control,
That Christ has regarded my helpless estate,
And hath shed His own blood for my soul.
Chorus
My sin, oh, the bliss of this glorious thought!
My sin, not in part but the whole,
Is nailed to the cross, and I bear it no more,
Praise the Lord, praise the Lord, O my soul!
Chorus
And Lord, haste the day when my faith shall be sight,
The clouds be rolled back as a scroll;
The trumpet shall resound, and the Lord shall descend,
Even so, it is well with my soul.

Spiritual and Social Health

The social component involves relationships with others within the context of culture. **Culture** encompasses many aspects but generally refers to the feelings, attitudes, beliefs, and values of a person or group. Such cultural factors often serve as common denominators between people who feel a kinship with one another. Examples include religion, race, ethnicity, education, socioeconomic status, age, and living arrangements. Thus, culture as a whole may help a person have a sense of belonging or identification with one group or another.

◖ Culture plays an important role in spiritual care because many people adhere to specific beliefs and ideals as a way of life, and these carry over into the most basic aspects of health and illness. A good example is end-of-life care. Each major religion has unique beliefs and practices related to death and dying and care of the dead body (see Chapters 5–12). For example, in Islam, the body must be cremated within days of death. Likewise, a culture may mandate specific ceremonies or rituals at the end of life for dying individuals and their families to promote a peaceful death and to free the spirit for the next life.

CONCEPTS RELATED TO SPIRITUALITY

A discussion of spirituality would be incomplete without the inclusion of key related concepts: suffering, hope, compassion, forgiveness, and grace. Although each concept can be defined uniquely, the human experience encompasses them all.

As providers of spiritual care, nurses will encounter people who are experiencing these aspects, particularly when they are facing a challenging health issue. As spiritual beings, nurses also bring these aspects to their encounters with patients. Nurses aware of how these concepts are interrelated can facilitate the healing process.

Suffering

Suffering is an ongoing state of distress that affects a person's sense of well-being. It can be physical, emotional, social, and/or spiritual in nature (O'Brien, 1999). "Suffering is a fact of human life and a very difficult one to understand" (Roach, 1992, p. 32). Inevitably, nurses encounter patients who are suffering. As Donley (1991) indicated, the mission of nurses includes being "with people who suffer, to give meaning to the reality of suffering" (p. 180).

As people experience suffering, they begin to question "Why me?" (O'Brien, 1999; Roach, 1992; Shelly & Miller, 1999). For many who believe in a loving God, the mystery of why that being would permit suffering in the world becomes paramount. O'Brien suggested that the essence of **spiritual care** is to be with patients when they ask "why me" and to "accept with them the mystery of human suffering, and that we [nurses] offer no false illusions" (p. 131). Eriksson (1994) noted that suffering alone has no meaning, but that people realize a unique meaning by living with suffering.

Little (1989) suggested that a significant purpose of societies is to organize suffering. Using political-legal, educational, and therapeutic institutions, societies legitimize suffering, which then becomes an instrument for restricting, punishing, caring, or avoiding greater pain. Manifestations include racism, incarceration, care of the sick, and advanced directives.

✛ Suffering frequently holds meaning for people in light of their faith traditions. Christians believe that suffering entered the world through sin and was not part of God's original creation. Despite this, God is with people in their suffering. Christians look forward to a time without suffering, made possible by the death and resurrection of Jesus Christ. They can respond to suffering in faith, trusting in God's mercy. The Roman Catholic Church recognizes the World Day of the Sick as a time to reflect upon the nature of suffering in light of God's plan while reflecting on the inspiration of Christian values on health care organizations (Vatican, 2001).

➕ In the book *Suffering into Joy* (Egan & Egan, 1994), the authors discussed what Mother Teresa taught about true joy. The quotes used from Mother Teresa in the book reflect the Catholic belief that Christians who endure suffering become closer to Christ. Many Catholics find meaning in crises by seeing their suffering as linked to the cross of Christ, believing that they then participate in Christ's redemption of the world. Many readers of Mother Teresa's writings express great comfort in the healing messages of her teachings.

➕ An interesting study of the Christian meaning of suffering is found in the novel *Silence* by Shusaku Endo. This story, based on historical fact, examines the horrendous persecution and torture of Japanese Christians in the 1600s. It traces the long and dangerous journey of a Catholic missionary priest who travels to Japan to provide encouragement for the remnants of small churches that have endured unspeakable persecution and torture for refusing to deny their faith. The priest eventually is forced to apostatize in an attempt to save the lives of many Christians. He then must deal with his own guilt and questions about his faith in the face of suffering. The theme of Endo's novel, the difficult question of why God is silent while his people suffer and how people must reconcile this idea with their own beliefs, is striking.

✡ The Hebrew Bible explains suffering as punishment for sin or as a test of character (Shelly & Miller, 1999). The book of Job tells about a man who feared God and lived a holy life but came under extreme suffering because of Satan's challenge to God. In his suffering, Job asked, "why me," but did not reject his faith. In the end, Job remained faithful to God, and God blessed him. Given their history of persecution and suffering in both ancient and modern times, many Jews believe that they must be strong to defend themselves against suffering, demonstrated in a stoic approach to problems they encounter on life's journey. Some Jews look toward a time when the Messiah (savior) will come and lead them to peace.

☾ Muslims believe that Allah (God) is all-powerful and that everything is under his control (Shelly & Miller, 1999). Thus, they accept suffering as part of living according to Allah's will. Islam teaches that Allah primarily uses suffering to build character in his followers, although some suffering may be a punishment. Zakat (alms giving), one of the Five Pillars of Islam, is a social practice that can help to alleviate suffering. In heaven, a place without suffering, there is sensuous delight, and Allah will determine a person's eternal destiny by weighing his or her deeds on a day of judgment.

☯ Buddhism maintains that suffering is central to life (Little, 1989). The first of Buddha's Four Noble Truths teaches that suffering is associated with human passions and greed. Retributive in nature, human suffering results from misdeeds in a previous life. To be free of suffering, a person must confront and embrace it, thereby removing himself or herself from human desires and achieving true understanding or enlightenment.

🕉 Hinduism teaches that suffering is linked to one's caste or station in life. The caste into which a person is born is based on the condition of his or her preceding life. To improve one's *karma* (destiny), the person must seek knowledge of the true self, known as *atman*. As long as a person focuses on his or her false self, suffering exists, and the Hindu will continue to experience the cycle of death and rebirth. Thus, knowledge of atman can help to eliminate suffering.

☯ Unlike Buddhism and Hinduism, Confucianism, derived from the teachings of Confucius, accepts suffering as reality (Taylor, 1989), with no attempts to explain its origin. The fundamental belief is to recognize the need to maintain a balance of yin and yang (positive/negative; male/female; hot/cold) for good life (O'Brien,

1999). Also central to Confucianism is the aim to create a moral society by transforming individuals into virtuous beings. Thus, people must respond to those who suffer because it is the moral thing to do.

While nurses will find it helpful to understand the different religious interpretations of suffering, they also must avoid assumptions. They need to assess each patient's particular perception of suffering. For instance, some authors suggest that the current trends of euthanasia and assisted suicide stem from desires to end suffering, especially when no meaning to the suffering is evident (Roach, 1992; Shelly, Miller, & Shelly, 1999). However, those who find meaning in suffering or accept that suffering cannot be fully understood may find euthanasia and assisted suicide unacceptable. In addition, nurses must recognize that their own perceptions of suffering may influence the way they provide nursing care and that nurses have the right to refuse to participate in actions that they find morally or religiously unacceptable.

Hope

One emotion that significantly helps people endure suffering is hope. **Hope** is an optimistic feeling, desire, or expectation (Burkhardt & Jacobson, 2000; Stoner, 1997). It can be as subtle and simple as wishing for nice weather for tomorrow's outing or as complex as praying for world peace. It can focus on a specific future outcome. It also can make a profound difference in whether one lives or succumbs to death. Viktor Frankl (1959) passionately described how hope contributed to his survival in a Nazi concentration camp, while others, giving in to hopelessness, died. Hope provides people with a sense that the future is in safekeeping (Burkhardt & Jacobson). This sense of optimism about the future is frequently grounded in a person's faith in his or her God.

Nurturing hope has been identified as an important responsibility for nurses as they care for patients (Gewe, 1994; Thompson, 1994). Not surprisingly, nurses have done significant research involving this concept, developing and refining several instruments to measure hope (Stoner, 1997). Findings from studies involving patients with cancer (Ebright & Lyon, 2002; Ersek, 1992; McGill & Paul, 1993), older adults (Herth, 1993; Hicks, 1999; McGill & Paul, 1993), patients with AIDS (Coleman & Holzemer, 1999), and patients with neurological diseases (Foote, Piazza, Holcombe, Paul, & Daffin, 1990) have indicated a strong correlation between hope and positive health outcomes and survival. Other findings have linked hope with spiritual well-being, high self-esteem, and self-transcendence (Carson, Soeken, Shanty, & Terry, 1990; Fehring, Miller, & Shaw, 1997; Haase, Britt, Coward, Leidy, & Penn, 1992; Mickley, Soeken, & Belcher, 1992; Piazza et al., 1991). Another link between spirituality and hope relates to belief in an afterlife. Hope in an afterlife can help individuals who are terminally ill by easing their transition to death because they have an expectation of a "world beyond." Chapter 15 includes strategies that nurses can use to instill hope in their patients.

Compassion

✛ When providing spiritual care to their patients, nurses must base their actions on **compassion**, or sensitivity to the suffering of others. Roach (1992) included compassion as the first of the "five Cs" of professional caring (Box 1.2) and described compassion as "a way of living born out of an awareness of one's relationship to all living creatures; engendering a response of participation in the experience of another; a sensitivity to the pain and brokenness of the other" (p. 58). The Greek word for compassion literally means "to feel in one's innards" (Prior, 1989, p. 35). Given this defi-

---

B O X 1 . 2   The Five Cs of Professional Caring

Compassion
Competence
Confidence
Conscience
Commitment

From Roach, S. M. S. (1992). *The human act of caring: A blueprint for the health professions.* Ottawa, Ontario: Canadian Hospital Association Press.

---

nition, one can easily see how compassion is part of spirituality and the life journey. Compassion can be a gift one receives in the presence of another. Through the role modeling of nursing instructors or spiritual leaders, others also can learn compassion. Compassion as a response to suffering is grounded in religion. Christians live compassion as a way of participating in the compassion of Jesus (Roach, 1992). For example, Mother Teresa led a life of compassion, walking with Jesus as she ministered and served others. Furthermore, Christians profess that the compassionate God the father sent Jesus as the savior for humans in their sin and brokenness.

Ⓢ Confucianists believe that *"jen,* goodness or humaneness, comes very close to our understanding of compassion and caring—one has a moral (and religious) responsibility toward others and cultivates an ability to empathize with their plight" (Taylor, 1989, p. 24). Thus, compassion is a stimulus motivating humans to act morally, to do what is right (Prior, 1989).

◑ In Buddhism, the Larger Self arises as people recognize their connectedness with others and nature. In becoming aware of the Larger Self, people divest themselves of separateness and embrace a self "which is no longer separate from but shared and involved with others, a self that becomes through and with others" (Sabatino, 1998, p. 87). This process invites *karuna,* compassion for all living things.

Compassion is critical to providing holistic nursing care. So often, compassion is neglected, especially in today's heavily economic and business-focused health care industry. The number of tasks that need to be done can overwhelm nurses, leaving little time for compassionate interventions. This also can drain the spirit of the nurse, leading to compassion fatigue (see Chapter 19). It is important that nurses learn to maintain compassion despite demands.

Grace

Compassion, a gift received in the presence of another, also is a gift received through grace. **Grace** is "a blessing that comes into one's life unearned" (Burkhardt & Jacobson, 2000). It empowers people to hope for things to which they are not otherwise entitled.

✚ Christians believe that grace comes to them ultimately from God (*Catechism of the Catholic Church,* 1997; Macquarrie, 1995). "Grace is *favor,* the free and undeserved help that God gives us to respond to his call to become children of God" (*Catechism of the Catholic Church,* 1997). Macquarrie wrote, "just as sin separates from God, so grace unites with God" (p. 13). Christians believe that through God's grace, they participate in the life of God through the death and resurrection of Jesus and the power of the Holy Spirit. Thus, through grace, Christians are liberated from sin and divinized in God's household (McDermott, 1995). The gift of God's Word, the Bible, is also a means of grace, which explains the public reading of scripture during worship (Evangelical Lutheran Church in America, 1996).

God's grace is experienced in interpersonal encounters "whenever there occurs authentic, loving self-transcendence" (McDermott, 1995, p. 8). For instance, in Victor Hugo's novel *Les Miserables* the bishop who forgives the thief is an agent of God's grace (Macquarrie). Grace occurs when a father continues to love his son, despite the son's imprisonment for murder. A woman experiences grace through authentic self-love when, as difficult as it may be, she leaves an abusive relationship and takes responsibility for her new way of life (McDermott). Sittser (1996) describes how his experience of suffering after the death of his wife and children led him to realize his need of and desire for God's grace through everyday living. Volf (1998) recognized through his experience of adopting a child that grace comes to individuals when they experience the ambiguities of life. Thus, grace comes to Christians through relationships with others during times of celebration and times of despair in life's journey.

✚ Sacraments are practices or rituals through which Christians experience God's grace in community (*Catechism of the Catholic Church*, 1997; Evangelical Lutheran Church in America, 1996). In many Christian denominations, the sacraments of baptism and eucharist (Holy Communion) are means of demonstrating God's grace. Baptism washes away sin, confers the righteousness of God upon believers, and fills them with the power of the Holy Spirit. Through Holy Communion, Christians receive forgiveness and salvation by partaking of bread and wine, the body and blood of Christ. Catholics recognize additional sacraments such as the sacraments of healing, which include the sacrament of penance and reconciliation and the anointing of the sick. One can readily see the relevance of the sacraments in situations involving health care professionals.

✪ The Jewish tradition views creation as an act of grace (Hertzberg, 1995). God bestowed his grace on his chosen people of Israel because he loved them. God's grace is linked with human merit; thus, grace can be blocked by human evil or evoked by human righteousness. God hopes that humanity will do good and conquer evil, and by striving to achieve what God wants them to achieve, Jews are graced by God with strengths and resources within themselves and the world around them. In Judaism, grace is the assurance that "the evil people do will fade and not live on; the good may be crushed to earth again and again, but it will rise and prevail, for God always helps" (Hertzberg, 1995, p. 22).

◑ ✚ The everyday world can be experienced as grace through our interconnectedness with others and nature. Based on the premise that caring is the underlying meaning of world, Sabatino (1998) writes:

> Especially in its possibility of care, spirituality allows us to approach God not as apart and separate, but as that grace of being which gathers us into the world in hope and promise of community. In doing so, it manifests God not as we look away from the everyday, but in its midst, especially in the healing touch by which we respond to those among us most in need, whether we do so in terms of the Buddhist symbol of the Larger Self, or the Christian symbol of the empowering, never the overpowering, presence of God. (p. 93)

Given this view, the relationship between caring for others, which is fundamental in nursing and other health care professions, and grace is twofold. First, from the patient point of view, the onset of illness can be a life-changing experience in which one may become aware of God's grace. People recognize grace because of its extraordinary nature. From the viewpoint of nurses, the work of caring for others can often be perceived as "just another day at the office." Thus, caring in the midst of ordinary life can be experienced as grace.

Forgiveness

Another way that grace and compassion are linked to spirituality is through forgiveness. **Forgiveness** is the internal release of emotions attached to past experiences (Burkhardt & Jacobson, 2000). It means abandoning grudges and recognizing that additional punishment of others will not promote healing. It has been said that forgiveness does not necessarily mean forgetting the wrong that has been done, but making a conscious choice not to hold that wrong against a person. Forgiveness is a healing process, regardless of whether one is the recipient or the giver.

✛ Forgiveness occurs in the context of relationships with God, others, and self. Christians seek forgiveness from God by confessing their sins and praying for mercy; they are granted forgiveness by God's grace. In the final steps of the 12-Step Program in AA, members ask for forgiveness from people they have hurt. Forgiving oneself for weaknesses and mistakes is also critical to maintaining a sense of spiritual well-being. Self-forgiveness opens one to receiving forgiveness from others. Forgiveness heals the spirit, allowing one to invest energies previously used for anger and guilt for growth, healing, and movement in a positive direction.

It is not unusual for nurses to encounter patients at the end of life who need assistance in resolving old differences with significant family members or friends. Forgiveness can resolve issues from the past and advance patients toward a peaceful state of mind as they approach death. Remaining family members and friends can find that forgiveness aids in healing during times of grief.

SPIRITUAL CARE IN NURSING

Given that the spirit is the core of a person's being, it certainly is essential to address spiritual care in nursing practice. But how do nurses and other health care professionals provide spiritual care to patients?

Wright (2002) states that "fundamentally, **spiritual care** seeks to affirm the value of each and every person based on nonjudgemental love" (p. 125). Other researchers posit that "the concept of spiritual care was also associated with the quality of interpersonal care in terms of the expression of love and compassion towards patients" (Greasely, Chiu, & Gartland, 2001, p. 629).

In a study using focus groups, Greasely, Chiu, and Gartland (2001) found that spiritual care "related to the acknowledgment of a person's sense of meaning and purpose to life which may, or may not, be expressed through formal religious beliefs and practices" (p. 629). Walter (2002) suggests that spiritual care often is restricted to the English-speaking world, and that other countries consider cure to be the provision of spiritual care. Walter further adds that not all nurses can provide spiritual care to all patients—such delivery depends on the situation and the nurse's spiritual background. Asking patients questions such as whether they believe in an afterlife and if they are a member of a formal belief system or church will help the nurse in planning spiritual care.

Several recent studies related to spiritual care and nursing practice shed light on some current issues. In her study, Vance (2001) found that nurses perceived themselves as highly spiritual, yet only "about 25% of those nurses provided adequate spiritual care to their patients" (p. 268). These nurses identified time constraints and lack of education as the most common barriers to providing spiritual care to patients. Nurses generally report feeling inadequately prepared to administer spiritual care. This is true even of advanced practice nurses. Stranahan (2001) surveyed 102 nurse practitioners with an average age of 50 years regarding their use of spiritual care interventions. The most commonly used interventions were praying privately for a patient and referring patients to clergy or other religious leaders (Stranahan, p. 90). More than 50% of the participants reported rarely or never providing such services. Advanced practice nurses thought they needed more formal education and coursework to provide adequate spiritual care.

In a critical incident study, Narayanasamy and Owens (2001) evaluated 115 nurses providing spiritual care. There was "an overwhelming consensus that patients' faith and trust in nurses produces a positive effect on patients and families, and nurses themselves derived satisfaction from the experience of giving spiritual care" (Narayanasamy & Owens, p. 446). The authors further found that spiritual care could be categorized as personal, procedural, culturalistic, or evangelical. Such categorizations may be helpful in exploring definitions of spiritual care (Box 1.3).

Much research done in the area of spiritual care has been with patients at the end of life. This is not surprising, given that this is often a time when patients and family members seek explanation for crisis and suffering while contemplating the meaning of their lives. Hospice nurses typically have been noted to be skilled at providing spiritual care to patients and families (Sheldon, 2000). Carroll (2001) conducted a phenomenological study of 15 hospice nurses who provided spiritual care to patients with advanced cancer. She found that "the spiritual dimension of care infiltrates all aspects of nursing care" (p. 81). Nurses were working in a spiritual context and had integrated spirituality into their practice.

BOX 1.3 Examples of Spiritual Care

Personal—The nurse uses listening, empathy, and reflective techniques to help the patient explore personal feelings about suffering. This approach can be nonreligious.

Procedural—The nurse uses a logical and technical approach to address spiritual needs by referring patients to the hospital chaplain. Nurses using this approach may have a tendency to stereotype patients.

Culturalistic—At the patient's request, the nurse incorporates cultural sensitivity into care by rearranging the Islamic patient's room so that his bed faces Mecca.

Evangelical—The nurse, who attends a Baptist church herself, relates a faith testimony to her patient who is also Baptist. In this approach, the nurse and patient generally share a common denomination or faith base.

Adapted from Narayanasamy, A., & Owens, J. (2001). A critical incident study of nurses' responses to the spiritual needs of their patients. *Journal of Advanced Nursing, 33*(4), 446–456.

**B O X   1 . 4   Web Sites for Professional Collaboration
About Spirituality and Health**

American Holistic Nurses' Association—http://www.ahna.org
George Washington Institute for Spirituality and Health—
http://www.gwish.org
Health Ministry Association—
http://www.healthmininstriesassociation.org
Interfaith Health Program—The Carter Center—http://www.ihpnet.org
International Center for the Integration of Health and Spirit—
http://www.nihr.org
International Parish Nurse Resource Center—http://www.ipnrc.
parishnurses.org
Nurses Christian Fellowship—http://www.ivcf.org/ncf
Stephen Ministries Foundation—http://www.stephenministry.org

Van Dover and Bacon (2001) developed a grounded theory by examining 20 nurses providing spiritual care in various settings. They found four key elements to be essential in the process of giving spiritual care:

1. Readiness and preparation to provide spiritual care

2. Recognition of spiritual concerns, including cues given by the patient or family

3. Experience in spiritual intervention

4. Ability to move the dialogue with the patient into dialogue with God through prayer (p. 26)

In addition, many studies have revealed prayer to be a common intervention (Dossey, 1996; Easton, 1999; Easton & Andrews, 1999; Easton, Rawl, Zemen, Kwiatkowski, & Burczyk, 1995; Van Dover & Bacon, 2001).

PERSONAL REFLECTIONS

- What is my concept of spirituality?
- How would I describe my current spiritual life? Where am I in my spiritual journey?
- What spiritual experiences have I had that I can use to better understand or relate to my patients having inner struggles?
- When difficult circumstances arise, how do I handle them?
- How would I rate my own spiritual wellness on a scale of 1 to 10? How does this relate to my physical, mental, and social wellness?
- How have I experienced suffering, hope, compassion, grace, and forgiveness?
- What single concept from this chapter is most meaningful to me as I think about providing spiritual care to my patients or family members?
- Name one strategy that I could use to increase my own sensitivity to the spiritual needs of my patients.

Examination of the mentioned studies and other existing literature on spiritual care reveals several common themes. First, nurses believe that providing spiritual care is part of their role, but many are confused about how to incorporate it into practice. Second, nurses at all levels of practice generally feel inadequately prepared to provide spiritual care. Those providing end-of-life care, such as hospice nurses, usually use more spiritual interventions and are more comfortable doing so than are nurses in other settings. Third, spiritual care may be defined in several different ways—nurses must adopt their own definition as well as a way to provide meaningful spiritual care for their patients. Prayer is one of the most commonly accepted forms of spiritual intervention, and the general public believes it effective in promoting healing and well-being. Finally, increasing the academic content related to spiritual care and providing continuing education workshops or classes for nurses in practice would be appropriate to address the concerns of nurses who wish to provide holistic care to their patients.

The nursing profession should promote the provision of spiritual care to patients and families as a fundamental nursing skill. In addition, it should pursue collaboration with health care providers through organizations indicated in Box 1.4 on issues involving spirituality and health. Through provision of spiritual care, nurses can provide both subtle and significant enrichments to the life journeys of their patients.

Key Points
- Spirituality is an abstract concept with many facets. It is the core of a person's being, involving one's relationship with God or a higher power.
- Religion, often confused with spirituality, is an organized set of beliefs.

CASE STUDY 1.1

Julie, a senior student in a baccalaureate program, is taking a course in community nursing. She is caring for a patient, Nancy, who has just started receiving hospice care. Nancy has advanced metastatic breast cancer, which was diagnosed about 9 months earlier. All medical interventions have proved futile, and Nancy has chosen to live her final weeks at home.

Nancy currently spends most of her time in bed and is taking large doses of pain medication. With the help of hospice staff, Nancy's pain is well controlled, and she can converse at intervals with family and friends, although she needs frequent rest periods.

Nancy confides some new concerns to Julie. Nancy has a teenage daughter from her first marriage and a 2-year-old son from her second marriage. Her current husband is very supportive and active in her care. Nancy expresses to Julie that she worries about how her husband will cope with caring for their son once she dies. She also is distressed about who will care for her teenage daughter, with whom Nancy's first husband has little or no contact. She does not want to ask her second husband, whose relationship with his stepdaughter is sometimes strained. Nancy fears that her daughter is not coping well with losing her. Nancy's parents are older, and she worries that they will not be able to handle a teenager.

(case study continues on page 16)

CASE STUDY 1.1 (continued)

Critical Thinking
- What actions does Julie need to take at this time?
- How are issues of suffering, hope, compassion, grace, and forgiveness involved?
- What spiritual interventions would be appropriate?
- What family members need spiritual interventions at this time?
- What resources can Julie use to help Nancy?
- Who can Julie herself go to if she feels inadequately prepared to handle this situation?
- How could this be a growing and learning experience for both Nancy and Julie?

- Human beings are holistic, with biopsychosocial and spiritual aspects.
- Spiritual health is balance between biopsychosocial and spiritual aspects of the person, promoting peace of mind and a sense of wholeness and well-being.
- Suffering, hope, compassion, grace, and forgiveness are concepts central to spirituality.
- Spiritual care in nursing is holistic and multidimensional. It is provided uniquely to each person.

References

Burkhardt, M. A., & Jacobson, M. G. N. (2000). Spirituality and health. In B. M. Dossey, L. Keegan, & C. E. Guzzetta (Eds.), *Holistic nursing: A handbook for practice* (3rd ed., pp. 91–121). Gaithersburg, MD: Aspen.

Carroll, B. (2001). A phenomenological exploration of the nature of spirituality and spiritual care. *Mortality, 6*(1), 81–98.

Carson, V., Soeken, K. L., Shanty, J., & Terry, L. (1990). Hope and spiritual well-being: Essentials for living with AIDS. *Perspectives in Psychiatric Care, 26*(2), 28–34.

Catechism of the Catholic Church, 2nd ed. (1997). Available at: http://www.vatican.va/archive/ccc/index.htm.

Coleman, C. L., & Holzemer, W. L. (1999). Spirituality, psychological well-being, and HIV symptoms for African Americans living with HIV disease. *Journals of the Association of Nurses in AIDS Care, 10*(1), 42–50.

Donley, R. (1991). Spiritual dimensions of health care. *Nursing and Health Care, 12*(4), 178–183.

Dossey, L. (1996). *Prayer is good medicine.* New York: Harper Collins.

Droege, T. (1991). *The faith factor in healing.* Philadelphia: Trinity.

Dunne, T. (2001). Spiritual care at the end of life. *Hastings Center Report, 31*(2), 22–27.

Egan, E., & Egan, K. (1994). *Suffering into joy: What Mother Teresa teaches about true joy.* Ann Arbor, MI: Servant Publications.

Easton, K. L. (1999). The post-stroke journey: From agonizing to owning. *Geriatric Nursing, 20*(2), 70–75.

Easton, K. L., & Andrews, J. C. (1999). Nursing the soul: A team approach. *Journal of Christian Nursing, 16*(3), 26–29.

Easton, K. L., Rawl, S. M., Zemen, D., Kwiatkowski, S., & Burczyk, B. (1995). The effects of nursing follow-up on the coping strategies used by rehabilitation patients after discharge. *Rehabilitation Nursing Research, 4*(4), 119–127.

Ebright, P. R., & Lyon, B. (2002). Understanding hope and factors that enhance hope in women with breast cancer. *Oncology Nursing Forum, 29*(3), 561–568.

Endo, S. (1980). *Silence.* Jersey City, NJ: Taplinger/Parkwest Publications.

Eriksson, K. (1994). Theories of caring as health. In D. A. Gaut & A. Boykin (Eds.), *Caring as healing: Renewal through hope* (pp. 3–20). New York: National League for Nursing.

Ersek, M. (1992). The process of maintaining hope in adults undergoing bone marrow transplantation for leukemia. *Oncology Nursing Forum, 19*(6), 883–889.

Evangelical Lutheran Church in America. (1996). *The use of the means of grace.* Chicago: Author.

Fehring, R. J., Miller, J. F, & Shaw, C. (1997). Spiritual well-being, religiosity, hope, depression and other mood states in elderly people coping with cancer. *Oncology Nursing Forum, 4,* 663–671.

Foote, A. W., Piazza, D., Holcombe, J , Paul, P., & Daffin, P. (1990). Hope, self-esteem and social support in persons with multiple sclerosis. *Journal of Neuroscience Nursing, 22*(3), 155–159.

Fowler, J. W. (1981). *Stages of faith development.* New York: Harper-Collins.

Frankl, V. (1959). *Man's search for meaning: An introduction to logotherapy.* Boston: Beacon Press.

Gewe, A. (1994). Hope: Moving from theory to practice. *Journal of Christian Nursing, 11*(4), 18–21.

Greasely, P., Chiu, L. F., & Gartland, M. (2001). The concept of spiritual care in mental health nursing. *Journal of Advanced Nursing, 33*(5), 629–637.

Haase, J. E., Britt, T., Coward, D. D., Leidy, N. K., & Penn, P. E. (1992). Simultaneous concept analysis of spiritual perspective, hope, acceptance and self-transcendence. *Journal of Nursing Scholarship, 24*(2), 141–147.

Herth, K. (1993). Hope in older adults in community and institutional settings. *Issues in Mental Health Nursing, 14*(2), 139–156.

Hertzberg, A. (1995). Grace in the Jewish tradition. *Living Pulpit, 4*(1), 22.

Hicks, T. J. (1999). Spirituality and the elderly: Nursing implications with nursing home residents. *Geriatric Nursing, 20*(3), 144–146.

Johnson, R. A., & Meadows, R. L. (2002). Older Latinos, pets, and health. *Western Journal of Nursing Research, 24,* 609–620.

Kaiser, L., Spence, L. J., McGavin, L., Struble, L., & Keilman, L. (2002). A dog and a 'happy person' visit nursing home residents. *Western Journal of Nursing Research, 24,* 671–683.

Larimore, W. L. (2001). Providing basic spiritual care for patients: Should it be the exclusive domain of pastoral professionals? *American Family Physician, 63*(1), 36–40.

Little, D. (1989). Suffering in comparative perspective. In R. Taylor & J. Watson (Eds.), *They shall not hurt: Human suffering and human caring* (pp. 53–72). Boulder, CO: Colorado Associated University Press.

Macquarrie, J. (1995). Grace in theology and life. *Living Pulpit, 4*(1), 12–13.

Maddox, M. (2002). Spiritual assessments in primary care. *Nurse Practitioner, 27*(2), 12–13.

McDermott, B. O. (1995). Grace in the authentically human. *Living Pulpit, 4*(1), 8–9.

McGill, J. S., & Paul, P. B. (1993). Functional status and hope in elderly people with and without cancer. *Oncology Nursing Forum, 20*(8), 1207–1213.

Mickley, J. R., Soeken, K., & Belcher, A. (1992). Spiritual well-being, religiousness and hope among women with breast cancer. *Image The Journal of Nursing Scholarship, 24*(4), 267–272.

Narayanasamy, A., & Owens, J. (2001). A critical incident study of nurses' responses to the spiritual needs of their patients. *Journal of Advanced Nursing, 33*(4), 446–456.

O'Brien, M. E. (1999). *Spirituality in nursing: Standing on holy ground.* Sudbury, MA: Jones and Bartlett.

Piazza, D., Holcombe, J., Foote, A. W., Paul, P., Love, S., & Daffin, P. (1991). Hope, social support and self-esteem of patients with spinal cord injuries. *Journal of Neuroscience Nursing, 23*(4), 224–230.

Prior, W. J. (1989). Compassion: A critique of moral rationalism. In R. Taylor & J. Watson (Eds.), *They shall not hurt: Human suffering and human caring* (pp. 33–51). Boulder, CO: Colorado Associated University Press.

Roach, S. M. S. (1992). *The human act of caring: A blueprint for the health professions.* Ottawa, Ontario: Canadian Hospital Association Press.

Sabatino, C. J. (1998). Spirituality: Experiencing the everyday world as grace. *Horizons, 25*(1), 84–94.

Sheldon, J. (2000). Spirituality as a part of nursing. *Journal of Hospice & Palliative Nursing, 2*(3), 101–109.

Shelly, J. A., Miller, A. B., & Shelly, J.A. (1999). *Called to care: A Christian theology of nursing.* Downers Grove, IL: InterVarsity Press.

Sittser, G. L. (1996). Why me? is the most natural human response to personal tragedy. But we might just as well ask: Why not me? *Christianity Today, 40*(3), 23–25.

Spence, L. J., & Kaiser, L. (2002). Companion animals and adaptation in chronically ill children. *Western Journal of Nursing Research, 24*, 639–656.

Stoll, R. I. (1989). The essence of spirituality. In V. B. Carson (Ed.), *Spiritual dimensions of nursing practice* (pp. 4–23) Philadelphia: W. B. Saunders.

Stoner, M. H. (1997). Measuring hope. In M. Frank-Stromborg & S. J. Olsen (Eds.), *Instruments for clinical health-care research* (2nd ed., pp. 189–201). Sudbury, MA: Jones and Bartlett.

Stranahan, S. (2001). Spiritual perception, attitudes about spiritual care, and spiritual care practices among nurse practitioners. *Western Journal of Nursing Research, 23*(10), 90–104.

Taylor, R. (1989). The religious response to suffering. In R. Taylor & J. Watson (Eds.), *They shall not hurt: Human suffering and human caring* (pp. 11–32). Boulder, CO: Colorado Associated University Press.

Thompson, M. (1994). Nurturing hope: A vital ingredient in nursing. *Journal of Christian Nursing, 11*(4), 11–17.

Vance, D. (2001). Nurses' attitudes towards spirituality and patient care. *Medsurg Nursing, 10*(5), 264–269.

Van Dover, L. J., & Bacon, J. M. (2001). Spiritual care in nursing practice: A close-up view. *Nursing Forum, 36*(3), 18.

Vatican. (2001). *Message of the Holy Father for the World Health Day of the Sick for the Year 2002.* Available at: http://www.vatican.va/holy_father/john_paul_ii/messages/sick/documents/hf_jp-ii_mes_2... Accessed October 18, 2002.

Volf, M. (1998). Ambiguity and grace. *Christian Century, 115*, 505–506.

Walter, T. (2002). Spirituality in palliative care: Opportunity or burden? *Palliative Medicine, 16*(2), 133–140.

Wright, M. C. (2002). The essence of spiritual care: A phenomenological enquiry. *Palliative Medicine, 16*(2), 125–132.

Wylie, L. J., & Solari-Twadell, P. A. (1999). Health and the congregation. In P. A. Solari-Twadell & M. A. McDermott (Eds.) *Parish nursing: Promoting whole person health within faith communities* (pp. 25–33). Thousand Oaks, CA: Sage.

Recommended Readings

Albom, M. (1999). *Tuesdays with Morrie.* New York: Doubleday.

Barnum, B. S. (1996). *Spirituality in nursing: From traditional to new age.* New York: Springer.

Daaleman, T. P., & VandeCreek, L. (2000). Placing religion and spirituality in end-of-life care. *Journal of the American Medical Association, 284*(19), 2514–2522.

Drayton-Hargrove, S., & Derstine, J. (2000). *Comprehensive rehabilitation nursing.* Philadelphia: WB Saunders.

Easton, K. L. (1999). *Gerontological rehabilitation nursing.* Philadelphia: WB Saunders.

Easton, K. L., & Andrews, J. C. (2000). The role of the pastor on the interdisciplinary team. *Rehabilitation Nursing, 26*(1), 320–322.

Eliopoulos, C. (2000). *Gerontological nursing* (5th ed.). Philadelphia: Lippincott Williams & Wilkins.

Ferrell, B. R. (1996). *Suffering.* Sudbury, MA: Jones and Bartlett.

Gastins, S., & Forte, L. (1995). The meaning of hope: Implications for nursing practice and research. *Journal of Gerontological Nursing, 21*(3), 17–24.

Honea, C. H. (Ed.). (1996). *A reader's companion to crossing the threshold of hope.* Brewster, MA: Paraclete Press.

Mauk, K. L., Russell, C. A., & Birge, J. (2003). *Congregational health.* Rockford, IL: Hilton.

Miller, J. F. (2000). Coping with chronic illness: *Overcoming powerlessness.* Philadelphia: FA Davis.

Orem, D. (2001). Nursing: *Concepts of practice* (6th ed.). St. Louis: Mosby.

Rawl, S. M., Easton, K. L., Zemen, D., Kwiatkowski, S., & Burczyk, B. (1998). Effectiveness of a nurse-managed follow-up program for rehabilitation patients after discharge. *Rehabilitation Nursing, 23*(4), 204–209.

Scandrett-Hibdon, S. (2000). Therapeutic communication: The art of helping. In B. M. Dossey, L. Keegan, & C. E. Guzzetta (Eds.), *Holistic nursing: A handbook for practice* (3rd ed., pp. 233–246). Gaithersburg, MD: Aspen.

Solari-Twadell, P. A., & McDermott, M. A. (Eds.). (1999). *Parish nursing: Promoting whole person health within faith communities.* Thousand Oaks, CA: Sage.

Weigel, G. (1999). *Witness to hope: The biography of Pope John Paul II.* New York: Cliff Street Books.

Young-Mason, J. (1997). *The patient's voice: Experiences of illness.* Philadelphia: FA Davis.

Resources

Catholic.net
432 Washington Avenue, North Haven, CT 06473
http://www.catholic.net
Provides documents and discussions relevant to the Catholic faith.

The Vatican
http://www.vatican.va
Official web site of the Vatican.

2

Spiritual Development Across the Lifespan

Freda Scales

LEARNING OBJECTIVES

At the end of this chapter, the reader will be able to:
- Recognize the stages of faith development.
- Integrate faith development with typical cognitive, socioemotional, and moral growth and development.
- Link faith development with cognitive domain and affective domain taxonomies.
- Identify generational influences on faith development.
- Respond to others in accordance with their stage of faith development.

faith development
Fowler's Stages of Faith
immanent
spiritual formation
transcendent

F or the purposes of this chapter, the term *faith development* will be used, rather than *spiritual development*. Most developmental theories of a spiritual nature are written to the concept of faith development. Most often **spiritual formation** is the choice of words for spiritual development, and this usually indicates a planned and deliberate spiritual development or spiritual "formation."

Faith development is similar to other types of human growth and development. There are stages and benchmarks, some of which are more noticeable than others. In addition, as with other types of growth and development, faith development is linear. Like other growth and development experiences, sometimes people can be in more than one developmental stage at one time. Sometimes, people step back into a stage or stages previous to the one they are in currently. For a good understanding of the various stages of spiritual development, one can examine growth and development theories and superimpose spirituality or faith development upon any of those theories.

This chapter is based heavily on the work of James W. Fowler, primarily from his texts *Faith Development and Pastoral Care* (1987) and *Weaving the New Creation* (1991). **Fowler's Stages of Faith,** from his classic text of the same name (1981), is referenced frequently in writings related to faith development. Fowler and his associates analyzed more than 500 2-hour interviews, which concerned, among other things, the faith journey or faith development of the interviewees. From those interviews, Fowler and his associates identified seven stages of faith development. Wing says of Fowler:

> His theory of faith development presented in his book, *Stages of Faith* (1981), has become the most popular and commonly accepted theory" of faith development. Fowler's faith development theory has been integrated into many adult research studies within the disciplines of psychology, theology, and... medical science (*Wing, 1997, p. 1*).

Throughout this chapter, references are made to Lawrence Kohlberg (Barger, 2000) and Jean Piaget (Atherton, 2002) in relation to their findings on moral development and cognitive development, respectively. Kohlberg recognized six stages of moral reasoning development; Piaget researched four stages of cognitive development. Erik Erikson's (Huitt, 1997) works are also referenced in relation to his research on socioemotional development. Integrated with Erikson's socioemotional developmental theory is a faith development theory by Larry Stephens (Stephens, 1996).

Fowler, Piaget, Erikson, and Kohlberg, despite the variations in the approaches of their theories, believe that the progression of developmental stages is linear—that is, a person does not skip stages as he or she develops. Nevertheless, all agree that people can be in more than one stage at one time. These four theorists also believe that the stages develop socially—that is, in and amongst contact with society. All the theorists believe that crises, conflicts, or dilemmas are instrumental in the progression from one stage to another. While people work through crises or dilemmas, they gain understanding and wisdom spiritually, cognitively, socioemotionally, and morally, moving them forward into the next developmental stage.

The cognitive domain and affective domain taxonomies of Bloom and Krathwold (Gronlund, 1985) have been included at the end of the chapter. These taxonomies demonstrate how growth and development and faith development are integrated into the levels of learning and the levels of valuing.

This chapter has relied upon another text, *Nurturing Faith Through the Stages of Life* (1998). This Augsburg Fortress manual on faith development not only provides specifics of faith development but also a synopsis by Poling-Goldenne (1998) of "generation" influences on faith formation, which is included at the end of the chapter.

FAITH DEVELOPMENT

Fowler (1991) proposes that faith develops through seven stages. Characteristics of these stages are related to the theories of Piaget, Erikson, and Kohlberg (Table 2.1). Fowler's seven stages develop sequentially, but not equally or completely, in all people. Beginning with the third stage, Mythic-Literal Faith, Fowler begins to attach the age group designation "and beyond" (e.g., Mythic-Literal Faith, Childhood and Beyond). In other words, someone much older than "childhood" may have a Mythic-Literal Faith. An example is an adult who believes in a literal or inerrant translation of the Bible or other sacred texts.

Primal Faith (Infancy)

Primal—original, first, primitive

At birth, or when a person is new to a faith, trust development is a necessity for faith to develop. This is Primal Faith. Infants learn trust through their experiences of taste, sight, sound, touch, smell, and motion. This sensorimotor cognitive stage identified by Piaget corresponds with the Primal Faith stage identified by Fowler. Infants begin cognitive development primarily with sensorimotor responses or reflexes. As children learn through reflexes and responses the predictability (or lack thereof) of their caregivers, they develop trust, again a basis for faith development.

Primal Faith coincides with Erikson's socioemotional developmental stage of trust versus mistrust, which according to him is totally emotionally oriented. Infants, or people new to faith, depend on the caregiver or nurturer, or sponsor, in the case of people new to faith. "Primal Faith forms in the basic rituals of care and interchange and mutuality.... It lays the foundation on which later faith will build," (Fowler, 1991, p. 103). When the caregiver, nurturer, or sponsor cares for infants and persons in the developmental stage of Primal Faith, the infants develop trust. If nurturing needs are not met, infants and persons in the stage of Primal Faith develop mistrust.

TABLE 2.1　Descriptions of Developmental Theories

Theorist	Infant	Early Childhood	Childhood and Beyond
Fowler (faith)	*Primal* First, original, primitive	*Intuitive-Projective* Without conscious reasoning Impulsive	*Mythic-Literal* Imagination of God in anthropomorphic terms Realistic, factual, black and white, no gray
Piaget (cognitive)	*Sensorimotor* Realizes that things continue to exist even when no longer present to the senses	*Sensorimotor* Realizes that things continue to exist even when no longer present to the senses	*Pre-operational* Thinking egocentric Has difficulty taking viewpoint of others Classifies objects by a single feather, e.g., inerrancy of the Bible
Erikson (socioemotional)	*Trust vs. Mistrust* Learns trust by having needs met Mistrusts if needs are met inconsistently or not at all	*Autonomy vs. Shame and Doubt* Expresses self by asserting will Shame develops if self is minimized	*Initiative vs. Guilt; Industry vs. Inferiority* Develops curiosity about the world Develops a sense of industry by successfully accomplishing tasks
Kohlberg (moral)	*Pre-Conventional* Obedience vs. Punishment	*Pre-Conventional* Obedience vs. Punishment	*Conventional* Good boy/girl Law and order

Trust development is the basis and foundation for faith development. Caregivers who consistently return to their children after any separation reduce anxiety in children and foster development of trust. If returns from parents have not been consistent and caring after separations from their children, then a break or dysfunction in the development of trust—and, subsequently, faith—can occur. Tension develops with the separations that infants and children experience. But if parents or caregivers predictably and consistently return, the development of trust and faith becomes greater than the development of mistrust.

The moral reasoning developmental stage of Kohlberg, Obedience and Punishment, coincides with Fowler's Primal Faith stage. During Obedience and Punishment, 2-year-old children react to authority based on reward and punishment, not on a cognitive, reasoned understanding of right or wrong, good or bad. As children are rewarded or punished, their faith begins to develop. Children begin to develop the concept of trust, and thus faith (albeit Primal Faith) based on when they are rewarded and when they are punished.

Primal Faith developmental tasks include the following:

• Separation without anxiety
• Consistent, loving, respectful responses from parents/caregivers/nurturers

Adolescence and Beyond	Young Adulthood and Beyond	Early Midlife and Beyond	Midlife and Beyond
Synthetic-Conventional Composed Ordinary and commonplace	*Individuative-Reflective* Unique, independent, distinct Thoughtful, considered	*Conjunctive* Connected	*Universalizing* Wholistic
Concrete Operational Thinks logically Classifies objects according to several features	*Formal* Operational Thinks logically about abstract propositions and tests hypothesis	*Formal Operational* Thinks logically about abstract propositions and tests hypothesis	*Formal Operational* Thinks logically about abstract propositions and tests hypothesis
Identity vs. Role Confusion Questions who one is Peers are frame of reference	*Intimacy vs. Isolation* Begins to develop intimate relationships with others or work Self-reflective	*Generativity vs. Stagnation* Finds meaning in paradoxes of life	*Ego Integrity vs. Despair* Self based on valued principles
Conventional Good boy/girl Law and order	*Conventional* Good boy/girl Law and order	*Social Contract* Not reached by majority of adults	*Principle Conscience* Not reached by majority of adults

Intuitive-Projective Faith (Early Childhood)

Intuitive—without conscious reasoning
Projective—impulsive

During early childhood, children are full of energy and curiosity. They are impulsive in actions, thoughts, and emotions. The boundaries that parents/caregivers provide or do not provide determine how children develop imaginative, intuitive, and projective faith. This stage shares similarities with the preoperational stage of Piaget's theory of cognitive development, coinciding with impulsive, unreasoned, and Intuitive-Projective Faith.

According to Erikson's socioemotional developmental stage of Autonomy versus Shame and Doubt and Kohlberg's moral development stage of Instrumental Relativist Orientation, young children in their impulsiveness learn with guidance what they can control. Within the development of self-control, they also develop a sense of free will. Children develop either a sense of regret as they receive punishment for acting on unacceptable impulses, or autonomy if they direct their impulsive energies into societally acceptable behaviors and self-control. Depending upon the responsiveness to their behavior by their caregivers, children can develop a view of the spiritual or God as warm, sensitive, and caring, thus encouraging their autonomy and impulsiveness, or as cold, uncaring, and judgmental, encouraging their shame and doubt.

Because children, as well as adults new in their faith, are in the stage of Intuitive-Projective Faith (without conscious reasoning), they develop a sense of their faith through sensations of watching, hearing, smelling, tasting, and touching. Children and those new in the faith accept what others tell them about faith. What they know about faith and spirituality is what they have experienced with others of faith.

When children begin to develop language skills and thus their imaginations, they often cannot tell the difference between what they imagine and what is real. Imagination is a fertile field during the child's faith development and plays a significant part in faith formation. Spiritual and faith stories create images, some of which remain throughout life. Religious symbols can provide good or evil images. The child can imagine a deity as something to fear or something to love. Children and those new in faith learn about faith through stories, simple repetitive songs, and religious celebrations of parents, caregivers, or others.

Intuitive-Projective Faith developmental tasks include the following:

- Reacting
- Listening to stories and fantasies

Mythic-Literal Faith (Childhood and Beyond)

Mythic—imaged
Literal—realistic, factual, black and white, no gray

Between 6 and 8 years of age, children begin to distinguish between make believe and not make believe, between what is imagined and what is real. Even though children of this age group still learn by doing, they have a longer attention span than in earlier years. Nevertheless, children are not yet reflective or deeply aware of an interior self of themselves or others. They act on their needs and wants.

These children are very literal and therefore have concrete images related to their faith. God is mythic and alive in the child's imagination, but is imagined literally. God is everywhere, but usually with a human-like image, and often with a voice.

Children are beginning to understand cause and effect and therefore have a sense of right and wrong in a reasoned but literal sense. They want to be rewarded when they do right and especially want others punished when they have done wrong. Children's spiritual and faith foundation therefore has a sense of right and wrong, reward and punishment, and thus children are in the beginning process of developing an understanding of forgiveness.

Because children have such a concrete image of God, concrete examples, such as examples of their parents or other adults, influence this image. If parents react restrictively and harshly, then children often sense that is how God reacts. If parents react restrictively and lovingly, then children may sense that is how God reacts, and incorporate that into their faith development.

For Piaget, the concrete operational stage of cognitive development begins between 6 and 8 years and beyond. During this stage, logical thinking is beginning to take shape. In Erikson's third stage, Initiative versus Guilt, children begin to take action, explore, and experience remorse for inappropriate actions. Erikson's stage of Accomplishment/Industry versus Inferiority may be involved in the Mythic-Literal stage of faith development, wherein the child begins to develop actions based on standards, rules, or laws. As a result of taking the initiative to act, children learn forgiveness or condemnation when they use initiative. When they make errors or do wrong things, they will experience scolding and then forgiveness (or condemnation without forgiveness).

Because children begin to develop an image of God during the Mythic-Literal stage, depending on the environment, the image of God can be a loving, personal, forgiving one or one of a demand for perfection. Kohlberg's fourth stage of moral development, Orientation Toward Authority, Law, and Duty, corresponds to Fowler's stage of Mythic-Literal Faith. According to Kohlberg, when one is oriented toward authority, law, and duty, then authority and law and duty determine morality.

Even though this stage involving law and order develops in childhood, it has been suggested that most adolescents and adults function primarily within Kohlberg's stages of "good boy/girl vs. bad boy/girl" and law and order (Muuss, 1975, p. 215). Fowler comments that "a fair number of persons—usually men—who may exhibit considerable cognitive sophistication in their occupational worlds, in their emotional and faith lives they are rather rigidly embedded in the structures of Mythic-Literal Faith" (1987, p. 86). In other words, adults cognitively functioning at Piaget's advanced Formal Operations stage might more often than not be functioning at Fowler's less advanced stage of faith development.

Mythic-Literal Faith developmental tasks include the following:

- Acceptance of the inerrancy of the book of faith
- Adherence to behavior codes that can be traced to a specific scripture verse or verses
- Possessing concrete mythical images of God, heaven, and hell

Synthetic-Conventional Faith (Adolescence and Beyond)

Synthetic—composed
Conventional—ordinary and commonplace, generally accepted

In adolescence, abstract and conceptual thinking begin to form. Adolescents still think of God but in human anthropomorphic terms. They often see God as an advisor and friend. However, simultaneously, because of the influence in abstract and analytical thinking, adolescents begin to have doubts about God or spirituality.

Although adolescents still accept much of their parents' attitudes toward faith, they are now going beyond written and verbal stories and are beginning to examine and question the relevance of their own faith in today's world. Sometimes, adolescents have difficulty connecting God or spirituality with the here and now. It is during adolescence that people often ask, "If there is a God, how can God permit floods, wars, and other calamities?" According to Piaget, the Formal Operational Stage of cognitive development (the final stage) begins when a person is approximately 11 years old and continues throughout life. During this stage, the person analyzes and thinks logically about the abstract. Because of this analytical and abstract thinking, he or she begins to question faith.

During adolescence, teens develop friendships that are more than just storytelling sessions. Friends begin to talk with, rather than to, one another. This is when long conversations occur between friends that are not just stories about each other but discussions of what each other thinks and feels. Adolescence is also when young people start seeing themselves as others see them, rather than seeing themselves based on their own needs and motivations. It is when they can form lifelong relationships, including spiritually. "These newly personal relations with significant others correlate with a hunger for a personal relation to God in which the adolescents feel themselves to be known and loved in deep and comprehensive ways" (Fowler, 1991, p.108).

Erikson categorizes the adolescent years as "identity crises" years. Adolescents develop a strong dependence on what others see them as being. Not only are adolescents sensitive to what close confidants and friends think about them, but also to comments and reactions from parents, teachers, and of course those in their faith community (e.g., pastors, rabbis, priests, teachers). What does God think about them? The identity crisis occurs as adolescents juggle what they sense as their self and what others see as who they are. The "self" is interpersonal. It is in this interpersonal stage that people experience God's love and companionship.

Kohlberg continues to characterize the moral development of adolescents as conventional. Adolescents may experience guilt when they fail to follow religious rules or laws.

Adolescents, unless they are questioning God's existence, begin to believe that God is the one who knows them most. It is God, their friends, and those whom they admire whom they think know and understand them. But it is God who truly can see them on the inside and on the outside.

Synthetic-Conventional developmental tasks include the following:

- Talking with friends about the meaning of faith or spirituality
- Believing that God is the only one who really knows them, yet at the same time . . .
- Questioning the existence of God

Individuative-Reflective Faith (Young Adulthood and Beyond)

Individuative—unique, independent, distinct
Reflective—thoughtful, considered

Young adults begin to view themselves beyond how others view them. More self-reflection and less other-dependence occur. Young adults are in charge of themselves, rather than determining themselves through interpersonal relationships with others. There is a relocation of authority from being other directed to more self-directed.

Faith becomes one's own. Analysis and reflection lead to a personal faith, not a faith that mimics someone else's. Faith is no longer based on interpersonal relationships, but more on reasoning, analysis, and questioning. However, in some respects basing faith in reason and analysis can cause faith to lose its mystery of symbol, myth, and ritual.

Because the spiritual analysis that began in the childhood and adolescence now takes "full flight," some young adults claim that they are now atheists. After analysis and reflection, some say it has become "obvious" to them that faith is something we human beings have invented as a crutch by which to live.

If young people remain somewhat active in a faith community, this may be a time that they withdraw from the faith, rather than declare themselves atheists. In their withdrawal, young people often state that they do not want to attend a service and be a "hypocrite like everyone else there."

It is during Individuative-Reflective Faith that "faith" issues become so crucial to young adults, crucial in that it is a struggle for them to form a faith identity. Their cognitive development of formal operational thinking allows them to think abstractly about their faith issues.

Erikson's coinciding personality stage is that of Intimacy versus Isolation. The conviction of this stage is that we are what we love, reflecting the intimacy of the relationship with another. We do not mimic what we love, as in adolescence, but we *are* what we love. In relation to faith, faith is a reflection of the intimacy of the relationship with God. The opposite outcome is isolation. Ironically, intimacy with God or the spiritual often is enhanced as people struggle with God or the existence of God. The resolution of the struggle may be withdrawal from or a denial of God or anything spiritual, or it may be an evolution into a mature intimate faith.

This struggle of faith also can be reflected in Conventional Moral Development. People in this stage may weigh their decisions based on being "good" in the eyes of their creator. Like adolescents, they may experience guilt about their decisions to not follow the laws of God.

Individuative-Reflective Faith developmental tasks include the following:

- Struggling with faith
- Developing an intimacy with or a withdrawal from faith

Conjunctive Faith (Early Midlife and Beyond)

Conjunctive—connected

Often in the mid-30s, as people become aware of changes in their lives, they begin to realize that something beyond their control has a meaningful part of their lives. Early midlife adults begin to accept life's paradoxes and learn to live their faith within that tension. They now recognize that not only is the spiritual **immanent** (within and personal) but also **transcendent** (beyond the personal).

Following the struggles of Individuative-Reflective Faith, those in early midlife regain an appreciation and an acceptance of symbol, myth, ritual, and the mystery of the spiritual, of God. Faith development transitions from analysis to a receptivity of God and spirituality. The early midlifers are realizing that their faith is not just something personal or impersonal, but something personal, interpersonal, intrapersonal, spiritual, mystical, and mysterious. Contemplative prayer marks the stage of Conjunctive Faith because those in early midlife are responsive to an integration, rather than an analysis, of faith and spirituality.

Faith becomes not just a development within which someone knows, but also one within which someone does not know. The confidence one has in self, self-control, and faith has been tested through emotional, psychological, sociological, physiological, and biological situations. Therefore, in Conjunctive Faith, faith and spirituality no longer thrive in the confidence of what is controlled, understood, or accepted, but what is always vulnerable. Faith and spirituality thrive in the confidence of what is always changing although always remaining the same.

Abstract thought associated with Piaget's stage of Formal Operations allows adults in the stage of Conjunctive Faith to ponder life's paradoxes and to reflect on their connectedness through faith. Erikson's personality development stage during midlife is Generativity versus Stagnation. Kohlberg's moral development stage, Social Contract and Obligation, also occurs midlife. Both in Erikson's and Kohlberg's developmental stages, midlifers are dealing with their polarities in life and society, confronting what is stable and what is vulnerable. In their personality and moral development, early midlifers are juggling whether to be active in their social environment or to withdraw, whether to explore the unexpected or to settle with the familiar. As early midlifers become receptive to their own faith, they become more open to nuances in it, as well as more open to other faith traditions. Although not necessarily embracing other faith traditions, early midlifers recognize other traditions as not totally distinct from their own, and in so doing strengthen their own.

Conjunctive Faith developmental tasks include the following:

- Discussions of early midlife in relation to faith
- Discussions of ecumenism and religious diversity/pluralism
- Prayers of contemplation and meditation

Universalizing Faith (Midlife and Beyond)

Universalizing—holistic

Faith becomes the person in the Universalizing Faith stage. Universalizing Faith is a transforming faith. People developed in Universalizing Faith identify with their faith.

By the time people reach a Universalizing Faith, they have identified themselves completely with it. They see themselves completely from the perspective of their faith. Faith, rather than self, drives their lives.

Abstract thinking, characterized by Piaget's stage of Formal Operations, allows people of Universalizing Faith to consider their actions in light of their values. The Ego Integrity versus Despair personality stage of Erikson and the Universal Ethical Principles Orientation stage of Kohlberg also coincide with the Universalizing Faith stage. In this stage, people make decisions of conscience based on ethical principles, placing the highest value on human life, equality, and dignity outside of self. Kohlberg suggests the following as probable participants in this highest stage of ethical, socioemotional, and faith-oriented behavior: Martin Luther King, Jr., Abraham Lincoln, and Joan of Arc (Muuss, 1975, p. 216).

Universalizing Faith developmental tasks include the following:

- Serving in social ministries, such as soup kitchens, food pantries, hospices, or prison ministries
- Living a lifestyle that places faith as the basis and framework for living

FAITH DEVELOPMENT AND THE COGNITIVE DOMAIN TAXONOMY

In addition to behavioral growth and development theories, one also can demonstrate connections between the developmental stages of faith and the cognitive domains. Bloom has identified six cognitive domains: knowledge, comprehension, application, analysis, synthesis, and evaluation (Gronlund, 1985) (Table 2.2).

Knowledge. The first level of Bloom's cognitive taxonomy is the task of *knowing*. Knowing does not imply understanding but simply knowing from experience. "Primal Faith" is knowing or trusting based upon experience. When a parent leaves and always returns, then children know and therefore trust that each time the parent leaves, he or she will return.

Comprehension. *Comprehending* or *understanding* is more than just knowing. Understanding occurs through experience and stories of everyday living. Children begin to understand faith from stories of faith and from experiences of trust and faith.

TABLE 2.2 Associations of Cognitive Domain and Affective Domain Taxonomies with Stages of Faith Development

Stages of Faith Development (Fowler)	Primal	Intuitive-Projective	Mythic-Literal	Synthetic-Conventional	Individuative-Reflective	Conjunctive	Universalizing
Cognitive Domains (Bloom)	Knowledge	Comprehension	Application	Analysis Synthesis Evaluation	Analysis Synthesis Evaluation	Synthesis	Evaluation
Affective Domains (Krathwohl)	Receiving	Responding	Valuing	Organization	Organization	Organization	Characterization by a Value

In Intuitive-Projective Faith, although children are impulsive and intuitive, they begin to understand or comprehend faith and trust through their behavior and subsequent reactions to it. Children in Intuitive-Projective Faith are also learning and comprehending through storytelling what it means to have faith.

Application. Once people develop an understanding of trust and faith, they begin to apply it. Examples include prayer and making life-altering decisions.

Children and adults with Mythic-Literal Faith are indeed at the "practical" or "application" stage of cognitive development. Mythic-Literal Faith is "functional" and rule oriented. Persons with Mythic-Literal Faith apply their faith literally to the way they live their lives.

Analysis. Eventually, people of faith begin to analyze their faith and to try to think it through logically (Synthetic-Conventional and Individuative-Reflective Faith). Some of faith's mysticism begins to disappear; in fact, the logical thinking of many adolescents and young adults removes them from faith and spirituality. For them, God does not fit logically into their interpretation of reality.

Synthesis. As people continue to think, reason, and work with life's dilemmas, they often find themselves returning to their faith (Conjunctive Faith) but not according to the standards that they followed previously. People return to their faith under the influence of their own mental, emotional, and social analysis and *synthesis*.

Evaluation. As people stay within their faith, dealing with conflicts and dilemmas, they are in the position to *evaluate* their faith and faith framework. They are secure enough in their faith that they can evaluate their own position within their faith and the rest of their world. Through evaluation, people realize that they are indeed secure in their faith and their faith in them (Universalizing Faith).

FAITH DEVELOPMENT AND THE AFFECTIVE DOMAIN TAXONOMY

Similar to Bloom's cognitive taxonomy, Krathwohl's taxonomy of the affective domain (Gronlund, 1985) also can be used as a framework for faith development (see Table 2-2).

Receiving. The first level in the affective domain is *receiving*. People must be receptive to something before they begin to process anything about it. Infants, children, adolescents, young people, and adults new to faith have become receptive to it. They do not understand it, but they sense something is in their presence, and they have identified it as faith (Primal Faith). People new to faith are aware of something new, something important to them, something in which they are developing trust.

Responding. The second level in the affective domain is *responding*. The response level of affective behavior is very much like Intuitive-Projective Faith, that of reacting, responding, and acting on impulses. Regardless of age, people new in faith respond to what they feel or sense. People at this second level are not just receiving faith, but are actually responding to it.

In the response level of the affective domain, people are participants in the faith, responding to their new belief. To superimpose Bloom's cognitive taxonomy, these people are developing an understanding or comprehension of faith. They begin to react to their faith by reading, praying, and participating in community faith gatherings; they are seeking more connection to their faith by responding to it.

Valuing. Once people new in the faith receive and then respond to it, they start developing a *value* in relation to it. In valuing their faith, they begin to apply their faith (Mythic-Literal Faith). Adolescents, young people, and adults beginning to value their faith are developing a personal meaning of their faith. Faith and spiritually begin to gain worth as people begin to value (or devalue) their faith. Those who value their faith want to own and hold on to it; they want to apply it to everyday life. Conscious valuing of faith usually leads to being able to explain their faith to others.

Organization. During the *organization* level in the affective domain, people begin to analyze faith into their own framework (Synthetic-Conventional Faith; Individuative-Reflective Faith; Conjunctive Faith). The organization level is when many adolescents and young adults begin to question their faith. As a result of such analysis, some may not continue in their faith. During this stage, people begin to realize that "faith" is not something that can be reasoned, calculated, or studied within an empirical framework. Many stop or abort their faith journey. However, those who continue realize that that is why "faith" is called faith; faith cannot be understood; faith cannot be reasoned.

As time and living circumstances progress, people begin to realize how life and death are paradoxical and mysterious. They begin to comprehend that there is something more than them in the world, universe, and beyond. They begin to regroup their faith journey. They return to the ritual and the mystery of their faith. In a sense, but not completely, people of faith during the organization level in the affective domain return to the receptive level, but now within a framework of faith as a journey of mystery, rather than as a passive recipient of something new.

A person's receptivity to faith is a renewed understanding of that to which he or she is responding. From here forward, the person begins to value and organize faith within his or her own framework, having been influenced not only by lived experiences, but also by analysis and organization of the experiences within a personal value system.

Characterization by a Value. Being *characterized by values* coincides with Fowler's faith developmental stage of Universalizing Faith; Kohlberg's moral development stage of Universal Ethical Principles Orientation; Erikson's personality development stage of Ego Integrity; and Bloom's cognitive domain taxonomic level of Evaluation. When people are characterized by their values, they are as one with their values. Values such as justice and peace characterized Gandhi and Martin Luther King, Jr. Mercy characterized Mother Teresa, whereas commitment and faith characterized Joan of Arc. There is no separation between people's values and themselves. People described as "godly" are often people who are a characterization of their faith. There is no separation of a person's faith and the person.

GENERATIONS

It has been documented that certain "generations" take on characteristics beyond the influences of general growth and development norms (Poling-Goldenne, 1998). Environmental forces unique to generations also have influenced faith development within each generation (Table 2.3). It is important to remember that these are gener-

TABLE 2.3 Generations Associated with Stage of Faith	
Generation (Poling-Goldenne)	**Stage of Faith Development (Fowler)**
GI	Mythical-Literal Faith
	Synthetic-Conventional Faith
Booster/Builder	Synthetic-Conventional Faith
	Individuative-Reflective Faith
Baby Boomers	Intuitive-Projective Faith
	Conjunctive Faith
	Universalizing Faith
Generation X	Individuative-Reflective Faith
Millennial Kids	Intuitive-Projective Faith

alizations and do not necessarily hold true for every individual in a particular generation.

The GI Generation. Members of the GI generation were born before 1930. The Great Depression and World War II shaped their attitudes. The GI generation trusts people in authority and accepts the tradition of chain of command. They enjoy traditional worship and have traditional faith values. Characteristics of those of the GI generation coincide with the characteristics of those who have a Mythic-Literal or Synthetic-Conventional Faith.

The Booster/Builder Generation. Members of the Builder/Booster generation were born between 1930 and 1945. The Depression and World War II have influenced this generation. The Builder/Booster generation is rooted in tradition and values hard work. They grew up with radio and the beginnings of television. Many of the characteristics of this generation resonate with those of Synthetic-Conventional Faith and somewhat with Individuative-Reflective Faith.

The Baby Boomer Generation. Born between 1946 and 1964, the Baby Boomers were influenced by social and political change in United States history. Assassinations, race and civil rights conflicts, political scandal, the women's rights movement, and the Vietnam War marked their formative years. Baby Boomers are suspicious of institutions, authority figures, and hierarchical chains of command. The generation gap became quite noticeable between the Baby Boomers and their parents; this gap has continued into adulthood and midlife.

Kohlberg's moral development study of Baby Boomers as college-age students who had been arrested in Berkeley in the 1960s reflected a typical dichotomy of characteristics of the Baby Boomers as students. The students who were arrested were primarily in either Stage Two (Instrumental Relativist, which is similar to Intuitive-Projective Faith) or in Stage Six (Universal Ethical Principles Orientation, which is similar to Universalizing Faith). Stage Two students stated that egoistic relativism and revenge motivated their protest. Stage Six students stated that their protest was a reflection of their principled morality (Muuss, 1975, p. 223).

Baby Boomers grew up watching television and listening to rock 'n' roll. They have a high degree of immediate gratification. They seek worship and a faith that is high energy and dynamic, wanting to be involved in a faith that "makes a difference" in the world (Conjunctive Faith).

The First Postmodern Generation. The first postmodern generation is often called "Generation X," and its members were born between 1965 and 1981. Key markers for Generation X are the Challenger explosion, the collapse of the Soviet Union and the Berlin Wall, acquired immunodeficiency syndrome (AIDS), and high divorce rates among their parents. National and international events in the lives of Generation X have enhanced a sense of insecurity in them.

Generation X values interpersonal experiences. They are very attuned to worship and spiritual experiences in small groups. They enjoy participating in congregational service projects. More so than previous generations, Generation Xers are more accepting of diversity and balance between genders. They consider themselves grounded in "real life" issues and thereby experience a "real life" faith and spiritual life, characteristic of an Individuative-Reflective Faith life.

The Millennial Kids Generation. The Millennial Kids generation was born in 1982 or after. They have a more frenetic pace of life, shorter attention spans, and less respect for authority than other generations. The Millennial Kids Generation, or "Twenty Somethings," is the first generation in which nontraditional families are common. One in 35 members of the Millennial Kids generation is multiracial (Poling-Goldenne, 1998).

Many of the Millennial Kids grew up with two working parents and thus assumed adult responsibilities at an early age. They have characteristics (impulsiveness, intuitiveness) that coincide with characteristics of those of Intuitive-Projective Faith.

SUMMARY

Anyone acquainted with the process of overall growth and development also is acquainted with the process of faith development. Faith development coincides with growth and development. Although the stages of growth and development are linear, persons progress uniquely through the stages, and their stage of faith development may not necessarily exactly correspond with their chronological age as indicated by the theorists. Like growth and development, the traditional trajectory of faith development is chronological, meaning that the older the person is, the more advanced his or her faith development will be as well. There are many reasons development of any sort, including faith development, is seldom linear. However, in all developmental processes, certain benchmarks indicate one's place, and such are the categories or benchmarks of Fowler's faith developmental stages.

Just as many aspects of growth and development depend heavily on environmental influences, so does faith development. However, regardless of negative influences, growth and development can continue quite healthily and within expected norms. The same is true with faith development. Sometimes, regardless of negative influences, faith development progresses according to a normative process, quite surprisingly and amazingly.

PERSONAL REFLECTIONS

- Where am I in my faith development journey?
- What have I witnessed in others that indicates where they are in their faith development?
- What reactions do I have when I assess someone in a particular level of faith development?
- In what do I see the influences of "the generation" in people's faith development?
- How do I use my understanding of faith development?

CASE STUDY 2.1

Melissa, 20 years old, is attending college. Course work has enhanced her critical thinking skills, and she begins to examine questions looking for evidence in the "real" world to support her answers. Reflecting on the events of September 11, 2001, she reasons that there is no God because a loving God would not have allowed that to happen. Furthermore, she wonders how people can use religious beliefs, typically based on concepts of peace, to justify harming others. She begins to see religions as social structures "constructed" by human beings to meet their desires for justification or their fears of death. She stops attending mass at the Campus Catholic Center, begins to withdraw from her "fanatically religious friends," and begins to become more involved in campus politics. While home on break, she gets into a heated debate with her parents, who are enmeshed in their faith as evidenced by their regular attendance at mass, daily praying of the rosary, and involvement in their parish's adult day care program. Melissa's parents are distressed by her radical views, blaming her "liberal" university for changing their daughter. They also ponder how their daughter, once very active in the parish's youth group, could now reject God.

Critical Thinking

- Identify Melissa's stage of faith development. Is Melissa's response to September 11, 2001, typical of that stage? Could her faith development take a different path?
- When might Melissa have developed the concept of a "loving God?"
- What stage of faith would you place her parents? Could they be in more than one stage? What hints are there to support your decision?
- Are you surprised by the disagreement between Melissa and her parents? Why or why not?

Key Points

- Everyone is in some level of faith development.
- Faith development may mean withdrawal from the faith. It also may mean advancement in the faith.
- Faith development follows normative growth and development patterns and expectations, coinciding with cognitive, socioemotional, and moral development.
- Faith development has similarities with cognitive domain and affective domain taxonomies.
- Faith development is vulnerable to generational environmental influences, from infancy onward.

References

Atherton, J. S. (2002). *Learning and teaching: Piaget's developmental psychology*. Available at: http://www.dmu.ac.uk/~jamesa/learning/piaget.htm. Accessed August 14, 2002.

Barger, R. N. (2000). *A summary of Lawrence Kohlberg's stages of moral development*. Available at: http://www.nd.edu/~rbarger/kohlberg.html. Accessed August 14, 2002.

Fowler, J. W. (1981). *Stages of faith*. New York: Harper & Row.

Fowler, J. W. (1987). *Faith development and pastoral care*. Philadelphia: Fortress Press.

Fowler, J. W. (1991). *Weaving the new creation: Stages of faith and the public church*. New York: HarperCollins Publishers.

Gronlund, N. W. (1985) *Stating objectives for classroom instruction*. New York: Macmillan Publishing Company

Huitt, W. (1997). *Socioemotional development*. Available at: http://chiron.valdosta.edu/whuitt/col/affsys/erikson.html. Accessed August 14, 2002.

Muuss, R. E. (1975). *Theories of adolescence*. New York: Random House.

Nurturing faith through the stages of life. (1998). Minneapolis: Augsburg Fortress.

Poling-Goldenne, M. (1998). You are generationally gifted. In *Nurturing faith through the stages of life* (pp. 30–31). Minneapolis: Augsburg Fortress.

Stephens, L. (1996). Faith development theories. In *Faith development theories*. Available at: http://www.youth.co.2a/model/faith2.htm. Accessed August 13, 2002.

Wing, K. A. (1997). *Adult faith development: Current thinking*. Available at: http://www.hope.edu/academic/psychology/335/webrep/faithdev.html. Accessed August 13, 2002.

Recommended Readings

Gronlund, N. E. (1999). *How to write instructional objectives* (6th ed.). New Jersey: Pearson Education.

Muuss, R. E. H., Velder, E., & Porton, H. (1995). *Theories of adolescence* (6th ed.). New York: McGraw-Hill Companies.

Resources

Augsburg Fortress Publishers
P.O. Box 1209, Minneapolis, MN 55440-1209
Phone: (800) 328-4648
Fax: (800) 722-7766
http://www.augsburgfortress.org
Publishing House of the Evangelical Lutheran Church in America.

Catholic Online
P.O. Box 9686, Bakersfield, CA 93389
Phone: (661) 869-1000
Fax: (661) 869-0461
http://www.catholic.org/

The Hindu Universe
Hindu Students Council, P.O. Box 9185, Boston, MA 02114-0041
Phone: (617) 698-1106
Fax: (617) 444-8725
http://www.hindunet.com

Union of American Hebrew Congregations (UAHC)
633 Third Avenue, New York, NY 10017-6778
Phone: (212) 650-4000
http://www.uahc.org/
The Union of American Hebrew Congregations is the central body of the Reform Movement in North America.

What You Need To Know About Islam
http://islam.about.com/mbody.htm

3

Development of Spiritual Care

LaVerna VanDan

LEARNING OBJECTIVES

At the end of this chapter, the reader will be able to:
- Trace the roots of spiritual caregiving through nursing and other disciplines while considering the Judeo-Christian world view.
- Identify major events that helped contribute to organized spiritual care within faith communities.
- Note the contributions of people who have greatly influenced the delivery of spiritual care in the context of health and faith integration.
- Describe current approaches that are contributing to a better understanding of spiritual care.

anointment; anointing   mysticism
charism   New Age
clergy   ordination
Common Era (CE)   parish
diaconal; diaconate; deacon/deaconess   parish nurse
ecumenical   pastoral
laity/layos   religious order
modern; postmodern   theology
Mosaic law   transcendence

T his chapter outlines the events and people who have created a system of caring for the body, mind, and spirit, especially as they relate to nursing. In addition, it explores the relationship between the development of organized religion and the delivery of spiritual care. The history of spiritual care as practiced throughout the world is rich and varied. Box 3.1 lists historical events that have greatly influenced spiritual care. This chapter focuses on a Judeo-Christian perspective of spiritual care. However, many other religions and traditions have provided significant contributions to the history of spiritual care. Chapters 5 to 12 discuss the contributions of various other religions and traditions.

HISTORICAL FOUNDATIONS OF SPIRITUAL CARE

In the Beginning...

People have practiced spiritual care since ancient times, long before the existence of organized religions. Rachel Naomi Remen claims in *Kitchen Table Wisdom* (1996) that people have been healing one another since the beginning of time. Ancient people who wondered about the origins of life, the mysteries of death, and the unexplained phenomena around them conducted "god talk" around open campfires. Perhaps 3000 to 4000 years ago, people believed that controlling forces were at work in the world, but few humans had the words to express how this "other" related to humans or nature. Ancient models of god and the spiritual world focused mostly on the natural and observable and served as the beginning of organized religion in the Middle East and Europe (Mills, 1998; Mitchell, 1977). Such models included stones, metals, foodstuffs, and other objects that ancient peoples needed for survival.

The ancient Greeks called the spirit *pneuma*, which means wind, breath, or an aspect of humanness making relationship with God (Shelly & Miller, 1999). Considering that wind is a natural phenomenon observable only by touch and a human experience apart from conscious control, it is easy to see the parallel.

BOX 3.1   Notable Dates in the Development
           of Spiritual Care

Advent of formal worship	@1868 BCE
Age of Mosaic law established	1462–1423 BCE
Rule of the Levite priests	@ 1423 BCE to 33 CE
Buddha dies	483 BCE
Confucius dies	478 BCE
Socrates born	471 BCE
Aristotle born	384 BCE
Alexander the Great ruled	336–323 BCE
Carthage-Roman war	152 BCE
The Essenes organized	150 BCE
Julius Caesar born	102 BCE
Age of Herod the Great	37–34 BCE
Birth of Jesus of Nazareth	5 BCE
The Ministry of Jesus of Galilee	26–29 CE
Buddhism reaches China	31 CE
St. Paul converted	36 CE
Justin Martyr born	103 CE
Early Christian Church	29–325 CE
Council at Nicea	325 CE
St. Jerome baptized	366 CE
Mohammed born	570 CE
Founding of many religious orders	325–1500 CE
Francis of Assisi lived	1181–1226 CE
Bubonic plague wipes out half the population of Europe	1347–1352 CE
Martin Luther ordained	1507 CE
Invention of the fork	@1600 CE
Vincent DePaul founds the Sisters of Mercy	1625 CE
75% of all children die before age 5 years	1741 CE
Florence Nightingale reforms Scutari hospital	1854–1857 CE
Westberg establishes Holistic Health Center	@1965 CE
Scope and Standards of Parish Nursing set	1998 CE

The religion of the ancient Egyptians combined both magical and medical cures. The Egyptians cared for dead bodies through embalming and burial rites. They cared for the living through practical therapeutic agents (O'Brien, 1999), such as poultices, simple medical regimens, and wound care; they also were the first culture to produce a medical textbook. However, caring for the living may have been secondary to preserving the dead.

✪ The ancient Hebrews claimed to have a long history and relationship with one God. They explained "spirit" through biblical texts, using the term "ruah." According to Shelly and Miller (1999), the Hebrews used *ruah* in several different ways, and interpretations depend on the translation. Examples of such interpretations include a "wind from God," "breath," "vital powers," "feelings," and "will." These things remain under God's control, but the *ruah* of God communicates with the *ruah* of humans to form a relationship. Biblical authors took the existence of an unseen spiritual world for granted. In fact, early in the Old Testament, God commands his people to avoid contact with other spirits (Exodus 20:1–6, Leviticus 19:31, Deuteronomy 18:9–14, I Samuel 28:3–19). The Hebrews believed that incessant curiosity and experimentation with other supernatural beings resulted in a broken relationship with God.

According to Kelsey (1995), the driving force of spiritual care rendered to humans has been God's word or will alone. All God has to do is say the word, and healing or destruction can occur. Therefore, one major tenet of all religions rooted in the Bible is the study and understanding of God's words as inspired, sent to men through the Holy Spirit and through angelic messengers (Shelly & Miller, 1999).

In the Old Testament, God is depicted as creator, judge, and redeemer, commonly understood perceptions of God. Perhaps less commonly understood are images of God as mother, lover, and friend (McFague, 1987). According to Mills (1998), to perceive these elements, the Hebrews claimed an intimate and personal relationship with the God revealed to them as "YHWH" or "YHWH-El," a being like them. Genesis begins the theme of "order and disorder," played on the stage of life in the presence of death. The rest of the Old Testament is written to provide a notion of who God is and how God will come to abide with humans again through those roles and images that the ancient Hebrews first described thousands of years ago.

The Governing Laws of Spiritual Care

The first attempt to rectify the broken relationship with the one God, first described in narratives about Adam and Eve, was through Abraham, the father of the Jewish, Christian, and Islamic religions. Abraham sought and developed a relationship with God, who provided Abraham with a vision of the blessings of a restored relationship (Genesis 17:1–8). This experience could be described as the first "spiritual healing" recorded by man.

⭘ Although other people who lived at the time of Abraham worshiped other gods, the Hebrews decided their God was the one true god–the creator of the universe. Contemporaries of Abraham may have adapted forms of spiritual healing through shamanism and object worship, but the Hebrews asserted that their way was the only way that had been blessed by God. They were so in awe of God that they did not even dare call God by name. Through Moses, God made his name known, explained that the God–person relationship was delicate and holy, and gave the Hebrews a set of laws to protect them so that they could survive in the perilous ancient world to fulfill the promise of the blessings given to Abraham. Some of those laws, found in Leviticus and Deuteronomy, could be considered the first public health laws. For example, in Leviticus 13, the Lord gave Moses and Aaron guidelines regarding isolation of those with certain types of skin disorders, describing in great detail the number of days a person was to be pronounced "unclean" according to the color and nature of the spots and scabs on the skin. God gave the people specific rules to follow, even treatments to be used for certain ailments. The priest was to check persons having skin plagues and was in charge of diagnosing leprosy, one of the most dreaded and contagious plagues of the day. Following these laws protected the people from these diseases.

Along with those laws, God established a hierarchy to keep the Hebrews from straying into spiritual danger. This plan revealed to Moses an established priesthood in the branch of the Hebrew family known as the Levites.

The Levites were responsible for strictly observing the physical and spiritual laws God gave to Moses (Numbers 1:53). The Levite male priests were well-educated scribes who guarded the Holy of Holies and the Ark of the Covenant, which housed the stone tablets that contained the initial Mosaic laws. The Levites maintained spiritual care through the ritual use of incense, reading, and interpretation of the *Pentateuch* (also referred to as the books of Moses or the Torah), ceremony (especially involving light), ritual washing, ritual animal sacrifice, fasting, and feasting events (Mitchell, 1977).

David built a city (Jerusalem) to house the government to uphold the religious hierarchy. His son Solomon built a temple, also thought to be the site of a significant event in the life of Abraham—where Abraham's son Isaac was spared becoming a human sacrifice. Thus, spiritual care was housed in Solomon's temple, under the auspices of the Levites.

Later, the prophets, thought to be divinely inspired by God, accused the Levites of a form of spiritual malpractice. Because the Hebrews would not listen and practice the strict religious code, the kingdom of Israel was plundered, and many of the Hebrew tribes were placed in bondage and exiled. God had warned them of this period of chaos. Many believed that this was the wrath of God's judgment on the people of Israel. The Hebrew tribes were restored to their promised land from Babylonian captivity to regain only partial political power and a fragmented religious system (Daniel 1–12).

A New Way of Spiritual Healing

✪ Several subgroups that arose in response to foreign invasion and influence over the Hebrew people maintained the regime of the Jewish priesthood after the period of the prophets and the restoration of Jerusalem. Largely, the Sanhedrin and the court of the Hebrew king carried out spiritual care and governance of the state of Israel. Conflicting groups began to exert political power to influence the delivery of spiritual care and religious worship in the face of Greek and then Roman occupation. These groups included the Sadducees, Pharisees, Essenes, and Zealots. All these groups believed a Messiah would come to restore Israel to its former glory and fulfill predictions of physical as well as spiritual healing for the people of Israel. Among those who arose at this time was a young rabbi who taught and corrected the people in and around Lake Galilee. This rabbi was named Y'shua or Jesus of Nazareth.

✪ Jesus clarified the Mosaic law and demonstrated great power by performing miracles (great works) in the areas of physical, psychological, social, and spiritual healing (see Chapter 1). Jesus is said to have broken many taboos and re-established precedents for healing, especially spiritual healing. He is known for his equity, compassion toward people whom Jewish culture otherwise shunned or abandoned, willingness to touch and be touched, wisdom, and even humor. Box 3.2 provides a list of incidences of healing in both the Old and New Testaments.

BOX 3.2 Scripture Related To Healing

OLD TESTAMENT

Ecclesiastes 3:1–11a	For everything there is a season
Isaiah 26:3–4	Trust in the Lord
Isaiah 35:1–10	Restoration of all that is broken
Isaiah 40: 28–31	The weak shall renew their strength
Isaiah 53:3–5	With his stripes we are healed
Isaiah 61:1–3	Good tiding to the afflicted
Psalm 13	A prayer of pain and sorrow
Psalm 23	Anointed head with oil
Psalm 27	God is the strength of my life
Psalm 30	Recovery
Psalm 41	Assurance
Psalm 51	A clean heart
Psalm 91	God's refuge
Psalm 103	God forgives
Psalm 138	Fulfilling a purpose
Psalm 146	God lifts the bowed down

NEW TESTAMENT

Matthew 5:1–12	Blessed are they...
Matthew 8:1–13	The healing of the leper and the servant
Matthew 10:1–8	Jesus sends disciples to heal
Matthew 11:28–30	Jesus will give rest
Matthew 15:21–28	A woman's faith
Matthew 26:36–39	Complying with God's will
Mark 1:21–28	The healing of the unclean spirit
Mark 5:1–20	The spirit named Legion
Mark 5: 21–43	Girl and woman healed
Mark 6:7–13	Anointing with oil
Mark 6:53–56	Bringing the sick to Jesus
Mark 8:22–26	The blind man
Mark 10:46–52	Take heart, rise
Luke 5:17–26	Take up your bed and walk
Luke 7:11–17	Jesus raises the widow's son
Luke 8:43–48	A woman healed of bleeding
Luke 17:11–19	Praise for healing
John 5:2–18	Do you want to be healed?
John 9	Healing of the man born blind
John 11:1–44	Lazarus raised
Acts 3:1–10	Peter and John heal the lame man
Acts 5:12–16	Jerusalem healings
2 Corinthians 1:3–5	God comforts the afflicted
2 Corinthians 4:16–18	All this is temporary
Colossians 1:11–29	Strengthened with God's power
James 5:13–15	Is any among you sick?
1 John 4:16–19	Fear succumbs to love
1 John 5:13–15	Our confidence
Revelation 21:1–4	God's kingdom is restored; a new earth

Jesus lectured through parables to the masses in great open air gatherings. He persistently taught that the old order of priests and interpreters of the law had become inharmonious with God. He began to draw large crowds and increasing criticism among the ruling Pharisees and Sadducees. These groups plotted to have Jesus brought to justice by the Roman procurator, Pontius Pilate, with the blessings of the ruling Jewish king, Herod (Luke 23:1–25).

✚ After the execution of Jesus, his followers reported seeing him alive again. They spread the word of his resurrection—the ultimate spiritual healing (Matthew 28:1–11; Mark 16:1–15; Luke 24:1–43; John 20:1–23). According to the Bible, Jesus remained with his followers for a brief time before his ascension into heaven, exhorting them to continue the mission of teaching about God, preaching the good news of the resurrection and the nearing kingdom of God, and healing those in need in his name. Soon after his ascension to heaven, Jesus' followers began to influence the practice of many of the rituals of the temple. They continued with baptism, anointing of the ill, washing of feet to show servitude and humility, and observing communion as a remembrance of the flight out of Egypt (Passover) but also as a commemoration of the life and death of Jesus (as Christ gave example with the Last Supper). Jewish-Christians began to grow increasingly separate from their Jewish brothers and sisters. Eventually, they were no longer regarded as Jewish, either by themselves or by non-Christian Jews.

✚ Spiritual Care in the Early Christian Church

The apostles and disciples of the early Christian church included many men and women who were known to deliver healing and spiritual care. These men and women were known as the diaconate, or deacons, from the Greek verb "diakonen," meaning "to serve" (O'Brien, 2003). Phoebe (mentioned in Romans 16:1–2), thought to be a woman of some means and stature in the community, attended to the needs of the poor and ill. At this time, because of the teachings and practices of Jesus (based on the foundations of the Hebrew faith), the diaconate delivered physical care in communal settings and to those other than near kin. They emphasized Jesus' model of compassion, kindness, gentleness, and service.

Although Jesus responded to people's needs holistically—he used all three approaches to healing, described by the Greeks as *Sozo* (salvation, rescuing), *holokeria* (restoring to wholeness), and *therapeuo* (treating the broken or ill)—the early Church began to partition roles and delegate responsibilities to those believers also considered caregivers. Men were responsible for bringing Eucharist, preaching, and teaching emerging doctrine. Women were given roles related to healing and caregiving.

Healers

The leading groups who delivered some spiritual and physical care to the congregation included women who worked in sacramental and teaching ministries, female prophets, female deacons, and widows. Widows were not only the providers but also the primary recipients of care. Widows were often called on to pray for the whole church (which was their benefactor). The practice of turning to widows for spiritual care is based on the belief that they were especially effective in praying for the sick and laying on hands. Widows were seen as just below presbyters and bishops and had great say in the governance of the church.

Roman Matrons

In the early Roman church, wealthy women, known as matrons, frequently supported the charitable work of caring for the sick. They founded hospitals and convents while living austerely. These women included St. Paula, St. Marcella, and St. Helena, known for their care of the sick and poor. After their lives, the work of nursing began to become institutionalized through the advent of abbeys and monasteries (O'Brien, 2003).

Medieval Spiritual Care

In medieval times, nursing continued through military orders and monastic nursing. Another important contribution was the establishment of "houses of God" or hotels Dieu in Lyon and Paris. These houses were designed to provide care for travelers, orphans, the needy, and the sick. Controversy exists regarding whether "hospitals" derived from these houses or whether these houses may have been based on Muslim models. These first hospitals demanded great sacrifice of the sisters who inhabited them: many made a vow to leave all parts of their former lives behind and not even receive visitors.

Military Orders

With the advent of the Crusades, men took vows to care for the fallen in battle. The three major groups, which included knights, priests, and deacons, were the Knights Hospitallers of St. John of Jerusalem, the Teutonic Knights, and the Knights of St. Lazarus. Some of the men who cared for the wounded Crusaders also cared for lepers and the ill in Jerusalem, at major battle sites, and along trade routes.

Medieval Monastic Nursing

Around 500 CE (Common Era), men and women began to be drawn to the practice of monasticism, which was guided by vows of poverty, chastity, and obedience. The monks' and nuns' daily routine included prayer and hard manual labor, but this began to change during the life of St. Benedict of Nursia, who began to focus ministry on the care of the sick. Later, monasteries and abbeys also became centers of learning.

Hildegard of Bingen (1098–1179 CE) was a German abbess, visionary, and musician. She is known primarily for her contributions to health, theology, nursing, and medicine. She wrote *Physica* and *Liber Composite Medicinae*, in which she described diseases of various organs and pointed to symptoms such as pallor, erythema, bad breath, and indigestion. She believed that all diseases and cures could be located in the four qualities of heat, dryness, moistness, and cold. For centuries her published and unpublished works remained virtually forgotten. Then her works were translated and are now appreciated for her thinking about the body–mind–spirit connection.

St. Radegunde (a daughter of a Thrungin king) took poor people into her own castle to care for them. She established Holy Cross Monastery, where more than 200 nuns lived and worked, especially with people who had leprosy. St. Hilda was a cultured and scholarly woman who also cared for lepers and housed others who followed her lead (O'Brien, 2003). St. Brigid founded the great monastery at Kildare, Ireland; she ministered to the indigent and especially to the lepers.

O'Brien (2003) notes that the early church and the monasteries often overlooked mental health care. Primarily, care came in the form of hospitality shown toward pilgrims. Care for the mentally ill began in Belgium during the monastic period and continues to this day. In fact, this care is known as a model for home health care of the mentally ill.

The Mystics

Hildegard, discussed previously, described profound spiritual experiences with God to justify her work. Yet the leaders of the church (perhaps out of jealousy for the love and devotion that some female spiritual care providers experienced or the social norms related to treatment of women) sought to restrict the movements and actions of these women. At the time, most women were subservient to and totally dependent on men. They could not own property in their own names or go out in public unaccompanied by men. Generally, they were not allowed to be educated. As such, they traditionally did not hold power in the church or the home. Often, they were thought incapable of doing the work of spiritual care and were relegated to delivering mundane and menial physical care.

Women mystics were those whose knowledge was based on intuition, meditation, and experience with God apart from human reason. They countered social inequalities and barriers with their profound experiences of God, which emboldened them and others who sought their help. These women, who (through visionary and prophetic mystical experiences with God) spoke with prophetic voices often heeded by male counterparts, include Julian of Norwhich, Mechthild of Magdeburg (Ruether, 2002), and St. Theresa of Avila (O'Brien, 2003).

Although most of the mystics in the medieval period were women, one notable exception is St. Francis of Assisi. Francis was a young man known for his compassionate care of the sick, poor, and dying. Stories of his generosity and healing touch abound. He cared for and lived with lepers, giving them hope and sympathy. One famous story concerns Francis giving his own garments to the poor around him until he was left nude. He often personally cared for the most difficult and unappreciative of the ill. He had many mystical experiences that seem to have motivated him.

St. Clare of Assisi, a follower of Francis, often tended to those who needed care but could not get to Francis because of the multitudes surrounding him. Often, Francis and Clare collaborated to maximize their caring potential. She, too, is considered a mystic.

MODERN SPIRITUALITY AND NURSING

Florence Nightingale

Most modern nurses consider Florence Nightingale (1820—1910) to be the mother of the nursing profession. Most know her as "the lady with the lamp" who almost single-handedly brought about sweeping changes in British medicine, care delivered on battlefields, and public health. But few understand her underlying motivations—the events that led to this life of activity—and the spirituality behind those actions.

Florence realized a call to care early in her life (some say as early as 6 years of age). She was a sickly child, and as the recipient of care from family members, she began to reciprocate in kind by nursing other sick relatives. She not only nursed people, but also pets and dolls. She enjoyed this work and began to think of it often. She realized her call into a life of purpose at 14 years of age while sitting under some trees in Embley, England (Dossey, 1998).

Several modern authors and historians attribute Nightingale's energy and commitment to caring for the ill to a life of mystical experiences (Dossey, 1998; Keighley, 1999). Nurse authors, upon reflecting on Nightingale's copious written work, suggest that she passed through the process of becoming a mystic, the phases of which include an awakening, purgation, illumination, surrender, and union (Dossey, 1998). Nightingale also is thought to have been heavily influenced by other mystics, such as St. Teresa of Avila, Blessed Angela of Foligno, St. Catherine of Siena, St. Gertrud of Helfta, and others who reported transcendental experiences and had a reputation of high regard for the poor, sick, and dying (Dossey, 1998).

Other thinkers may have influenced Nightingale toward social activism: the Brownings, George Eliot, and John Stuart Mill, to name a few (Keighley, 1999). These thinkers led Nightingale to conclude that industrial society was leading people away from God and one another as sources of hope.

Florence sought places where she could learn to care for the sick and dying in a way that distinguished what she did from that of common chambermaids. She attended the Institution of Deaconesses at Kaiserwerth in Dusseldorf, Germany. This place was known as a Protestant training hospital that taught something akin to nursing as a call from God and a diaconal function. Through her time at Kaiserwerth and her contacts from there, she learned that all persons on a mission or quest to become Christ-like are given certain gifts and talents. She learned that people who functioned in the diaconal role were considered to be "enlightened conductors" who were able to distinguish truth from error and to root out growing agnosticism, and that they were placed in a position to advance knowledge. Some say Nightingale was a modern prophet of God and saw herself as a liberated human being.

Nightingale has been compared to other mystics and saints in Western tradition: St. Francis of Assisi, St. Joan of Arc, and George Fox (the founder of the Quakers). These people were sometimes thought of as odd, because they claimed to receive visions and other forms of revelation of God's power.

Nightingale wrote the three-volume work *Suggestions for Thought* and was quickly identified as a person with good ideas and abundant personal resources. She was given her first professional position in 1854 and quickly improved the small 27-bed charity hospital. Others saw her as divinely inspired. During the Crimean War, she was the one person from England who was effective at the hospital in Scutari, where the mortality rate was 42%, with most deaths resulting from infections and poor sanitation. In 6 months she lowered the mortality rate to 2.2% (Dossey, 1998). She is the first to be credited with organizing and training nurses for duty in both field hospitals and individual homes.

Nightingale was a catalyst for change into the 20th century and has had a global influence on medical and nursing care. She was an avid writer who produced thousands of letters, journal entries, and several notable published works, including *Suggestions* and *Notes on Nursing: What It Is and What It Is Not*. From her legacy springs modern nursing science and education. Many people consider her a Protestant "saint of the people." Her family grave marker harkens to the life she led: a very simple cross bears the words "F. N. Born 12 May, 1820. Died 13 August, 1910." She refused a burial in Westminster Abbey (Dossey, 1998; Keighley, 1999).

The Clergy as Spiritual Caregivers

The clergy have a role and responsibility for spiritual caregiving. Throughout the centuries, many theologies of healing were developed through ordained clergy. St.

Basil the Great, St. John Chrysostom, St. Augustine, St. Martin of Tours, St. Jerome, St. Gregory the Great, St. Thomas Aquinas, St. Boniface, St. Bernard of Clairvaux, John Calvin, Martin Luther, John of Beverly, John Wesley, George Fox, and Dietrich Bonhoeffer practiced physical as well as spiritual healing. Groups that splintered from traditional churches also included spiritual caregivers: Phineas Quimby, Mary Baker Eddy, A. J. Gordon, Dr. Elwood Dorchester, Kathrynn Kuhlman, Edgar Cayce, David Wilkerson, Paul Cho, and Oral Roberts, to name a few (Kelsey, 1995).

Healing comes from various sources: liturgy, words, rituals, and specific counseling. The Roman Catholic Church has a Sacred Liturgy (III.73 ff.) that makes it quite clear that the church expects healing, and not just during extreme unction (the point of death). Not all with the *charism* (gift) of healing have been widely accepted (e.g., St. Catherine of Siena); some have been chastised for not "keeping their place" within an order.

Nelson (2001) asserts that nuns, as members of the ordered clergy, have long been unrecognized in their roles as nurses and spiritual caregivers. Long before Florence Nightingale influenced and reformed nursing in the modern era, nuns established a quiet and often unappreciated presence throughout the world, beginning in Europe and spreading to the far reaches of European empires.

Modern pastoral care is remarkably similar to the spiritual care that nurses provide. Open communication is greatly desired; to be therapeutic, the pastor must remain nonjudgmental. Pastoral counseling is seen as relatively short term, client driven, and goal oriented (Clinebell, 1992).

Pastoral counseling often includes detecting and intervening in spiritual distress; counseling families, engaged couples, and people in grief; and giving spiritual guidance, development, and direction. Unless they have a license and are certified in a specific area of counseling, pastors usually refer those needing long-term counseling to counseling centers.

Pastors have begun to use the structure of scientific investigation to be more effective in their counseling and delivery of spiritual care. They are relying more heavily on research findings and instruments with high reliability and validity to measure progress toward a goal and to accurately assess for signs and symptoms of disease (Clinebell, 1992).

The Laity in Spiritual Care

✚ The *layos*, or the members of the church who are believers but not necessarily clergy, also are being permitted to define, develop, and use their individual charisms toward healing and spiritual care. Movements such as Lay Witness Missions (in which members give personal testimony to their faith in Jesus Christ), the Walk to Emmaus, and the Great Banquet and Charismatic Movements (in which people are allowed to express their individual spirituality and explore their gifts of the spirit, including the gifts of healing), as well as Stephen Ministry, Hands of Christ, Helping Hands, Habitat for Humanity, Christmas in April, and Elizabeth Ministry, provide care to people in need. Box 3.3 lists many notable caregiving organizations. These ministries are founded on the belief that God encourages self-care and the "priesthood of all believers." Although these caregiving groups are popular among the laity, most are administered in conjunction with and under the direction of a pastor. Training and ongoing education are necessary, although not extensive or cost prohibitive.

BOX 3.3   Internet Links to Lay Caregiving Organizations

Christmas-in-April, http://www.rebuildingtogether.com
Deaconess Foundation, http://www.deaconess.org
The Elizabeth Ministry, http://www.dcfl.org/eliz.htm
Florence Nightingale Foundation, http://www.florence-nightingale-foundation.org.uk
Habitat for Humanity, http://habitat.org/
Health Ministries Association, http://www.hmassoc.org
International Parish Nurse Resource Center, http://ipnrc.parishnurses.org
Salvation Army, http://www.salvationarmy.org
Society of St. Vincent DePaul, http://www.vincenter.org/tree/svdp/index.html
Stephen and Christ Care Ministries, http://www.christcare.com

Modern Nursing Models

In addition to the work of Florence Nightingale, several models and influences have shaped modern nursing. Some researchers have criticized the nursing profession as being too dependent on and easily influenced by other disciplines, which they view as hindering the profession's ability to achieve status and regard. Others state that the inability to adopt and adhere to a single model has hampered nursing. Most analysts of the nursing profession tend to evaluate nursing effectiveness on physical (and perhaps to a lesser degree psychosocial) care, resulting in less emphasis on spiritual care (Box 3.4). Several models which have influenced the development of spiritual care in nursing are described below.

Military Model

Although Nightingale envisioned nursing as a largely spiritual movement, her time with the military was influential, and the military model of nursing care persists even today. The military influence largely accounts for why nurses have been socialized to promote a specific hierarchy and rules of protocol. Other examples of the military influence include the abolitionist, temperance, and women's suffrage movements, which churches often supported and administered.

Before the 1950s in the United States, nurses often sought to preserve a "starchy" image promulgated by military hierarchy. The military model continues in the provision of spiritual care today in the form of the Salvation Army Movement and the DeMolay.

Medical Model

The medical model has heavily influenced the delivery of nursing care. Its effects are seen today in the layers of proficiency and specialization that are identified commonly with nursing, often fragmenting care. The public often confuses nursing with medicine, viewing nurses as physician "assistants" or "helpers."

BOX 3.4   Research: Spiritual Care Among Nurse Practitioners

Stranahan, S. (2001). Spiritual perception, attitudes about spiritual care, and spiritual care practices among nurse practitioners. **Western Journal of Nursing Research, 23(1), 90.**

Susan Stranahan found several references in her literature review that led her to question how nurses perceived and provided spiritual care in settings in which one would expect such practices to abound. As she points out in her problem statement, nurses do not always feel comfortable providing spiritual care, even though doing so is well within nursing's domain.

Stranahan decided to study a sample of nurse practitioners to measure their spirituality and the spiritual care practices they employed. The sampling group was composed of 296 nurse practitioners in Indiana; 40% responded to the inquiry. Her purpose was to examine attitudes, perceptions, and practices of nurse practitioners regarding spiritual care. Stranahan used Pearson R techniques to find the relationships. She used Reed's Spiritual Perspective Scale* and a modified version of Nurses' Spiritual Care Perspectives Scale developed by Taylor, Highfield, and Amenta.† (Both instruments have been found to have adequate reliability and validity, and both use Likert-type scales.)

The study found that 57% of responders stated they rarely or never included spiritual care in their daily work. Forty-five percent stated that their ability to provide spiritual care was weak or limited. And 34% were uncomfortable providing spiritual care, compared with 32% who reported feeling very comfortable.

These nurses most often used very basic spiritual care interventions, such as using standard documentation, reading religious material, praying (both privately and with clients), and reporting spiritual needs to colleagues. The nurses who scored high on the spirituality scale employed more complex interventions and provided spiritual care more frequently.

Other researchers have concluded that nurses most frequently pray privately for clients or refer them to religious leaders for support. Stranahan indicated that responders might have been measuring religiosity in addition to, or rather than, spirituality. As the Stranahan states, "rarely did they provide direct or visible spiritual care." The nurses in the study also noted the lack of educational foundations in spiritual care at the graduate and the undergraduate levels. This study mentions that 70% report the absence of this educational experience.

*Reed, P. G. (1987). Spirituality and well-being in terminally ill hospitalized adults. *Research in Nursing and Health, 10,* 335–344.

†Taylor, E., Highfield, M., & Amenta, M. (1994). Attitudes and beliefs regarding spiritual care. *Cancer Nursing, 17,* 479–487.

Business and Scientific Models

As nursing has passed through and paused within the medical model, it also has had an affinity for and alliance with the business and scientific models. Business operates on the law of supply and demand; therefore, its most important outcome is profit. The scientific model operates largely on empiricism (what can be seen and is observable) in the world view. Both models have helped develop and organize nursing into a profession and an occupation based on evidence. Scientific models of nursing have emphasized the life sciences (such as biology and biochemistry) and the social sciences (such as psychology and sociology). But those views are often radically and diametrically opposed to spiritual care; some nurses may perceive that "if it isn't really there (in material fashion), you can't really care." Nurses who seek nursing as a vocation or a calling often criticize these models of nursing. They consider nursing using the business or scientific model as being too materialistic and reductionistic. They think the spiritual world is not measurable under the laws of economics and science but does indeed exist. They see their practice in terms of art versus science (Shelly & Miller, 1998).

Currently, nursing scientists are busy constructing tools of measure, articles of description, and textbooks describing religion and spirituality (Carson, 1989). Most have written about or tried to explain spirituality in terms of distress or deviation from "normal." Only a few have tackled explaining spiritual wellness. Table 3.1 lists nursing and other research related to spiritual care, and helps to identify leaders in this subject area. Chapter 18 describes in greater detail some of this literature and its importance to the nursing profession.

Postmodern Models and Theories

Partially in response to criticisms of the military, medical, business, and scientific models of nursing, nursing theorists have attempted to view the person from a spiritual vantage point. These theorists include Martha Rogers and her protégé Rosemarie Parse. Rogers and Parse have attempted to extend the scientific view of nursing to include the unknown and perhaps the spiritual. These nurses, who have been heavily influenced by quantum physics and mechanics and Eastern religious and spiritual practices, envision nursing care bringing patients and nurses into a new realm of being through transcendental experience. They have aspired to bring nursing out of the realm of religion per se and into the realm of the spiritual in a way that is different from traditional Judeo-Christian thought. Those who have engaged in theories related to explanations of the time–space continuum and the subparticulate material world often describe concepts infinite in scope. They perceive God to be the Being distinct to those who practice Judeo-Christian faiths (Martsolf & Mickley, 1998; Stevens-Barnum, 1995, 1996).

Ⓢ So-called New Age religions and traditions engage heavily in a wide variety of Eastern and nontraditional Western practices and concepts. Practices such as energy medicine (including therapeutic touch and Reiki), music therapies, aromatherapy, and other "alternative" therapies have made their way into the mainstream of nursing practice.

Not all nurses who practice spiritual care are exuberant about this blend of East and West, especially when crossing religious boundaries. Shelly and Miller (1999) caution against the use of New Age practices, and view them as a form of pagan worship and idolatry. However, other nurses have envisioned a happy medium between the traditional and nontraditional worlds. According to Stevens-Barnum (1996), nurse theorists such as Watson have attempted to explain nursing practice based on

TABLE 3.1 Literature Review of Recent Articles on Spiritual Care

Topic	Author and Year
Spirituality and chronic illness	Landis, 1996
	O'Neill & Kenny, 1998
	Sterling-Fisher, 1998
Terminal illness and cancer	Babler, 1997
	Bay, 1997
	Belcher, Dettmore, & Holzemer, 1989
	Burton, 1998
	Carson & Green, 1992
	Coward, 1991, 1993, 1994, 1997
	Coward & Lewis, 1993
	Coward & Reed, 1996
	Fehring, Miller, & Shaw, 1997
	Kaczorowski, 1989
	Kazanjian, 1997
	Ley & Corless, 1988
	Martsolf, 1997
	Messenger & Roberts, 1994
	Mickley, Soeken, & Belcher, 1992
	Nowotny, 1989
	Owen, 1989
	Reese & Brown, 1997
	Seely, 1999
Spirituality and the elderly	Beggren-Thomas & Griggs, 1995
	Coward & Reed, 1996
	Holstein, 2000
	Reed, 1991
	Ross, 1997
	Trice, 1990
Spirituality and women	Miller, 1995
Spirituality and children	Hart & Schneider, 1997
Spirituality in community clients	Burkhardt & Nagai-Jacobson, 1985
	Chapman & Pepler, 1998
Spirituality in orthopedic patients	Clark, 1997
Spirituality among caregivers	Carson, 1997
	Kaye & Robinson, 1994
Spirituality and the mentally ill/substance abusers	Catalano, 1998
	McGee, 2000
	Mickley, Carson, & Soeken, 1994
	Mitchell & Lunney, 2000
	Nolan & Crawford, 1997
Spiritual care interventions and concepts	**Hope**
	Benzein, Saveman, & Norberg, 2000
	Dufault & Martocchio, 1985
	Hall, 1994
	Herth, 1990, 1993
	Kylma & Vehvilainen-Julkunen, 1997
	Penrod & Morse, 1997
	Rees & Joslyn, 1998
	Rustoen & Wang, 2000

(continued)

Topic	Author and Year
Spiritual care interventions and concepts	**Hope**
	Rustoen, Wiklund, Hanestad, & Moum, 1998
	Wang, 2000
	Zorn, 1997
	Meditation and Guided Imagery
	Brown-Saltzman, 1997
	Art Work
	Bailey, 1997
	Forgiveness Facilitation
	Davidhizar & Laurent, 2000
	Festa & Tuck, 2000
	Bibliotherapy
	Cress-Ingebo & Chrisagis, 1998
	Dream-Telling
	Dombeck, 1995
	Prayer
	Castledine, 1998
	Lewis, 1996
	Meraviglia, 1999
	Murray & Stoner, 1998
	O'Mathuna, 1999
	Silva & DeLashmutt, 1998
	Stolley, Buckwalter, & Koenig, 1999
	Story-Telling
	Taylor, 1997
Combined review of interventions	Emblen & Halstead, 1993
	Hall & Lanig, 1993
	Messenger & Roberts, 1994
	Nagai-Jacobson & Burkhardt, 1989
	Sellers & Haag, 1998
	Tuck, Pullen, & Lynn, 1997
Instrument of measure for spirituality and spiritual wellness	Hungelmann, Kenkel-Ross, Klassen, & Stollenwerk, 1996
	Treloar, 1999
Diagnosing in the spiritual domain	Engebretson, 1996
	Highfield, 1997
Descriptions of spiritual care	Burkhardt, 1989
	Emblen, 1992
	Govier, 2000
	Haase, Britt, Coward, Leidy, & Penn, 1992
	Halstead & Mickley, 1997
	Lane, 1987
	Stevens-Barnum, 1995
	Treloar, 1999
	VandeCreek, 1997

some of each of the two worlds. Indeed, Watson envisions a world in which nurses, rather than completely ignoring religious beliefs or pretending faith is not a part of what they do, embrace spirituality and use it not only as a personal resource of the client, but also a personal resource of the nurse, and one to be mutually shared while engaged in the nursing process.

Integrated Care Models

The integration of new and traditional religious views with new ways of providing care through multidisciplinary approaches has launched several new ways of providing spiritual and physical/psychosocial care. Westberg, through an experiment conducted by Lutheran General Hospitals in Chicago, attempted to revisit the old way of providing care through congregations yet with the advances of modern science and empirical knowledge to guide practice. He did not really envision a new model or theory of nursing, but instead a new delivery model for nursing care through churches. This movement has formed the basis for what is now parish nursing (Solari-Twadell, Djupe, & McDermott, 1990; Solari-Twadell & McDermott, 1999; Westberg & McNamara, 1990).

Shelly and Miller (1999) have also developed a model of nursing care based on some of the work of Westberg, using the integration of faith and health through nursing practice in faith communities with a stronger emphasis on fundamental Christianity. This model, which explains spiritual care as the duty of all nurses, but especially parish nurses, harkens back to concepts from the Hebrew tradition of shalom as wholeness.

✚ Parish Nursing

The integration of health and faith also is the integration of science and religion. Based on the work of Westberg and others in the parish nurse movement, as well as the works of scientific investigators, the worlds of the spiritual and empirical are no longer considered mutually exclusive, stand-alone concepts. Indeed, through parish nursing and similar models of care, the spiritual and the scientific work together toward healing others.

Parish nurses usually are defined as nurses who carry out the central mission of integrating faith and health within a faith community (Solari-Twadell & McDermott, 1999). Parish nursing evolved through the work of Granger Westberg and Lutheran General/Advocate Health Care, who saw that compartmentilization of the client's needs (as with the medical model) and the movement of health care toward a business model left many people in need of service that they either did not get or got too late to be effective. They also saw that nurses are in an ideal position to deliver holistic and preventive services to the congregation. No other institution reaches people from cradle to grave and through all phases of health and well-being. No other institution can influence the beliefs and daily lifestyle practices of people as much as the church. Because churches have great influence and a wide span of control, they are ideal places to promote health and healing without the pitfalls of care delivered through health maintenance organizations.

These ideas have not been accepted without question, however. First is the issue of the perception of the parish nurse. Are parish nurses clergy or, at least, pastoral care providers because the entire scope of their practice is within the realm of the congregation? If so, does that imply that the parish nurse be placed in a covenant agreement with the church and fully financially supported by the congregation who is considered the client-at-large? How should parish nurses be prepared for this new role, which often is perceived as a very advanced and independent practice? Who should supervise and mentor the practicing parish nurse? How will the parish nurse continue to improve the quality of his or her work without the benefits of peer review and direct nursing supervision?

The roles of parish nurse are, for the most part, comfortable and familiar to most nurses: health educator, counselor, advocate, referral agent, developer and facilitator of support groups, and volunteer supporter. The setting and the autonomy of practice are unique features of parish nursing (Solari-Twadell & McDermott, 2000).

What is sometimes awkward to the novice parish nurse has been described as the parish nurse's chief mission, as stated earlier—to integrate faith and health. Nurses who have been socialized into the military, medical, business, and scientific models are not always prepared for what bringing faith and health together means while implementing changes in the client's internal or external environment.

During the rapid development of parish nursing as a cost-effective and holistic way of delivering care to a client, the question of whether parish nursing was a professional nursing practice was often debated, because so many parish nurses were volunteers and did not want to be confined by the heavily regulated climate of the modern practice of nursing. They envied their clerical counterparts who have different ways of being accountable for their practices. Early parish nurses sometimes complained that by focusing too much on "the nuts and bolts of practice" (i.e., documentation and evaluation), the joy of providing nursing service was somehow diminished.

As a result, through focus group study and a series of events, the International Parish Nurse Resource Center and the Health Ministries Association agreed that parish nursing was not just a delivery model, but a subspecialty of nursing akin to community health nursing, and thus a professional model of nursing, even for the unpaid parish nurse. This has great implications for anyone who uses the title of parish nurse.

In 1998, the Health Ministries Association in conjunction with the American Nurses Association developed the *Scope and Standards of Parish Nursing*. This document helps to define, guide, and limit practice (although some criticize that it does not contain enough about what parish nurses are *not* allowed to do). Because parish nursing is defined so broadly, some potential conflicts exist within the role of the parish nurse as health minister and the pastor or governing clergy. In addition, because there is an emphasis on what skills a parish nurse can employ (no invasive measures), it makes parish nursing (in the mind of some) relatively undervalued. Legal questions of authority, autonomy, and potential liability remain unanswered and await a legal test before parish nurses clearly understand their scope and span of practice because most parish nurses do not practice under the authority of a medical provider.

Parish nursing has grown quickly throughout the world but continues to predominate in the Midwest of the United States. Other areas where parish nursing is thriving include Korea, parts of Africa, Europe, and Australia.

Conflicts with clergy are inevitable as the parish nurse grapples with the organizational structure of the church and denomination in question, and his or her place within that structure. Clergy often misunderstand the role of the nurse, viewing him or her as an extension of the physician or as a provider of physical care only. Some clerics may envy the nurse who can bring clients to a greater understanding of health and who often develops warm and long-lasting relationships with clients. Others may contend that the spiritual care of the congregation is solely their domain. Nurses also struggle with the old problem of becoming "an extender," this time not a physician extender, but a clergy extender. For a list of current literature describing how advance practice nurses perceive spiritual care in general and parish nursing in particular, see Table 3-1.

Congregational Health Programs

For churches that do not have a parish nurse, starting a congregational health program is another alternative to addressing health needs within a group. Many smaller churches have nurse volunteers who may organize themselves to meet some of the health care needs of their congregation. Activities that might be offered range from services such as blood pressure screenings to health fairs or educational programs. Those who work in health professions and affiliate with a particular church may offer individual services (such as a physician in the congregation offering free sports physicals to church members) or band together to plan and implement a more structured and comprehensive plan for their congregation. A recent consumer reference book that may be used as a guide for those interested in organizing a health program for their churches is *Congregational Health* (Mauk, Russell, & Birge, 2003).

INTO THE FUTURE

At the beginning of the new millennium, spiritual care theorists already are working hard to conceptualize the future of spirituality. Books expound on a future of "spiritual machines," a "spiritual" society (Bave, 2001), postnuclear-age spirituality (McFague, 1987), a new theology for those who embrace the scientific age (Peacocke, 1993), and "quantum" theology (O'Murchu, 1997). The meaning of these conceptualizations, combined with the effects of non-Western spirituality, is uncertain yet exciting.

Indeed, some scientists propose the possibility of mathematically and statistically proving God's existence. Astrophysicists, wrestling with theories such as uncertainty and relativity, have proposed theories to either support or weaken the argument for or against the empirical challenge of God's existence. These debates are important to nurses who perform spiritual care because a person's belief system may ultimately dictate choice of health behaviors. Those who doubt God's existence may use these debates to validate an unhealthy lifestyle, rejecting arguments to care for themselves out of obedience to God.

The marriage of faith and science is a dubious one for many, who approach these ideas with a healthy skepticism. The ideas of Stephen Hawking may profoundly influence the person who is trying to understand the meaning and purpose of life and death. In *A Brief History of Time*, Hawking (1988) attempts to explain the creation of the universe, black holes, and quarks as ideas that lend themselves to a spiritual ramification of the existence of God. He further proposes that God was not just at the beginning during the "Big Bang," but that all matter may go back to God periodically, resulting in creation and re-creation.

So here we are, coming full circle, still pondering the great questions of the ancients. In the meantime, people live, care for one another, and find hope at the end of life through acts of mercy, kindness, gentleness, and compassion—the acts of nursing practice through spiritual care.

PERSONAL REFLECTIONS

- How important is theology to the practice of nursing?
- Are faith and science compatible or diametrically opposed?
- How does a Christian religious community practice innovation? How does it maintain orthodoxy and tradition? Why?
- How have the ancient and modern Christian churches treated women (especially nurses)? How have women responded?
- Many practicing parish nurses volunteer their labor. How do you think nursing leaders such as Nightingale, Orem, Roy, Newman, Parse, and Watson would respond to that practice?
- How are the roles of priest/pastor and nurse/deaconess different? How are they the same?
- Are parish nurses clergy or laity? Support your argument.
- Some New Age scholars suggest that Jesus of Nazareth may have studied Buddhist philosophies. Is that possible? If so, is it important? Why?
- What is postmodernity? What do people mean by New Age religion? Explain why some Christian nurses oppose using integrated care techniques such as therapeutic touch.

CASE STUDY 3.1

Jo is an advanced practice nurse who wants to use her knowledge and talents to promote health within her congregation. Her area of expertise is gerontology, and she attends a synagogue with a large elderly population. The congregation is in a lower socioeconomic area, and the people have many chronic health needs. Jo realizes that the people could never afford to hire a nurse but that the faith community could greatly benefit from her services.

Critical Thinking
- What are some strategies that Jo might use to begin helping to promote health within her congregation?
- How would knowledge of past and future trends of spiritual care in nursing assist Jo in starting a program within her synagogue?
- What information should Jo obtain before starting any type of ministry in her local congregation?
- Are there any models that might help Jo?
- What resources would be of use in this situation?

Key Points

- Various individuals and groups have delivered spiritual care for a long time.
- Many of humanity's advances in social order, technology, and artful expression are also responses to faith.
- Spiritual care is an indispensable aspect of holistic care.
- Most Judeo-Christian faith communities, while based on a respect of the traditional, are constantly trying to be innovative when addressing age-old questions relating to death, suffering, and the meaning of life.
- Some people experience God in very profound, sometimes controversial ways.
- Various models of organizing care for the body, mind, and spirit have been and continue to be used in the world today.
- The provision of the care of the body has largely been relegated to women, whereas the provision of the care of the mind and the spirit has largely been relegated to men.
- The provision of spiritual care has been a key component of professional nursing since its inception.
- People can have high spirituality and low religiosity and be healthy; conversely, people can have high religiosity and low spirituality and also be healthy.
- Leaders in the spirituality movement and "new age of nursing" often use a combination of traditional and nontraditional interventions.

References

Babler, J. E. (1997). A comparison of spiritual care provided by hospice social workers, nurses, and spiritual care professionals. *The Hospice Journal, 12*(4), 15–27.

Bailey, S. S. (1997). The arts in spiritual care. *Seminars in Oncology Nursing, 13,* 242–247.

Bave, F. W. (2001). *The spiritual society.* Wheaton, IL: Crossway.

Bay, M. J. (1997). Healing partners: The oncology nurse and the parish nurse. *Seminars in Oncology Nursing, 13,* 275–278.

Benzein, E. G., Saveman, B. I., & Norberg, A. (2000). The meaning of hope in healthy, nonreligious Swedes. *Western Journal of Nursing Research, 22,* 303–319.

Brown-Saltzman, K. (1997). Replenishing the spirit by meditative prayer and guided imagery. *Seminars in Oncology Nursing, 13,* 255–259.

Burkhardt, M. A. (1989). Spirituality: An analysis of the concept. *Holistic Nurse Practitioner, 3*(3), 69–77.

Burkhardt, M. A., & Nagai-Jacobson, M. G. (1985). Dealing with spiritual concerns of clients in the community. *Journal of Community Health Nursing, 2,* 191–198.

Burton, L. A. (1998). The spiritual dimension of palliative care. *Seminars in Oncology Nursing, 14,* 121–128.

Carson, V. B. (1989). *Spiritual dimensions of nursing practice.* Philadelphia: WB Saunders.

Carson, V. B. (1997). Spiritual care: The needs of the caregiver. *Seminars in Oncology Nursing, 13,* 271–274.

Carson, V. B., & Green, H. (1992). Spiritual well-being: A predictor of hardiness in patients with acquired immunodeficiency syndrome. *Journal of Professional Nursing, 8,* 209–220.

Castledine, G. (1998). The value of prayer in modern-day nursing. *British Journal of Nursing, 7,* 1290.

Chapman, K. J., & Pepler, C. (1998). Coping, hope, and anticipatory grief in family members in palliative home care. *Cancer Nursing, 21,* 226–234.

Clark, C. C. (1997). Recognizing spiritual needs of orthopaedic patients. *Orthopaedic Nursing, 16*(6), 27–32.

Clinebell, H. (1992). *Basic types of pastoral care & counseling: Resources for the ministry of healing & growth.* Nashville: Abingdon.

Coward, D. D. (1991). Self-transcendence and emotional well-being in women with advanced breast cancer. *Oncology Nursing Forum, 18,* 857–862.

Coward, D. D. (1994). Meaning and purpose in the lives of persons with AIDS. *Public Health Nursing, 11,* 331–336.

Coward, D. D. (1997). Constructing meaning from the experience of cancer. *Seminars in Oncology Nursing, 13,* 248–251.

Coward, D. D., & Lewis, F. M. (1993). The lived experience of self-transcendence in gay men with AIDS. *Oncology Nursing Forum, 20,* 1363–1368.

Coward, D. D., & Reed, P. G. (1996). Self-transcendence: A resource for healing at the end of life. *Issues in Mental Health Nursing, 17,* 275–288.

Cress-Ingebo, R., & Chrisagis, X. (1998). Try a good book: Bibliotherapy as spiritual care. *Journal of Christian Nursing, 15*(2), 14–17.

Davidhizar, R. E., & Laurent, C. R. (2000). The art of forgiveness. *Hospital Materiel Management Quarterly, 21*(3), 48–53.

Dombeck, M.-T. B. (1995). Dream telling: A means of spiritual awareness. *Holistic Nurse Practitioner, 9*(2), 37–47.

Dossey, B. M. (1998). Florence Nightingale: A 19th-century mystic. *Journal of Holistic Nursing, 16*(2), 111–164.

Dufault, K., & Martocchio, B. C. (1985). Hope: Its spheres and dimensions. *Nursing Clinics of North America, 20,* 379–391.

Emblen, J. D. (1992). Religion and spirituality defined according to current use in nursing literature. *Journal of Professional Nursing, 8*(1), 41–47.

Emblen, J. D., & Halstead, L. (1993). Spiritual needs and interventions: Comparing the views of patients, nurses, and chaplains. *Clinical Nurse Specialist, 7,* 175–182.

Engebretson, J. (1996). Considerations in diagnosing in the spiritual domain. *Nursing Diagnosis, 7,* 100–107.

Fehring, R. J., Miller, J. F., & Shaw, C. (1997). Spiritual well-being, religiosity, hope, depression, and other mood states in elderly people coping with cancer. *Oncology Nursing Forum, 24,* 663–671.

Festa, L. M., & Tuck, I. (2000). A review of forgiveness literature with implications for nursing practice. *Holistic Nursing Practice, 14*(4), 77–84.

Govier, I. (2000). Spiritual care in nursing: A systematic approach. *Nursing Standard, 14,* 32–40.

Haase, J. E., Britt, T., Coward, D. D., Leidy, N. K., & Penn, P. E. (1992). Simultaneous concept analysis of spiritual perspective, hope, acceptance and self-transcendence. *Image: The Journal of Nursing Scholarship, 24,* 141–147.

Hall, B. A. (1994). Ways of maintaining hope in HIV disease. *Research in Nursing & Health, 17,* 283–293.

Hall, C., & Lanig, H. (1993). Spiritual caring behaviors as reported by Christian nurses. *Western Journal of Nursing Research, 15,* 730–741.

Hart, D., & Schneider D. (1997). Spiritual care for children with cancer. *Seminars in Oncology Nursing, 13,* 263–270.

Hawking, S. (1988). *A brief history of time.* New York: Bantam.

Health Ministries Association, Inc. and American Nurses Association. (1998). *Scope and standards of parish nurse practice.* Washington, DC: American Nurses Publishing.

Herth, K. (1990). Fostering hope in terminally ill people. *Journal of Advanced Nursing, 15,* 1250–1259.

Herth, K. (1993). Hope in the family caregiver of terminally ill people. *Journal of Advanced Nursing, 18,* 538–548.

Highfield, M. F. (1997). Spiritual assessment across the cancer trajectory: Methods and reflections. *Seminars in Oncology Nursing, 13,* 237–241.

Holstein, M. (2000). A spiritual role for the elderly. *Health Progress,* March-April, 12–16.

Hungelmann, J., Kenkel-Rossi, E., Klassen, L., & Stollenwerk, R. (1996). Focus on spiritual well-being: Harmonious interconnectedness of mind-body-spirit—use of the JAREL Spiritual Well-Being Scale. *Geriatric Nursing, 17,* 262–266.

Kaczorowski, J. M. (1989). Spiritual well-being and anxiety in adults diagnosed with cancer. *The Hospice Journal, 5,* 105–116.

Kaye, J., & Robinson, K. M. (1994). Spirituality among caregivers. *Image: Journal of Nursing Scholarship, 26,* 218–221.

Kazanjian, M. A. (1997). The spiritual and psychological explanations for loss experience. *The Hospice Journal, 12*(1), 17–27.

Keighley, T. (1999). A woman of mystery. *Nursing Standard, 13*(34), 14–15.

Kelsey, M. (1995). *Healing and Christianity.* Minneapolis: Augsburg.

Kylma, J., & Vehvilainen-Julkunen, K. (1997) Hope in nursing research: A meta analysis of the ontological and epistemological foundations of research on hope. *Journal of Advanced Nursing, 25,* 364–371.

Landis, B. J. (1996). Uncertainty, spiritual well-being, and psychological adjustment to chronic illness. *Issues in Mental Health Nursing, 17,* 217–231.

Lane, J. (1987). The care of the human spirit. *Journal of Professional Nursing, 3,* 332–337.

Lewis, P. J. (1996). The review of prayer within the role of the holistic nurse. *Journal of Holistic Nursing, 14,* 308–315.

Ley, D. C., & Corless, I. B. (1988). Spirituality and hospice care. *Death Studies, 12,* 101–110.

Martsolf, D. (1997). Cultural aspects of spirituality in cancer care. *Seminars in Oncology Nursing, 13,* 231–236.

Martsolf, D. S., & Mickley, J. R. (1998). The concept of spirituality in nursing theories: Differing world-views and extent of focus. *Journal of Advanced Nursing, 27*(2), 294–304.

Mauk, K. L., Russell, C. A., & Birge, J. (2003). *Congregational health.* Rockford, IL: Hilton.

McFague, S. (1987). *Models of God.* Philadelphia: Fortress.

McGee, E. M. (2000). Alcoholics Anonymous and nursing: Lessons in holism and spiritual care. *Journal of Holistic Nursing, 18*(1), 11–26.

Meraviglia, M. G. (1999). Critical analysis of spirituality and its empirical indicators. *Journal of Holistic Nursing, 17*(1), 18–33.

Messenger T., & Roberts, K. T. (1994). The terminally ill: Serenity nursing intervention for hospice clients. *Journal of Gerontological Nursing, 20*(11), 17–22.

Mickley, J. R., Carson, V., & Soeken, K. L. (1994). Religion and adult mental health: State of the science in nursing. *Issues in Mental Health Nursing, 16,* 345–360.

Mickley, J. R., Soeken, K., & Belcher, A. (1992). Spiritual well-being, religiousness, and hope among women with breast cancer. *Image: Journal of Nursing Scholarship, 24*(I), 267–272.

Miller, M. A. (1995). Culture, spirituality, and women's health. *JOGNN, 24,* 257–263.

Mills, M. E. (1998). *Images of God in the Old Testament.* Collegeville, MN: Liturgical Press.

Mitchell, L. L. (1977). *The meaning of ritual.* Ridgefield, CT: Morehouse.

Murray, C. K., & Stoner, M. (1998). Say a little prayer. *Nursing 98,* June, 55.

Nagai-Jacobson, M. G., & Burkhardt, M. A. (1989). Spirituality: Cornerstone of holistic nursing practice. *Holistic Nurse Practitioner, 3*(3), 18–26.

Nelson, S. (2001). *Say little, do much: Nursing, nuns, and hospitals in the nineteenth century.* Philadelphia: Pennpress.

Nolan, P., & Crawford, P. (1997). Towards a rhetoric of spirituality in mental health care. *Journal of Advanced Nursing, 26*(2), 289–294.

Nowotny, M. L. (1989). Assessment of hope in patients with cancer: Development of an instrument. *ONF, 16,* 57–61.

O'Brien, M. E. (2003). *Spirituality in nursing: Standing on a holy ground* (2nd ed.). Boston: Jones and Bartlett.

O'Mathuna, D. P. (1999). Prayer research: What are we measuring? *Journal of Christian Nursing, 16*(3), 17–21.

O'Murchu, D. (1997). *Quantam theology.* New York: Crossroad.

O'Neill, D. P., & Kenny, E. K. (1998). Spirituality and chronic illness. *Image: Journal of Christian Scholarship, 30,* 275–280.

Owen, D. C. (1989). Nurses' perspectives on the meaning of hope in patients with cancer: A qualitative study. *Oncology Nursing Forum, 16,* 75–79.

Peacocke, A. (1993). *Theology for a scientific age.* Minneapolis: Fortress Press.

Penrod, J., & Morse, J. M. (1997). Strategies for assessing and fostering hope: the hope assessment guide. *Oncology Nursing Forum, 24,* 1055–1062.

Reed, P. G. (1991). Self-transcendence and mental health in oldest-old adults. *Nursing Research, 40,* 5–10.

Rees, C., & Joslyn, S. (1998). The importance of hope. *Nursing Standard, 12*(41), 34—39.

Reese, D. J., & Brown, D. R. (1997). Psychosocial and spiritual care in hospice: Differences between nursing, social work, and clergy. *Hospital Journal, 12*(1): 29–41.

Remen, R. N. (1996). *Kitchen table wisdom.* New York: Riverhead.

Ross, L. A. (1997). Elderly patient's perceptions of their spiritual needs and care: A pilot study. *Journal of Advanced Nursing, 26,* 710–715.

Ruether, R. R. (2002). *Visionary women: Three medieval mystics.* Minneapolis: Fortress Press.

Rustoen, T., Wiklund, I., Hanestad, B. R., & Moum, T. (1998). Nursing intervention to increase hope and quality of life in newly diagnosed cancer patients. *Cancer Nursing, 21,* 235–245.

Seely, J. F. (1999). [Review of the book *Facing death and finding hope: A guide to the emotional and spiritual care of the dying*]. *Journal of Palliative Care, 15*(1), 56–57.

Sellers, S. C., & Haag, B. A. (1998). Spiritual nursing interventions. *Journal of Holistic Nursing, 16,* 338–354.

Shelly, J. A., & Miller, A. B. (1999). *Called to care: A Christian theology of nursing.* Downers Grove, IL: InterVarsity.

Silva, M. C., & DeLashmutt, M. (1998). Spirituality and prayer: A new age paradigm for ethics. *NursingConnections, 11*(2), 13–17.

Solari-Twadell, P. A., Djupe, A. M., & McDermott, M. A. (Eds.). (1990). *Parish nursing: The developing practice.* Oak Brook, IL: Advocate Health Care.

Solari-Twadell, P. A., & McDermott, M. A. (Eds.). (1999). *Parish nursing: Promoting whole person health within faith communities.* Thousand Oaks, CA: Sage.

Sterling-Fisher, C. E. (1998). Spiritual care and chronically ill clients. *Home Healthcare Nurse, 16,* 243–250.

Stevens-Barnum, B. (1995). Spirituality in nursing: Everything old is new again. *Nursing Leadership Forum, 1*(1), 24–29.

Stevens-Barnum, B. (1996). *Spirituality in nursing: From traditional to New Age.* New York: Springer.

Stolley, J. M., Buckwalter, K. C., & Koenig, H. G. (1999). Prayer and religious coping for caregivers of persons with Alzheimer disease and related disorders. *American Journal of Alzheimer's Disease, 14,* 181.

Stranahan, S. (2001). Spiritual perception, attitudes about spiritual care, and spiritual care practices among nurse practitioners. *Western Journal of Nursing Research, 23*(1), 90.

Taylor, E. J. (1997). The story behind the story: The use of story telling in spiritual caregiving. *Seminars in Oncology Nursing, 13,* 252–254.

Treloar, L. L. (1999). Spiritual care: Assessment & intervention. *Journal of Community Nursing, 16*(2), 15–18.

Trice, L. B. (1990). Meaningful life experience to the elderly. *Image: Journal of Nursing Scholarship, 22,* 248–251.

Tuck, I., Pullen, L., & Lynn, C. (1997). Spiritual interventions provided by mental health nurses. *Western Journal of Nursing Research, 19,* 351–363.

VandeCreek, L. (1997). Collaboration between nurses and chaplains for spiritual caregiving. *Seminars in Oncology Nursing, 13,* 279–280.

Wang, C. H. (2000). Developing a concept of hope from a human science perspective. *Nursing Science Quarterly, 13,* 248–254.

Westberg, G. E., & McNamara, J. W. (1990). *The parish nurse: Providing a minister of health for your congregation.* Minneapolis: Augsburg.

Recommended Readings

Belcher, A. E., Dettmore, D., & Holzemer, S. P. (1989). Spirituality and sense of well-being in persons with AIDS. *Holistic Nurse Practitioner, 3*(4), 16–25.

Bonhoeffer, D. (1982). *Spiritual care.* Minneapolis: Fortress.

Carlson-Catalano, J. (1998). Nursing diagnoses and interventions for post-acute-phase battered women. *Nursing Diagnosis, 9,* 101–110.

The Field Museum. (1993). *Scrolls from the Dead Sea.* Washington, DC: Archetype Press.

Fuller, M. (1994). *The theology of the hammer.* Macon, GA: Smyth & Helwys.

Halstead, M. T., & Mickley, J. R. (1997). Attempting to fathom the unfathomable: Descriptive views of spirituality. *Seminars in Oncology Nursing, 13,* 225–230.

Haugt, K. (1991). Stephen series caring ministry workshop participant manual. St. Louis: Stephen Ministries.

Mitchell, E. R. (2000). The case management plan for a chemically dependent homeless man. *Nursing Diagnosis, 11,* 80–83.

Shelly, J. A. (2000). *Spiritual care.* Downers Grove, IL: InterVarsity.

4

Introduction to Influences of Religion and Culture on Nursing

Christoffer H. Grundmann, David G. Truemper, and Theodore M. Ludwig

LEARNING OBJECTIVES

At the end of this chapter, the reader will be able to:

- Discuss why and how religious attitudes of patients become topics for nursing care.
- Discriminate between spirituality, religiosity, and religion.
- Describe how religion functions in the culture of people's lives.

KEY TERMS

religion
religiosity
spiritual distress
spirituality

While researchers "know surprisingly little about the" actual and precise "impact of religion and spirituality on health" (Smith, 2001, p. 356), they do know that religious as well as spiritual orientation certainly plays an important role in coping with diseases and getting well again (Koenig, Bearon, Dayringer, 1989; Koenig et al., 1992; Maton, 1989). It is from this perspective that these topics are important in nursing practice. For example, experiencing chronic illnesses, suffering from severe bodily mutilation caused by an accident or an aggressive medical treatment, or sensing the shadow of impending death call for a heightened awareness of and attention to those spiritual and religious factors in life that, under normal circumstances, are regarded as medically insignificant and viewed as mere personal preferences. These factors are strongly apparent in times of personal crisis involving serious illness and disease because they threaten a person's earthly existence. Another reason for being consciously aware of spiritual and religious matters in nursing is the consumer oriented health-care setting in the United States, which demands a nondiscriminating respect for personal preferences as one element of quality care management (Carson, 1989).

However, serious ethical concerns call for extreme sensitivity in these matters and health care professionals are cautioned not to address religious issues in times of health crisis without obvious need. These concerns include the respect for personal privacy as a vital part of patient autonomy, the desire not to inflict harm upon patients or to exercise coercion, and the need to discriminate between religious and nonreligious patients (Sloan, Bagiella, & Powell, 2001). When addressing spiritual issues in nursing practice, a competence is needed to know how to discern the appropriate from the inappropriate in matters affecting **spiritual distress**, an approved and well established nursing diagnosis (Carpenito-Moyet, 2003; Kim, McFarland, & McLane, 1987; Stoll, 1979).

This and the following chapters in this unit try to pave a way into the highly complex interdependencies of religion, health, and healing, with special reference to elements of importance for nursing professionals, so this discussion focuses only on the basics. Readers who want more detail are advised to make ample use of the multivolume reference works *Encyclopaedia of Religion and Ethics* (Hastings, 1908–1926) and *The Encyclopedia of Religion* (Eliade, 1987) in addition to the literature given in the chapters' various references and recommended readings.

THE BASICS OF RELIGION AND SPIRITUALITY

Although spiritual attitudes and religious convictions do have an impact on the day-to-day lifestyles of people, religion and spirituality, as such, are neither just personal options nor therapeutic elements. To use them like special therapies or drugs whenever it seems appropriate to achieve a specific goal is to distort them totally.

Speaking of **religion** means speaking of the distinctive and all-encompassing central expression of a person's very way of life. People live what they believe in, whether they consciously articulate it or not. What people cherish most, they spend their time, energies, and money on, and what they disrespect, they show their disgust for clearly. Therefore, it is appropriate to speak of a religious dimension in humans as an anthropological given, for people cannot help but act out what they believe.

However, a distinction needs to be made here. In light of the general statement made, one should speak more precisely about the **religiosity** of people. This religiosity gets appropriated by individuals by means of their **spirituality**—which turns into formal religion only at that point when it gets articulated within a distinctive cultural and social framework. The hallmark of "religion" is the corporeal and collective acknowledgment of and abidance by a set of values, norms, and regulative behavior based on a formulated set of teachings, often the "holy texts" or "holy traditions" of the respective religion. Regular and frequent public services, as well as the exercise of private piety, keep these traditions alive, thereby fostering a distinctive, overarching attitude toward life. Each of the established classical religions thrives in a particular language, which it takes care to preserve, even though this language may no longer be a spoken one: ancient Hebrew for the Jews, Koine Greek for the Christians, Quranic for the Muslims, or Pali for the Buddhists. And it is language that shapes culture, just as culture finds its most succinct expression in its language (Crystal, 1987). Because language and religion are so intimately intertwined, it is not surprising to find religion permeating all of culture via the medium of language—even without people being aware of it.

To speak of religion is to speak of the very basic orientation of a multitude of people, an orientation manifest far more in common habits and manners than just in explicitly religious exercises. The observance of certain festivals or diets, the way of dress, and how the significant events of life such as birth, puberty, marriage, and death are celebrated all reflect a religious dimension. The same holds true of attitudes toward the body and the appreciation of life unimpeded by health crises. Religion is the result of the commonly accepted order of life of a community to quite an extent (Durkheim, 1912, 1975), albeit religion represents only one aspect of it. Religion does reflect personal maxims too, and often very much so (Allport, 1950; Hill et al., 1998; Pargament, 1997). Because of this, and considering the vast diversity of existent religions—naturalistic, theistic, and nontheistic ones—religion can be appropriately defined as a lived relationship toward an ultimate.

Lived relationship points to the fact that religion is more than just the consciously acknowledged content of any belief or faith in an ultimate, often not verbalized at all but detected in the lifestyle of the individual. *Toward an ultimate* is used to accommodate the broad variety of ways in which the ultimate is perceived by different traditions, be it a personal God, as in Judaism, Christianity, and Islam; a specific enlightenment, as in Buddhism; or the realization of the basic principle of the world, as in Daoism (Grundmann, 1999). This definition implies that religion cannot simply be equated with "belief in God" or involvement in church or communal activities. Speaking of religion in these terms reflects only a particular perception of religion.

Divisions are found within each and every religion, divisions that sometimes are called sects, movements, or denominations. Without delving into the sociology of religion now (Niebuhr, 1960; Troeltsch 1912/1949), it is good and helpful to be aware of it in order to avoid speaking fictitiously of Christianity, Judaism, Islam, or Buddhism.

There are no such monolithic religions. All religions are lived in a variety of ways because segregation occurs in the course of any development. Although a certain set of holy scriptures and practices are held in common by all who might be called Christians, Muslims, or Buddhists, the interpretations of these respective traditions and scriptures differ significantly, as does the observance of religious duties. When it comes to the implementation of religious demands by individuals, differences are unavoidable. Once these differences aggregate into tensions that reach a certain level, they give rise to a spin-off, starting a new tradition of that particular religion. As long as the connection between the root tradition and the offspring is still visible, both are still counted as one religion, at least by outsiders, but religions too have a life of their own, sprouting, branching out, blossoming, and bearing fruit. Sometimes they dry up and fade away, like the ancient religions of Mesopotamia or Egypt.

Thus, to relate meaningfully to individuals, nurses should realize that patients are not just Muslims, but Shiite or Sunnites; not just Jews, but Orthodox, Conservative, Reformed, or Reconstructionist; not just Christians, but Roman Catholics, Lutherans, or Reformed. The general labeling of a patient as "Christian," "Jew," "Muslim," "Buddhist," or "Native/Indigenous American" can serve only as a general identification of a particular root-tradition, which needs to be more precise to do justice to the individual patient. The aspects of peculiar diversity within a given religion are addressed in each of the following chapters in Unit 2.

Because the term *religion* addresses predominantly a collectively shared perception of life and world, norms and values, tradition and habits, the term *spirituality* is used to express the religiosity of individuals. These individuals might or might not be members of established and formal religious bodies, such as a local congregation, church, synagogue, or mosque (Burkhardt, 1989; King, Speck, & Thomas, 1994; Stoll, 1979). Spirituality need not necessarily be linked to religious commitment at all, but can be perceived of in a totally irreligious way, as an indicator of the decisive human capability to transcend life beyond the merely vital vegetative and materialistic spheres. It is the spiritual capacity that enables humans to make sense out of the chaotic mass of sensual experiences during their lifetime. Spirituality is the brain power, the mental capacity, and the "spirit" by which humans master life. In this sense, every human being has a spirituality of his or her own (Beland & Passons, 1975; Simson & Weiner, 1989). Most adherents to established religions have a kind of religiously informed spirituality, imparted to them by their upbringing and religious practice. But the same holds good for humanists, philanthropists, and agnostics. Only within this broad perspective does the diagnosis of spiritual distress become intelligible against the background of a pluralistic society.

OVERVIEW TO THE CHAPTERS ON WESTERN RELIGIONS

To help readers easily find relevant information, each chapter about Western religions is structured as follows:

- A brief historical overview of how the religion came about and how its main branches developed
- A sketch of the religion's basic features and teachings
- A paragraph about how the religion's perceptions of life, body, diseases, and dying affect nursing

A selected bibliography marks the end of each subsection within this unit.

The chapters on Western religions are listed chronologically according to their appearance in history to avoid any value judgment. Thus, discussion begins with Judaism and its movements; followed by Christianity, with its many denominations; and Islam, with its respective branches. Discussion then moves to Native American and African-American religious traditions, which deserve special attention.

OVERVIEW TO THE CHAPTERS ON EASTERN CULTURES AND RELIGIONS

The intimate connection between health and spiritual wholeness has been known and cultivated since ancient times by people in the various Eastern cultures and religions. Systems of traditional medicine that rely on spiritual as well as physical factors have flourished in India, China, and elsewhere. Today, of course, peoples of the Eastern cultures make use of Western allopathic medicine, especially for acute sicknesses. But traditional healing practices, closely linked with their religious traditions, still play an important supplementary role alongside Western medicine. Even for those who have immigrated to Western countries, traditional attitudes toward health and healing, rooted in their long-standing religious world views, continue to be influential. A significant number of non-Asians, including Western health practitioners, have become interested in the spiritual outlook and therapeutic practices that come from these Eastern cultures.

Of course, there is much diversity among the peoples of the East. In general, the term "Eastern" is used to refer to the peoples of the eastern segment of Asia. More specifically, this includes South Asia (India, Sri Lanka, Nepal, Bhutan, Pakistan, Bangladesh, and Afghanistan), Southeast Asia (Thailand, Myanmar, Cambodia, Laos, Vietnam, Malaysia, Indonesia, and the Philippines), and East Asia (China, Taiwan, Korea, Japan, and Mongolia). These peoples make up more than half of the world's population and consist of many distinct ethnic groups, cultures, and religious traditions. Among South Asians, Hindus greatly predominate in India and Nepal, but Indians are Muslim, with smaller communities of Sikhs, Jains, Buddhists, Christians, and Parsis. Pakistan, Bangladesh, and Afghanistan are strongly Muslim, and Sri Lanka and Bhutan have Buddhist majorities. In Southeast Asia, Buddhism is dominant in some of the countries (Thailand, Myanmar, Cambodia, Laos, and Vietnam), whereas Islam is by far the most dominant in others (Indonesia and Malaysia), although there are significant Hindu, Buddhist, and Chinese communities. Philippine people are predominantly Christian, with a significant Muslim population. Pervasive throughout all the lands of East Asia are the Buddhist, Confucianist, and Daoist traditions, as well as localized indigenous traditions, such as Shinto in Japan; again, there are minority Christian and Muslim communities as well.

Thus, to speak of the influence of Eastern religions and cultures in the sphere of spirituality and health is an enormous topic. Later chapters focus on the larger influences of Hindus and Buddhists, together with Chinese and Japanese religions and practices, bringing in influences from Jains, Sikhs, and others.

Despite the diversity in these Eastern cultures and religions, some areas of convergence do exist among these peoples that are distinct from common Western attitudes and values. In contrast to Jewish, Christian, and Muslim ideas of an almighty creator God who determines events from outside the world, as it were, Eastern perspectives generally see the world as self-contained and self-governing. Forces that determine events, whether understood as gods, spirits, karmic forces, gunas, yin-yang forces, operational phases, or human volition, are all part of the interdependent functioning of life. The underlying sense of correspondence between the macrocosm and the microcosm, the great sacred cosmos and the local community or human body, posits an organic identity that includes physical, social, mental, and spiritual entities. Individual health and wholeness is understood within the larger fabric of cosmic forces, nature, family, ancestors, and human society.

Maintaining human health requires understanding these patterns of forces, based on longstanding experience and tradition in a particular culture. It also requires practicing the techniques, rituals, arts, and methods devised through centuries-long human experimentation for integrating human life most appropriately and healthfully with these various forces. Various spiritual practices of healing abound: prayer, chanting, rituals, meditation, yoga, bodily exercises, and ethical disciplines. The distinctive medical therapies that have evolved in these cultures, such as herbal remedies, acupuncture, physical exercises, and massage, are based on the underlying religious worldviews.

CONCLUSION

The nursing diagnosis "spiritual distress" is defined as the "state in which the individual experiences or is at risk of experiencing a disturbance in his [or her] belief or value system that is the source of strength and hope" (Carpenito-Moyet, 2004, p. 743). One other definition explains it as "distress of the human spirit ... a disruption in the life principle which pervades a person's entire being and which integrates and transcends one's biological and psychological nature" (Kim et al., 1987, p. 314). Both of these definitions are wide enough to avoid any religious specifics.

While it would be too much to expect nurses to be proficient in the highly diverse realm of religion, it rightly can be expected of them to recognize if their patients do experience spiritual distress. Once they have diagnosed it accordingly, nurses should attempt to get the spiritual counselors or other representatives of the respective religious tradition involved, provided the patient consents to this. Nurses leave the decisions to patients out of respect for their personal autonomy and dignity. This should be the standard procedure, but if patients do not want a priest, rabbi, imam,

PERSONAL REFLECTIONS

- Begin to observe your interactions with others. Can you identify ways in which religion has permeated your culture?
- Will it be difficult for you to see patients beyond the label of their "root-tradition" religion?
- Do you agree with the authors when they claim that it was a wise decision to avoid religious specifics in the definition of "spiritual distress?" Why or why not?
- Why are nurses obligated to accurately "discern the appropriate from inappropriate in matters affecting" the spiritual care of patients?

or other religious representative at their bedside, nurses and patients will have to manage on their own. Because spirituality exists as an integral part of the whole person, nurses should acquaint themselves with the various religious traditions to be able to provide holistic and culturally sensitive care. And it is in this respect only that the orientations on the various religious traditions in Chapters 5 through 12 are provided.

CASE STUDY 4.1

During report, the nurse from the afternoon shift describes the woman with a new diagnosis of cancer who has been admitted to the oncology unit as "Jewish." The afternoon shift nurse goes on to say that she "ordered the patient a Kosher diet" but that the day nurse will need to "call the rabbi to let him know the woman was admitted." The nursing colleague, who will be caring for the woman overnight, asks "to which branch of Judaism" the patient belongs. The afternoon shift nurse replies, "I don't know. I didn't have time to ask her about her religion. It just says Jewish on her admission form."

Critical Thinking
• Is the nursing assessment adequate?
• Which assumptions has the afternoon shift nurse made? How did the nurse make these assumptions? Why might these assumptions be false?
• Which ethical principle has the afternoon nurse violated? Which ethical principles have the potential of being violated? How can the night nurse act as a patient advocate while increasing her colleague's cultural sensitivity?
• Why would this be an important time for the patient in terms of examining her religious beliefs?

Key Points
• Illness, suffering, and impending death heighten awareness about life factors that are usually not considered medically significant.
• Ethical principles are involved when health care professionals address religious issues.
• Religion speaks of the distinctive and all-encompassing central expression of one's very way of life. Religion permeates all of culture, although people may not be aware of this.
• Religion can be defined as a lived relationship toward an ultimate. It predominately addresses a shared perception of life and the world.
• Divisions, known as sects, movements, or denominations, can be found within each religion.
• Although Judaism, Christianity, and Islam are traditionally known as Western religions and Hinduism, Buddhism, Confucianist, and Daoist traditions are typically labeled Eastern religions, these religions are pervasive throughout the world.
• Traditional healing practices in Eastern cultures are closely linked with religion.

References
Allport, G. (1950). *The individual and his religion.* New York: Macmillan.

Beland, I. L., & Passons, J. Y. (Eds.). (1975). *Clinical nursing* (3rd ed.). New York: Macmillan.

Burkhardt, M. A. (1989). Spirituality: An analysis of the concept. *Holistic Nursing Practice, 3,* 69–77.

Carpenito-Moyet, L. J. (2003). *Nursing diagnosis: Application to clinical practice* (3rd ed.). Philadelphia: Lippincott Williams & Wilkins.

Carson, V. B. (1989). *Spiritual dimensions of nursing practice.* Philadelphia: WB Saunders.

Crystal, D. (1987). *The Cambridge encyclopedia of language.* New York: Cambridge University Press.

Durkheim, E. (1912). *Les formes élementaires de la vie religieuse.* Paris: Alcan.

Durkheim, E. (1975). *Durkheim on religion* (ed. and intro. by W. Pickering). London: Routledge and Kegan Paul.

Eliade, M. (Ed.). (1987). *The encyclopedia of religion,* 16 vols. New York: Macmillan.

Grundmann, Ch. H. (1999). *Wahrheit und Wahrhaftigkeit: Für einen kritischen Dialog der Religionen.* Hannover, Germany: Lutherisches Verlagshaus. (American edition in press.)

Hastings, J. (Ed.). (1908–1926). *Encyclopaedia of religion and ethics,* 12 vols. Edinburgh: T & T Clark.

Hill, P. C., Pargament, K. I., Swyers, J. P., Gorsuch, R. L., McCullough, M. E., Hood, R. W., & Baumeister, R. F. (1998). Definitions of religion and spirituality. In D. B. Larson, J. P. Swyers, & M. E. McCullough (Eds.), *Scientific research on spirituality and health: A consensus report* (pp. 14–30). Rockville, MD: National Institute for Healthcare Research.

Kim, M. J., McFarland, G. K., & McLane, A. M. (1987). *Pocket guide to nursing diagnosis* (2nd ed.). St. Louis: Mosby.

King, M., Speck, P., & Thomas, A. (1994). Spiritual and religious beliefs in acute illness: Is this a feasible area for study? *Social Science and Medicine, 38,* 631–636.

Koenig, H. G., Bearon, L. B., & Dayringer, R. (1989). Physician perspectives on the role of religion in the physician-older patient relationship. *Journal of Family Practice, 28,* 441–448.

Koenig, H. G., Cohen, H. J., Blazer, D. G., Pieper, C., Meador, K. G., Shelp, F., Goli, V., & DiPasquale, B. (1992). Religious coping and depression among elderly, hospitalized medically ill men. *American Journal of Psychiatry, 149,* 1693–1700.

Maton, K. (1989). The stress-buffering role of spiritual support: Cross-sectional and prospective investigations. *Journal for the Scientific Study of Religion, 28*(3), 310–323.

Niebuhr, H. R. (1960). *Radical monotheism and Western culture: With supplementary essays.* New York: Harper.

Pargament, K. I. (1997). *The psychology of religion and coping: Theory, research, practice.* New York: Guilford Press.

Simson, J., & Weiner, E. (Eds.). (1989). *Oxford English dictionary* (2nd ed.). New York: Oxford University Press.

Sloan, R. P., Bagiella, E., & Powell, T. (2001). Without a prayer—Methodological problems, ethical challenges, and misrepresentations in the study of religion, spirituality, and medicine. In T. G. Plante & A. C. Sherman (Eds.), *Faith and health: Psychological perspectives* (pp. 339–354). New York: Guilford Press.

Smith, T. W. (2001). Religion and spirituality in the science and practice of health psychology—Openness, skepticism, and the agnosticism of methodology. In T. G. Plante & A. C. Sherman (Eds.), *Faith and health: Psychological perspectives* (pp. 355–380). New York: Guilford Press.

Stoll, R. (1979). Guidelines for spiritual assessment. *American Journal of Nursing, 79,* 1574–1577.

Troeltsch, E. (1912/1949). *The social teaching of the Christian churches,* 2 vols. Translated by O. Wyon, with an introductory note by C. Gore. London: G. Allen & Unwin. New York: Macmillan (original: Die Soziallehren der christlichen Kirchen und Gruppen, Tübingen, 1912).

Recommended Readings
Barret, D., Kurian, G., & Johnson, T. (Eds.). (2001). *World Christian encyclopedia,* 2nd ed., 2 vols. New York: Oxford University Press.

Bonvillain, N. (1996). *Native American religion*. New York: Chelsea House Publishers.

Brannigan, M. C. (2000). *Striking a balance: A primer in traditional Asian values*. New York: Seven Bridges Press.

Cragg, K. R., & Speight, M. (1980). *Islam from within: Anthology of a religion*. Belmont, CA: Wadsworth.

Dorff, E. N. (1986). The Jewish tradition. In R. L. Numbers & D. W. Amundsen (Eds.), *Caring and curing health and medicine in the Western religious traditions* (pp. 5–39). New York: Macmillan.

Eck, D. L. (2002). *A new religious America: How a Christian country has become the world's most religiously diverse nation*. New York: Harper.

Hinnells, J. R., & Porter, R. (Eds.). (1999). *Religion, health and suffering*. London: Kegan Paul International.

Raboteu, A. J. (1986). The Afro-American traditions. In R. L. Numbers & D. W. Amundsen (Eds.), *Caring and curing—Health and medicine in the Western religious traditions* (pp. 539–562). New York: Macmillan.

Resources

Buddhanet
Buddha Dharma Education Association, Inc., P.O. Box K1020, Haymarket, Sydney NSW 2000, Australia
http://www.buddhanet.net
Buddhist information and education network.

The Hindu Universe
Hindu Students Council, P.O. Box 9185, Boston, MA 02114-0041
Phone: (617) 698-1106
Fax: (617) 444-8725
http://www.hindunet.com

The Pluralism Project
Harvard University, 201 Vanserg Hall, 25 Francis Avenue, Cambridge, MA 02138
Phone: (617) 496-2481
Fax: (617) 496-2428
http://www.pluralism.org/index.php
The Pluralism Project was developed by Diana L. Eck at Harvard University to study and document the growing religious diversity of the United States, with a special view to its new immigrant religious communities.

The Vatican
http://www.vatican.va
Official web site of the Vatican.

Wabash Center Guide to Internet Resources for Teaching and Learning in Theology and Religion: World Religions
Wabash Center, 301 W. Wabash Avenue, Crawfordsville, IN 47933
Phone: (765) 361-6047; (800) 655-7117
Fax: (765) 361-6051
Hinduism—http://www.wabashcenter.wabash.edu/Internet/hinduism.htm
Sikhism—http://www.wabashcenter.wabash.edu/Internet/sikhism.htm
Buddhism—http://www.wabashcenter.wabash.edu/Internet/buddhism.htm
Religion in China—http://www.wabashcenter.wabash.edu/Internet/china.htm
The Wabash Center for Teaching and Learning in Theology and Religion seeks to strengthen and enhance education in North American theological schools, colleges, and universities.

5

Judaism and Its Branches

Christoffer H. Grundmann and David G. Truemper

LEARNING OBJECTIVES

At the end of this chapter, the reader will be able to:

- Meaningfully distinguish between the beliefs of Judaism and Christianity.
- Identify the basic tenets of Judaism.
- Relate certain aspects of health behavior to the religious attitudes of those of the Jewish faith.
- Recognize issues of spiritual and religious concern within the distinctive beliefs and practices of the Jewish religion.
- Gain confidence in referring patients to the appropriate religious counselors.

Conservative Judaism	Old Judaism
Davidic kingdom	Orthodox Judaism
Hebrew	rabbi
Hellenistic Judaism	Rabbinic Judaism
kosher	Reconstructionist Judaism
Modern Judaism	Reform Judaism
Mt. Sinai	Torah

HISTORICAL OVERVIEW

✪ "It is history that provides the clue to an understanding of Judaism, for its primal affirmations appear in early historical narratives" (Baron & Silberman, 1990, p. 402). The principal, though not the only, realm of revelation of the ultimate to the Jews is history, namely the Exodus, the miraculous liberation from bondage in Egypt under the leadership of Moses, which took place in the 13th century BCE, and the covenanting of YHWH ("the living God") with his people at **Mt. Sinai.** On occasion of this covenant, the Jews received the **Torah** ("teaching"), the God-given order of life and law. In a restricted sense, Torah refers exclusively to the five books of Moses, called the *Pentateuch*. But in its broader sense the "written Torah" includes all of Jewish sacred scriptures (to most Christians commonly known as the Old Testament), whereas the "oral Torah" includes authoritative rabbinical teaching from over the centuries, which was codified in the Talmud ("study; learning") and other codes of law.

Four major epochs can be identified within the historical development of Judaism from its very beginnings to today:

1. **Old Judaism** (Ancient Israel) —20th to 4th centuries BCE
2. **Hellenistic Judaism**—4th century BCE to 2nd century CE
3. **Rabbinic Judaism**—2nd to 18th century CE
4. **Modern Judaism**—1750 to the present

Biblical texts tell us much about the Judaism of old—the Exodus, Torah, **Davidic kingdom**, division of Judah and Israel (926 BCE), Babylonian exile, return to Israel (about 522 BCE), and the reconstruction of the temple (515 BCE). But they tell only a little about the later periods, and these, too, were of similar importance to what Judaism is today.

During the Hellenistic period, which some researchers call the period of "Early Judaism," the elements of Jewish identity were established: mandatory commitment to the Torah, Sabbath sanctification, ritual and ethnic purity, and living as God's holy people in the Holy Land. But with the raid of Jerusalem and the destruction of the second temple in 70 CE, the Jews lost their political, as well as their religious, center. To compensate for this loss, they turned to scriptures as never before, making Judaism an exemplary "religion of the book," while at the same time nurturing the idea of a final restoration of their holy place in the holy city when the Messiah comes. Consequently, the synagogue emerged as the place of Jewish public worship, and a new kind of religious profession developed of those learned in the scriptures, the **rabbi** ("my teacher"). The rabbis became the principal figures, dominating Jewish life in all of the countries to which Judaism spread in the more than 1¹/₂ millennia that followed. Their major discussions were collected in the voluminous Talmud and some other canonical books, which are still referred to when religious counsel is sought (Werblinsky, 1992; Neusner, 1999).

Throughout the centuries, Jews migrated all over Europe and to many places in Asia, Africa, America, and Australia, mainly as a result of numerous persecutions, which often were explicitly motivated by the religious concerns of those in power. This caused Jews to internalize the idea of having to live as a people in exile among hostile peoples until the Messiah comes. But this concept was challenged during the time of Jewish enlightenment, called Haskala, in the 18th century. Now, because "the end of the doctrine of the Exile" is assumed, "Jewish modernity for most scholars ... is marked by the end of a passive waiting on the Messiah and the beginning of an active pursuit of personal or national fulfillment on this earth and preferably in one's lifetime" (Hertzberg, 1990, p. 422). To better assimilate into the dominant cultures, reform movements boosted by the intellectual aftermath of the American (1776) and French (1789) Revolutions advocated limiting the use of **Hebrew** and changes in liturgy, dietary laws, and ritual customs, which caused counter-reactions that brought about the multifaceted Judaism of today. In the United States, four movements or main branches of Judaism can clearly be discerned: the Orthodox, Conservative, Reconstructionist, and Reform.

BASIC FEATURES AND DOCTRINES OF JUDAISM

Common to all observant Jews is the high reverence for the Torah, the celebration of the major religious festivals, and the veneration of the weekly Sabbath as a 24-hour period of almost complete rest between Friday and Saturday evening. But special dietary laws, strict religious ruling of daily life, and abiding by the Jewish religious law by consulting the Rabbinic tradition as found in the Talmud are binding to only certain movements.

To be the elected people of the only true and living God because of God's covenanting with Israel at Mt. Sinai marks the core religious element of Judaism. This covenant mainly implies the observance of the "law" given to the Jews, the Torah. God promises protection and redemption of his people and their permanent settling in the Holy Land, with Zion in its center, at the end of times (see Deuteronomy 11:26–31). Consequently there is an untiring hope and expectation in God's final rulings, along with a loving appreciation of the law, which becomes obvious even to non-Jews in the gesture when the scrolls are taken from the shrine and carried in a procession through the synagogue during worship. Belief in creation of all the world by God is also common to all Jews. Differences are manifested in the way in which these basics are interpreted by the various movements, which lead to very different attitudes and behavior.

Orthodox Judaism. The Orthodox Movement, which gained momentum in the second half of the 20th century, is distinguished by a literal belief in the Torah as the ultimate word of God, and the belief "that Jewish law is to be determined by reference to the codes and responsa [the answers given by the rabbis] of the past" (Dorff, 1986, p. 7). Thus, in Orthodox Jewish circles, Torah, Talmud, and the teachings of the rabbis play a role for Orthodox Jews that is hardly to be overestimated.

Conservative Judaism. Recognizing that Judaism has changed during the course of time, the Conservative movement closely and critically scrutinize the tradition in order to carefully discern the will and mood of the current Jewish generation. However, for Conservative Jews, the use of the Hebrew language in Jewish worship and life is of vital importance because it "represent[s] the spirit of Judaism" (Hertzberg, 1990, p. 424). When being asked about giving advice in critical matters such as medical ethics, Conservatives tend to be more conventional in their counsel than are progressive Jews because the "law" is binding to them. However, this law can be understood properly only when interpreted in its historical setting. This belief makes Conservative Judaism the most scholarly movement and one which is more inclined to adjust to modern needs than the Orthodox, as can be seen in the Conservative ordination of women rabbis since 1985.

Reconstructionist Judaism. The Reconstructionist movement developed in reaction to the earlier Conservative movement. To the Reconstructionists, the Torah and the Talmud are important too, but not just as religious documents. They are important as sources for determining the Jewish "culture" common to all Jews, religious or not (Kaplan, 1967). Jews should "reconstruct" their lives in a new cultural covenant on the foundation of their existence as an historical people, for which the existence of the state of Israel (since 1948) is of vital importance because it represents the focal point of the cultural roots of Judaism. The religious law is not ultimately binding, but the cultural bonds are. Thus, Reconstructionist Jews cultivate the sense of belonging to an old and well-established cultural body of global dimensions while showing a fairly liberal religious attitude toward the challenges of the day.

Reform Judaism. The oldest and most influential Jewish movement in the United States is Reform Judaism, which began early in the 19th century. Driven by the desire to overcome their marginalizing ghetto existence, in part caused by their peculiar religious observances, Jews abandoned many of their practices and teachings to better adapt Judaism to the modern world. The binding force of Jewish ritual law was declared void, and the use of Hebrew was restricted to certain liturgical prayers. The Philadelphia Platform (1869) declared that Jews should no longer expect to return to Palestine; this stand was re-emphasized by the Pittsburgh Platform (1885), which stressed the need for deorientalization of Judaism, viewing Judaism as an evolutionary rather than a national faith. The liturgy was changed accordingly, omitting all references to animal sacrifices and the physical return to the Holy Land. The scriptures (i.e., Torah, Talmud) may serve as one among many other sources that an individual or congregation may consult when a critical decision is to be made, but are in no way binding because they are not understood as the final and authoritative word of God. Jews of the Reform Movement are the most liberal and modern.

DOCTRINAL DISTINCTIONS AFFECTING NURSING

Anyone caring for patients of Jewish faith has to be mindful of three general elements that might differ from what is usually taken for granted:

1. Jewish perception of the body as being created by God, given on loan throughout lifetime to the individual
2. Significance of the Jewish calendar, especially the observation of Sabbath and particular festivals
3. Importance of visiting the sick, especially the very sick

Because visiting the sick is regarded as an important meritorious religious duty, irrespective of social standing, and as a factor contributing to bringing about comfort and healing, nurses should be hospitable to a patient's visitors. Large congregations tend to organize the visitation of sick people by establishing a Visiting Society, which often also serves as the Burial Society. Family members and representatives of these societies should not be hindered from being with the diseased person, especially when death draws near, for Jews should never die alone, but surrounded by the people of Israel to whom they belong. Proper nursing of a Jewish patient requires making sure this is possible.

Care should be taken as well to respect special religious rulings regarding Sabbath keeping. Turning lights on and off or riding in a car on the Sabbath is looked at as improper work for most Orthodox and Conservative Jews, as are the handling of money and the use of telephones, radios, or televisions. Nursing planning should be farsighted enough to avoid unnecessary interference with these rulings.

The perception of the human body as a God-created entity entrusted to or on loan for the lifelong stewardship of the individual has many implications for nursing, affecting mainly the handling of the sick and diseased body but also affecting how to deal with a corpse. The body should be retained in all its integrity and not mutilated (in autopsy or cremation) as long as it lasts; mutilating a body is tantamount to destroying God's creation. Death should be neither hastened nor hindered, rendering active euthanasia an impossibility, but leaving "passive euthanasia"—palliative care and allowing a person to die without interference—acceptable to most Jews. Although Reform and Reconstructionist Jews show a permissive attitude toward organ transplantation and vasectomies, Orthodox Jews prohibit them explicitly, and Conservative Jews hesitate to allow them on the basis of the integrity of the body. In critical cases, nurses should advise their patients to seek the advice of their respective rabbis.

Bodily cleanliness and purity also are important, for they are viewed not merely as a hygienic matter but also as a religious duty to honor God's good creation. Thus, in addition to caring for the overall cleanliness of bedbound or homebound patients according to general nursing standards, certain additional precautions are to be observed, especially with regard to the care of women. Orthodox women, for example, won't be touched by their husbands while they have their menses, not even assisted in and out of bed. Thus, nurses have to be prepared to do this themselves or with the help of other women around, a situation they most probably will not encounter with patients of the Reform or Reconstructionist movements. In addition, a male nurse would in principle not likely be permitted to care for an Orthodox Jewish woman according to these traditions.

The dead body (the corpse) is the most impure of all bodies. In an Orthodox environment, the deceased patient should by no means be left alone until buried and should not be touched or washed by medical personnel, but only by members of the Burial Society. If the patient dies on the Sabbath, these activities should be postponed until the next day, for Orthodox Jews will not violate the "Day of the Lord." Nurses should enable relatives or other "people of Israel" to be present at all times and should avoid bringing in flowers, which are regarded as improper on such an occasion.

Nurses also need to observe special practices with regard to the care of newborns when attending Jewish patients, especially Orthodox and Conservative Jews, because Jewish infants are named a few days after birth, rather than immediately. A boy is named on the 8th day after delivery when his ritual circumcision is performed. A girl receives her name on the next Sabbath after her birth during the reading of the Torah. Thus, Jewish newborns are without a name for several days, a situation to which nurses should be sensitive. When they need to speak about the infant, they may refer to him or her as "the son" or "the daughter" of the patient. In case of an abortion, permissible to Orthodox Jews only under certain clearly defined circumstances, but allowed more liberally by other movements (Dorff, 1986), the fetus should be prepared to be buried, not just disposed of, because it too is God-created.

Finally, nurses caring for Jewish patients should be mindful of certain dietary peculiarities. As a general rule, food served to Orthodox and Conservative Jews should be kosher, meaning that it is prepared according to the Jewish religious code, whereas Reform or Reconstructionist Jews usually do not require kosher food. Because the kosher regulations are highly complex, food should be ordered from religiously approved stores, or relatives should be asked to provide it. Nurses should address this issue because doing so makes their patients aware of the nurse's sensitivity and thus eases the mind and soul. Leaving sufficient time for prayer before and after meals is another important gesture, especially when a nurse has to feed the patient.

PERSONAL REFLECTIONS

- Have I ever provided nursing care to a person of the Jewish faith? If so, to which branch of Judaism did they belong?
- What have I done to educate myself about providing spiritually and culturally competent care to Jewish patients? What could I do to improve my knowledge in this area for the future?
- What changes in planning nursing care would I make the next time I have a patient who is Jewish? What questions should I ask him or her about dietary practices? About religious observances?
- What would I do if faced with a situation in which, to support the spirituality of a patient, I had to violate some traditional hospital rules, such as allowing kosher food to be brought in from home or allowing a large number of visitors in the room at the same time? If I were in a supervisory capacity and a family asked me to make concessions such as these, how would I handle the situation?
- If I were in an educational role in a teaching hospital, what strategies might I use to enhance the knowledge of my staff about religious practices of Jewish persons?

CASE STUDY 5.1

The nurse is caring for Rabbi Rubenstein, an Orthodox Jew admitted to the county hospital for treatment of prostate cancer. He does not often communicate verbally to the female nurse who is caring for him but seems more comfortable talking with the male nursing assistant. There are frequent visitors to the room throughout the day, and although they are quiet and respectful, their presence seems to upset the patient's roommate. The nurse is concerned that Rabbi Rubenstein is becoming depressed and that his health care environment is not ideal for his recovery.

Critical Thinking
- What changes could the nurse make within this health care system to provide spiritually competent care for this patient?
- In a typical county hospital system without religious affiliation, what limitations are presented to the nurse in providing spiritual care for a patient of Jewish faith?
- What religious practices would the nurse expect to see in this case?
- What dietary practices would be expected?
- What accommodations could immediately be made to make the patient feel more comfortable? How should the nurse approach teaching the patient about his condition?

Key Points
- History is the principal realm of revelation of the ultimate to the Jews, especially the liberation from bondage in Egypt under the leadership of Moses in the Exodus and the covenanting of YHWH, the living God, with his people at Mt. Sinai.
- The four main branches of Judaism are Orthodox, Conservative, Reconstructionist, and Reform.
- Special dietary laws, strict religious ruling of daily life, and abidance by the Jewish religious law by consulting the Rabbinic tradition are binding to only certain movements.
- The Jewish perception of the body is that it is created by God.
- The observation of Sabbath and particular festivals may be especially significant to patients.
- Visiting the sick is an important part of the Jewish tradition.

References

Baron, S. W., & Silberman, L. H. (1990). The history of Judaism. In *Encyclopedia Britannica*, Vol. 22, 15th ed. (pp. 402–403). Chicago: Encyclopaedia Britannica, Inc.

Dorff, E. N. (1986). The Jewish tradition. In R. L. Numbers & D. W. Amundsen (Eds.), *Caring and curing health and medicine in the Western religious traditions* (pp. 5–39). New York: Macmillan.

Hertzberg, A. (1990). Modern Judaism. In *Encyclopedia Britannica*, Vol. 22, 15th ed. (pp. 422–427). Chicago: Encyclopaedia Britannica, Inc.

Kaplan, M. M. (1967). *Judaism as a civilization: Toward a reconstruction of American-Jewish life.* New York: Schocken Books.

Neusner, J. (1999). *The encyclopaedia of Judaism*, (3 vols.). Leiden/Köln: Brill. (Reprint of 1934 ed.)

Toruschka, U. (1992). Judentum. In M. Tworuschka & U. Tworuschka (Eds.), *Bertelsmann Handbuch Religionen der Welt: Grundlagen, Entwicklung und Bedeutung in der Gegenwart* (pp. 20–24). Gütersloh/München: Bertelsmann Lexikon Verlag.

Werblinsky, Z. (Ed.). (1992). *The Oxford dictionary of the Jewish religion.* New York: Oxford University Press.

Recommended Readings

Glazer, N. (1987). *American Judaism.* Chicago: University of Chicago Press.

Martin, B. (Ed.). (1978). *Movements and issues in American Judaism: An analysis and sourcebook of developments since 1945.* Westport: Greenwood Press.

6

Christianity and Its Branches

Christoffer H. Grundmann and David G. Truemper

LEARNING OBJECTIVES

At the end of this chapter, the reader will be able to:
- Meaningfully distinguish between the beliefs of Judaism and Christianity.
- Identify the basic tenets of Christianity.
- Relate certain aspects of health behavior to the religious attitudes of those of various denominations within Christianity.
- Distinguish the major differences in religious beliefs among many Christian denominations.
- Recognize issues of spiritual and religious concern within the distinctive beliefs and practices of the major divisions of Protestantism.
- Gain confidence in referring patients to the appropriate religious counselors.

KEY TERMS

Anabaptists
Anglican Church
Amish Church
Assemblies of God
Baptist
Calvinists
charismata
Christian Science Church
Church of God
Church of the Nazarene
Congregationalists
Disciples of Christ
Episcopal Church
evangelicals
fundamentalists

Hutterian Brethren
Jehovah's Witnesses
Lutheran
Mennonites
Methodism
Pentecostal
Presbyterians
Puritans
Quakers
Reformed tradition
Roman Catholic Church
Salvation Army
Seventh-day Adventist
Society of Friends
United Church of Christ

HISTORICAL OVERVIEW

✝ Christianity dates its origin to the life and ministry of Jesus of Nazareth, who after his resurrection, was acknowledged by his followers as the Christ (the Anointed One; the Messiah, see John 1:41). Interpreting Christ's resurrection from the dead as breaking the power of death once and for all and as a token of what will happen to all people who believe (John 11:25f; Romans 6:9), Christians believe that this meant a complete reversal of the human condition. Eventually, because of the historical significance of this event, they began counting years using the birth of Jesus Christ as the starting point. This eventually became the standard reference for the modern globalized Common Era (CE).

✡ ✝ When Jesus of Nazareth was approximately 33 years old, the Roman authorities then in power in Palestine crucified him. Only after encountering the crucified Jesus as the risen Christ did the small group of his disciples, so far regarded as just one among other deviant Jewish sects, begin to openly proclaim Jesus as the Messiah and risen Savior. Peter and Paul became the dominant representatives of the nascent church, each in his particular way (Acts 15; Galatians 2). While Peter stressed the importance of the Jewish religious law for Christians, Paul advocated liberation from it. He thus made the Gospel, the good news of salvation to all who recognize Christ as Lord, acceptable throughout the Roman Empire and its capital (see Romans). By the time the collection of holy scriptures called "The Book of Books" or simply "The Bible" was finalized in the 4th century, Christianity had become the official religion of the Roman Empire (Edict on Religion of 380 by Theodosius the Great). From this time, the church was regarded as "catholic" (literally, universal), encompassing all subjects of the then-known world.

✝ The unity and catholicity of the church disappeared when the Latin church formally broke with the Eastern church in 1054 CE by means of mutual excommunication.

Afterward, both the Catholic and the Orthodox churches developed independently. The **Roman Catholic Church** became the dominant cultural factor in the West, whereas Orthodoxy became the dominant cultural factor in the East (Norwich, 1988–1995). The idea of the papacy, a central leadership in the church, developed systematically by Leo the Great in the 5th century, applied to the Latin speaking church only. In the Greek and Syriac speaking churches of the East, the emperors were the heads of the church. Monks served as theological and spiritual leaders, a feature still existing in most of Orthodox Christianity, with its outspoken loyalty to the respective national government. The Orthodox churches tended to affiliate with the respective national leadership, bringing about a Russian, Greek, Serbian, and Ethiopian Orthodoxy, to name a few.

Various reform movements during and after the Middle Ages challenged the Roman Catholic Church in the West. One of the most significant was the Reformation, initiated by the biblical scholar and former Augustinian monk Martin Luther in 1517, when he posted his *95 Theses* on indulgences at the Castle Church at Wittenberg. The Augsburg Confession of 1530 not only gave a clear account of the differences in core matters of faith, doctrine, and practice the Lutherans held, but also refuted those teaching otherwise, as was the style of the day. This Confession, along with the religious and political conflicts that followed during the next 125 years, set into motion a movement of secessions from the Roman Catholic Church, which ultimately resulted in numerous Protestant denominations (Hudson, 1955; Niebuhr, 1929). The **Reformed tradition** emerged after the Lutherans, led by the Huldreich Zwingli and John Calvin, both of whom were Swiss, expressed the basics of their faith in the *Confessio Helvetica* (Swiss Confession) in 1536. The **Calvinists**, as those of the Reformed tradition are sometimes called, evolved into **Congregationalists** and **Presbyterians** in Anglo-Saxon countries (e.g., England, Scotland). The so-called **Puritans** in the 17th century were all members of these churches that challenged yet another reform church, such as the Church of England or **Anglican Church** (known in the United States as the **Episcopal Church**), which came about by royal decree in 1534. The King of England replaced the Pope as the head of the church and gave it the *Book of Common Prayer* for its liturgy and, in 1563, the *39 Articles* as its doctrinal basis.

Mennonites, or **Anabaptists**, date their origins to the Protestant Reformation and take their name from the 16th century Dutch priest Menno Simons, who opposed any authority in the church other than Christ. The communal living **Hutterian Brethren** and the **Amish Church**, which were founded later, belong to this tradition as well. Today Mennonites are known especially for their outspoken and dedicated social and pacifist concerns, which they have in common with the **Society of Friends**, the Quakers.

An offspring of the Puritans, **Quakers** did away with any kind of organized church government, liturgy, and ministry to provide opportunity for the workings of the indwelling Holy Spirit. Thus, Quakers have no special church buildings, ordained clergy, or outward observance of sacraments or liturgy. They advocate the all-encompassing binding relevance of Christ's teachings in communal as well as private life (*The Mennonite Encyclopedia*, 1955–1959).

In the 18th century, another important Protestant movement, which became known as **Methodism**, emerged from the Church of England. Concerned about the personal piety of every Christian, especially those on the margins of the established church, the Anglican clergyman John Wesley and his brother Charles adopted a new method of itinerant ministry: going out to the people where they lived, preaching to them in the open air, and providing them with new songs. First conceived as a "society" within the Church of England, a formal break took place in 1795, making the

Methodists an independent body. At the same time, vigorous missionary/evangelistic work brought Methodism into the New World beginning in 1769 after an attempt by the Wesley brothers in Georgia in 1736 made no impact. By the middle of the 19th century, Methodism had more members than any other American denomination because of its appeal to the masses of the industrial labor force whom the other established churches did not reach. By the end of the 19th century, after Methodism became well established, the Holiness Movement separated from it in the United States. Parts of this movement later merged with independent Pentecostal congregations and led to the formation of the **Church of the Nazarene** (Barrett, Kurian, & Johnson, 2001).

One important Methodist minister was William Booth, who founded the **Salvation Army**. Building on his work among the least privileged in East London, in 1865 Booth founded an organization based on strict military principles; the church is still renowned for its committed social work, brass bands, and hospitality to all. A number of other unique church-like religious organizations emerged in post-Civil War America that show a strong emphasis on either the dawning end of time, such as the **Seventh-day Adventists** (1863) and **Jehovah's Witnesses** (1879), or on healing, such as the **Christian Science Church** (1879). These organizations are discussed later in this unit.

The roots of **Baptist** churches, which hold that only conscious believers should receive baptism and this by total immersion, also are found in 17th century English Puritanism. Spreading to the United States that same century, the Baptist church today is a multifaceted phenomenon with a variety of Conventions, numerous independent congregations, and a very influential, dominant contemporary evangelist, Billy Graham. The African-American Baptist churches, which were organized after the Civil War by freed slaves, have made significant contributions to African-American life, with Rev. Martin Luther King, Jr. and Rev. Jesse Jackson among their most prominent representatives.

Pentecostalism, a revivalist spin-off of the Holiness Movement, emerged early in the 20th century, thriving especially among the socially marginalized as Methodism once did in the 18th century. Sparked in 1906, in a church led by Pastor William Seymour on Azura Street in Los Angeles, it was first known as the "Azura Street Revival"; it was soon called "Pentecostal." Its name refers to the first Pentecost, when the church received the gifts of the Holy Spirit (see Acts 2). These gifts, also called *charismata*, are mainly speaking in tongues, healing, and prophesying (see 1 Corinthians 12:4–11). According to **Pentecostals**, all Christians should seek to receive these gifts as an empirical proof of their baptism in the Holy Spirit. It was initially a revitalizing movement within the existing churches, but it soon became obvious that the established churches could not cope with it. Thus, Pentecostalism became independent, spread rapidly beyond the United States, and today represents one of the fastest growing branches within Christianity (Woodward, 2002).

Another comparatively recent branch of Christianity that has gained much influence is that represented by the evangelicals or fundamentalists. **Evangelicals**, who organized themselves in 1942 by forming the Association of Evangelicals, are antimodernist as far as Bible interpretation is concerned: the Bible is the Word of God and neither its text nor its content is to be critiqued. Evangelicals lobby for their cause with all of the modern means of high-tech communication, such as television, radio, and the Internet. Whatever is taught as God's word is to be believed. Belief is understood as an act of obedience by the pious, who then are expected to object to anyone saying otherwise. Defending their beliefs to others who would question that the Bible is the holy and infallible Word of God is a means of witnessing to the truths of their faith.

Since the church's founding in 1932, the intention of the **Disciples of Christ** has been to overcome denominational segregation by returning to simple and primitive Christianity as found in the New Testament. Currently, three major bodies comprise the Disciples of Christ: the Churches of Christ, the Christian Church (Disciples of Christ), and the nondenominational Fellowship of Christian Churches and Churches of Christ. Simplicity of worship and working toward unity of the church are the typical features of these denominations. The **United Church of Christ** (not related to the Churches of Christ), which is a U.S. body only, resulted in 1961 from a merger of the Evangelical and Reformed Church with the General Council of Congregational Christian Churches and represents the concern for Christian unity and especially unity among Protestants.

In summary, Christianity consists of a highly diverse group of denominations, most of them called "churches." To complicate the matter further, most of these denominations have branched and divided, thus making the number of distinct Christian denominational entities more than 30,000 according to a recent global survey (Woodward, 2002). This somewhat disturbing phenomenon is an indication that Christianity, which is still the largest among the religions of the world, with more than 2 billion adherents (Barrett & Johnson, 2002), is still vibrant and very much alive, although suffering from extreme individualism in the enlightened postmodern West.

BASIC FEATURES AND DOCTRINES OF CHRISTIANITY

✝ Despite the broad spectrum of Christian denominations, certain commonalities can be discerned. These concern the Bible, especially the story of Jesus the Christ as told in the Gospels, and the importance of worship in the local congregation, which is understood as a manifestation of the church. Christians see themselves as the "new people of God." This is why all of the Jewish holy scriptures are also found in the Bible, where they are commonly designated as the "Old Testament." Christianity thereby acknowledges the Jewish tradition as being part of the history of salvation, which came to fruition definitively in Jesus Christ. The Gospels and Apostolic letters contained in the "New Testament" give an ample account of Jesus Christ and reflect that Christianity transcended ethnic and nationalistic boundaries at an early stage of its existence (see Romans 5).

The acknowledgment of the crucifixion and resurrection of Jesus Christ is the core of what Christians have in common across all the numerous denominations. However, the denominations differ greatly in how this is to be interpreted and shared with people outside of the Christian fold. Because of the predominance of the Bible, Christianity, especially its Protestant branches, shows a significantly higher concern for scriptural interpretation and theological discourse than do other religions. Controversies about the meaning of scripture and the perception of the life and ministry of Jesus of Nazareth and questions about church government are some of the reasons for the extremely high incidence of dissenting groups and denominations within Christianity. Potentially, there are as many conflicting views on various subjects as there are individual believers.

Communal worship is vitally important to Christianity. Although the large number of Christian denominations indicates the influence of modern and secular individualism and of vested interests in material gain or institutional power, Christian faith is not merely religious individualism but is bound to be social as well. The Good

News needs to be shared with others because faith, at least in the Christian sense, is not just a matter of individual belief. The community of believers, the church, is important as well, for it is the church that hands down the tradition and relevant content of faith in as unadulterated a way as possible. To safeguard their heritage, churches have developed such institutions as the papacy, departments of doctrine and theology, a specially trained ministry and officially appointed or ordained clergy, and a particular order of service and liturgy. All of these institutions are open to variations and interpretations. The extremes may range from declaring the church to be the institute of salvation per se to declaring it unimportant for salvation at all. Questions of church government have been disputed throughout the centuries, as have issues about the ministry, the sacraments, the Holy Spirit, and the proper Christian life, with these disputes eventually leading to further separations. Because this divisiveness contradicts the very intention of the New Testament (John 17:21; 1 Corinthians 3:1ff), the 20th century witnessed the emergence of the Ecumenical movement as a conscious effort toward Christian unity in diversity, finding its ultimate expression in the formation of the World Council of Churches (WCC) in Amsterdam, The Netherlands, in 1948.

The veneration of the Bible, especially the narration of the life, ministry, suffering/passion, and resurrection of Jesus, and the appreciation of worship in a community are the two distinctive elements of Christianity. Other elements might be distinctively Christian, of course, but not necessarily held in common by all. This situation makes familiarity with the specifics of each particular denomination all the more imperative for nurses seriously concerned about the spiritual welfare of their patients. Nursing competence requires being able to discern critically between appropriate and inappropriate care for the individual Christian patient. Because of the number of variations, nurses should seek the patients' or their relatives' advice and guidance to avoid increasing spiritual distress.

DOCTRINAL DISTINCTIONS AFFECTING NURSING

Jesus of Nazareth, renowned for his healing miracles (Wilkinson, 1980), charged his disciples with the unselfish and unconditional care of the sick, most impressively in the parables of the Good Samaritan (Luke 10:25–36) and the great Judgment Day (Matthew 25:30–46). Caring for the needy to ease their suffering and thereby glorify God has become a hallmark of Christianity.

As an expression of genuine love for God, nursing care is first an outcome of the commitment to something greater than just a means of earning a livelihood. In providing nursing care to the sick, one is understood to be offering a service to God. Nursing care exemplifies acts of kindness and comfort for which Christianity is known. Thus, for Christians who feel called to serve, the profession of nursing may be a logical career choice that embodies their ideas of vocational calling and ministry to God.

In principle, Christians, like Jews, believe that they are created beings and therefore accountable to God for how they care for their bodies. This is not just confined to the welfare of the body, but also implies an explicit ethical connotation, which is described in the admonition of the Apostle Paul to Christians in Corinth: "Don't you know that your body is a temple for the Holy Spirit within you, given by God? ... Therefore glorify God with your body!" (1Corinthians 6:19–20). While almost all Christians perceive beauty and well-being as gifts of God, in cases of disease and suffering, Christians show a considerable diversity, finding its ultimate expression in the formation of the World Council of Churches (WWC) in Amsterdam, The Netherlands, in 1948.

The truly bewildering diversity of Christian denominations makes it imperative for any quality nursing care that seeks to ease spiritual distress to be based on the respective information and data as precisely and as early as possible so that a plan of care specific to each patient can be devised. This might be achieved by a separate section within the patient file that lists not just the religious affiliation but also the observation of a special religiously informed calendar (Sunday or Saturday Sabbath) and diet (ovo-lacto or strict vegetarian; avoidance of "unclean" foods), information on certain religious articles of worship (rosary, icons, Bible, hymn book, prayer book), and church or congregational particulars concerning visits and clerical administrations.

Roman Catholics

For observant Roman Catholic patients, administration of the sacraments, in most cases by a priest, is very important. The first sacrament to consider is baptism. In the case of a difficult delivery in which a newborn is in acute danger of dying, any attending Christian nurse, midwife, or physician may baptize the child by applying water to the infant's head and saying, "I baptize you in the name of the Father, and of the Son, and of the Holy Spirit." Although it may happen only in exceptional circumstances, stillborn and even aborted fetuses also are to be baptized in this way. A note made in the patient's register will relieve greatly the spiritual distress of affected mothers and fathers.

The Anointing of the Sick is the sacrament most commonly encountered by nurses attending Catholic patients. This sacrament, a gift of the church for the spiritual consolation and healing of those in sickbed, must be administered by a priest and may even be given to a person who is already dead if the priest was called in too late (O'Connell, 1986). The sacrament of anointing, once called the "sacrament of the dying," is extremely important for those in acute agony. Nurses should speak with their Catholic patients as long as the patients are conscious and should ask for the address of the nearest Catholic church (or the parish in which the patient is a member), keeping a record of this in the patient's file.

Holy Communion is another sacrament commonly encountered by the nurse. Catholics observe this practice at every Mass and may wish to receive communion during the hospital stay. The hospital priest or deacon, if Catholic, may administer the sacrament; nurses should excuse themselves from the room when possible when the priest visits to offer communion. The nurse should consult with the hospital priest regarding patients with special dietary considerations, or those who are to receive nothing by mouth, in the event that the patient wishes to receive communion at the bedside.

Attendance at Mass is also important in the Catholic faith. If the hospital or health care facility has a chapel that offers Catholic services, nurses should offer patients the opportunity to participate. Many facilities offer a closed-circuit television channel to which patients may tune and watch the service.

If the Catholic patient is very rigorous in his or her observance, nurses should be sensitive to special dietary or fasting habits, especially during Lent. Lent is the 6½ weeks before Easter; eating meat on Fridays during Lent is regarded as improper (McCormick, 1987). Although these fasts have become less common, observant Catholics, especially at a time of spiritual crisis, may find the practice of fasting helpful and reassuring.

Finally, nurses should be conscious of making all the religious artifacts Catholic patients wish to have available, including a rosary (which should be always close at hand) and images or statutes of preferred saints and of Mary. The nurse should place articles in such a way that the patient can establish eye contact easily or even touch them. During cleaning of the room, the nurse takes care to handle these items respectfully and put them in their appropriate place immediately afterward.

Orthodox Christians

Nurses caring for patients of the Orthodox tradition should be mindful of factors very similar to those already referred to in the discussion of Catholicism (Douropulos, 1975; Harakas, 1996). Orthodox Christians perceive their religious life as an ongoing participation in a sacramental-liturgical worship of divine origin. To them, the administration of sacraments such as Holy Communion and Anointing of the Sick by a priest is very important. Orthodox priests visit the sick frequently, even when patients are not in a critical condition, to let them share in liturgical prayer and to read to them from the Service Book (Harakas). This might take quite some time; nurses should not rush the rituals and should provide an appropriate allotment of time if possible. Nurses serving on neonatal care units should know that a newborn of Orthodox parents should be baptized within 40 days after birth, preferably by complete immersion and pronouncing it to be done "in the Name of the Father and of the Son and of the Holy Spirit." If this is not possible, sprinkling of water over the head is acceptable. In any case, the priest must be notified.

When an Orthodox patient's situation becomes serious, a priest must be called, for it is he who will perform the last rites, which are regarded as very important. If a patient dies, it cannot be taken for granted that relatives will consent to autopsy or organ donation, certainly not if they belong to the Russian Orthodox tradition, which abhors euthanasia, abortion, and cremation as well.

The dates of Orthodox observation of the Christian festivals differ from those of the common calendar, another important distinction from Catholicism. The main Orthodox Christmas celebration is the Feast of the Epiphany (January 6th), and Easter normally is celebrated 2 weeks or so later than the Easter of the common calendar. Thus, it is advisable to become well informed about the specifics of the Orthodox calendar when providing nursing care to Orthodox Christians.

Lutherans

When caring for Protestant Christians, one can generally assume that liturgical activity is less a concern than is the case with Roman Catholic and Orthodox Christians, but that counseling is more important. However, as far as Lutherans are concerned, a broad variety of practices is to be expected, ranging from very liturgical to nearly nonritualistic (Marty, 1983). For some Lutheran patients, especially when they are in critical condition, confession and Holy Communion at the bedside are of vital importance, but others might care more for someone praying with and for them or reading passages from the Bible (such as Psalm 23, Romans 8:31–38), or singing familiar hymns in the sick room.

An important sign of sensitivity by nurses is to be sure that a Bible and a hymn book or prayer book are easily accessible for the patients as well as for their visitors. If no visitors are present, nurses might offer to read to their patients a favorite biblical text or say a prayer at the close of the day. Because the priesthood of all believers is a basic tenet of the Lutheran confession, any believer is entitled to pray for and to bless a patient as desired; in addition, nurses may baptize newborns, and anyone may pray and read. If no ordained clergy is available, deaconesses or deacons or someone else from the congregation may bring the sacrament, conduct prayers and devotions, and bless the sick or anoint them (a practice fairly recently observed by Lutherans).

Committed Lutherans will not concede to active euthanasia and will not endorse artificial prolongation of life by all means. Organ donation might be acceptable to some, whereas others will object to it, as is the case with cremation (Lindberg, 1986). In principle, Lutherans have no dietetic restrictions. However, during special seasons of the church year, such as the important festivals of Christmas, Easter, and Pentecost and the weeks preceding Christmas (Advent) and Easter (Lent), some adjustments might be required.

Calvinists

Broadly speaking, patients of the Reformed or Calvinist tradition, which in the United States includes Congregationalists and Presbyterians, are distinguished by their pragmatic attitude toward illness (Vaux, 1984). To them, God is the Great Physician who grants the gift of healing to those who qualify for a healing ministry, be it as physicians, nurses, or counselors. Medicine thus becomes a *doxological science* (i.e., a science that gives praise to God) (Smylie, 1986, p. 217), and Presbyterians have become renowned for their hospital work in the United States as well as abroad in medical missions (Dodd, 1934; Wanless, 1911). Wherever medical or nursing help is available, it should be made use of and not neglected. It is a means and sign of God's continuing concern for the well-being of the people with whom He has formed a covenant. Thus, Presbyterians and Congregationalists alike are open to any medical advancement, provided it serves the purpose of doing good and not inflicting harm (Vaux, 1984). This openness enables nurses to do whatever is necessary without feeling hampered by a strict religious regimen. Engaging in one's chosen vocation makes it religious in the sense of obedience to one's calling. Besides this typically Calvinist attitude, which elevates and dignifies the nursing profession far beyond mere professionalism, nothing particular is to be observed in nursing. If patients require it, provision should be made for receiving Holy Communion or for letting the Elders and Presbyters come for prayer and the laying on of hands. Members of the United Church of Christ, who are heirs to the Reformed and Congregationalist tradition, hold to the same maxims and practices, as do those within the Disciples of Christ tradition (Harrell, 1986).

Episcopalians

Patients of the Episcopal Church share in the Anglican tradition and its liturgical way of worship as found in the *American Book of Common Prayer*. The rite of holy unction is part of their fairly extensive ministrations for the sick, which also includes visitation and prayer (Smith, 1986). They endorse ordinary healing but also are open to so-called faith healing and have been engaged in ministry to the aged for a long time (Booty, 1986). Thus, nurses can count on strong support and assistance from the respective congregation when caring for an Episcopal patient. Most Catholic, Orthodox, Lutheran, and Episcopal patients will seek to observe the principal Christian festival times. Sometimes, such as during Lent and Advent, this might require dietary restrictions about which nurses should inform themselves by asking. As strong advocates of human dignity and the individual's right of informed choice, Episcopalians do not condemn controversial though responsible medical decisions, provided they do not demean the dignity of patients by reducing them to mere objects of treatment, trials, or research. Nurses may assist patients in arriving at well-informed decisions, such as whether to terminate a pregnancy or carry it to term or whether to stop artificial life support or organ donation, because "when it comes to difficult questions concerning medical ethics ... virtually every possible point of view can be found ... in Anglicanism" (Booty, 1986, p. 260). Although nurses are entitled to baptize a newborn in an emergency and to notify the local priest afterward, they should call the priest for all other religious ministrations.

Methodists

Methodism is characterized by its stress on sincere, straightforward personal piety gained from Bible study as a sign of holy living. It also shows across its diverse branches a remarkable reverence for its founder, John Wesley (1703–1791) and his teachings (Vanderpool, 1986). When attending to Methodist patients, nurses should ensure that a Bible, a Methodist hymnal, and, if possible, a selection of John Wesley's sermons are always available for the patient, if these materials are not provided by relatives or friends. Methodists favor a healthy lifestyle as an expression of love for God and of responsibility toward the corporeal life given by God. This makes them receptive to the request of organ donation (Holifield, 1986). They advocate simple and plain remedies and show an openness for healing brought about by prayer, "that medicine of medicine," as John Wesley called it (Vanderpool, p. 328). Nurses should be prepared for their patients to ask for Deacons or Elders to pray and anoint them, for this is seen as obedience to scriptural testimony (James 5:14–15). In addition, because saintly dying, consciously accepting death without fear by looking ahead to what will come in the world thereafter, has been an element of Methodism from its very beginning, nurses should be alert that it might be a goal for many contemporary Methodists (Vanderpool, 1981). Appropriate passages from scripture should be read and prayers said, preferably by an officially ordained minister of the church, who always should be informed when a situation turns critical. This applies to a life-threatening delivery as well because the minister (Deacon or Elder) is regarded as the person most appropriate to perform baptism or to anoint the sick.

Nazarenes

The Methodist considerations hold true for members of the Salvation Army and the Church of the Nazarene, but some distinctive variations are to be observed when patients belong to these Methodist spin-offs. These variations pertain to dietary regulations, especially the consumption of alcohol and smoking, which are strictly forbidden for Nazarenes. Regarding the baptism of infants, while Salvation Army members do not observe a particular ceremony when a child is born, except for a dedication to Christ, Nazarenes place much emphasis on baptism. But because to them baptism means the baptism of believing individuals, they face some difficulty in reconciling this belief with their desire to be faithful to the scriptural testimony, which does not have a definite ruling on this point. Thus, they leave the option to parents who are anxious about their newborn in serious condition. Newborns may be baptized, if death is imminent, or "dedicated" to the triune God, if there is genuine hope for overcoming the crisis, whichever seems most appropriate in the situation. Nazarenes also make it a point to bury a stillborn (Geradi, 1989).

Mennonites

Most Mennonite patients will have no difficulties in accepting traditional modern medical treatment and nursing. However, those belonging to the Old Order Mennonites, the Amish, and the Hutterites show a certain restraint and prefer older remedies, and in remote areas they may sometimes resort to indigenous folk medicine, called *powwowing* (Klaassen, 1986). Nurses should be prepared to meet with a certain resistance to "modern techniques," especially when making home visits. Because the local congregation represents the factual presence of God's kingdom for Mennonites, nurses should seek the counsel of the "sisters and brethren" of their patients, who are generally well disposed to listen to the community's voices sympathetically (Snyder, 1995). An inviting, hospitable attitude toward visiting community members eases much of the spiritual distress of those afflicted with a disease. Although there may be a concern that visitors might disturb the professional rhythm, they also provide a source of consolation and comfort, thereby helping patients to cope with diseases. Nurses should draw on this community support and make it an ally in their provision of quality care, because dying in isolation, sometimes even in a separate room on a hospital ward, would be detrimental to people religiously socialized in a tradition bound to a community and would likely increase their spiritual distress.

The Mennonite churches, unlike other religious traditions with a strong emphasis on a consecrated or ordained ministry, stress the aspect of sharing the meal together, rather than the sacramental aspect; for example, Holy Communion is not normally asked for during hospitalization, but anointing the sick with oil might be requested. In addition, because surrender to the will of God is paramount for Mennonites, a heroic, disciplined acceptance of a terminal disease or the conscious acceptance of imminent death puts a halt to unrestrained application of medical means to extend or to terminate life and to medicalize the process of dying. However, this attitude often is accompanied by a depressive state because Mennonites rarely can be certain as to having really fulfilled the "law of Christ" (Klaassen, 1986, p. 282).

Virtually all Mennonites honor the dignity and sanctity of life and thus oppose abortion. Mennonites do not practice infant baptism but do practice a dedication. Mennonites baptize their youth only after they have attained knowledge of good and bad and have become responsible for their personal actions; they may be baptized as grown adolescents of about 18 to 20 years of age, as among the Hutterites, Amish, and Old Order Mennonites, but they are sometimes baptized in their younger teen years, as among the majority of the acculturated, modern Mennonites (Hostetler, 1974; Klaassen, 1986, p. 282). Mennonites, especially those who are the least acculturated, may demand to always wear their traditional head covering, even when confined to bed by illness.

Quakers

When caring for patients belonging to the Religious Society of Friends (also called Quakers), nurses might expect a principled openness to any provision necessary for quality nursing. The Friends' abnegation of any outward representation of religion and waiting for the Holy Spirit to speak makes any sick visit a fairly quiet and solemn one; nurses should not disturb this atmosphere and should provide sufficient room for it when planning patient care. Because they regard baptism and communion as purely spiritual happenings, Friends do not celebrate or administer these sacraments. Thus, nurses need not worry about asking if baptism or Holy Communion are desired. But because certain Friends would like to have their baby baptized (Geradi, 1989) nurses should be sensitive toward these expectations. Friends do not have particular religious requirements for terminally ill patients.

Baptists

Most of the patients from the multifaceted Baptist tradition are favorably disposed to modern medicine and nursing, provided that they do not destroy a God-given life by means of abortion or euthanasia (Lippard & Sharp, 1975; Weber, 1986). The absolute authority of the Bible and a fairly strict church discipline and lifestyle regimen are elements to which nurses should be sensitive. Church members visit the sick to pray over them for strength to endure such "times of trial" or for healing and sometimes to anoint patients with oil. Nurses in certain geographical areas might encounter a strong belief in faith healing, which may add to or ease the spiritual distress of the patients. If the nurse perceives that the patient has increased spiritual distress, he or she should contact the respective clergy and talk to the people concerned, advocating the case of the patient. Nurses also should inform the clergy if patients ask for Holy Communion. The ready availability of a Bible at the bedside at all times relieves much mental agony of Baptist patients, especially those who suddenly find themselves hospitalized as the result of an accident. If time permits, nurses may offer to read a biblical text to those who are not visited by Baptist "brothers and sisters"; if this is not possible, the nurse may ask a hospital volunteer to do so, especially if the situation turns serious and the sick person is dying.

Because Baptists believe that only genuine believers should receive baptism, which excludes infants, nurses need not be concerned about special regulations while assisting in delivery. Except for a ban on alcohol, at least among members of the Southern Baptist Convention, and restrictions on smoking in certain other congregations (Tyler, 1944; Tyrrell, 1979), Baptists do not have religious rules concerning diet. Thus, nurses are at liberty to set up menus for Baptist patients according to the nursing plan. If Baptist patients have to be fed, care should be taken to leave them sufficient time for prayer before meals, after meals, or both.

Pentecostals

Pentecostal Christians, such as members of the **Assemblies of God** or the Church of God in Christ, can be expected to have a certain pragmatic and unbiased approach to contemporary medicine and nursing. Because Pentecostalism is in part indebted to the Holiness Healing Movement that occurred at the turn of the 20th century, the eager expectation of instant healing as God's response to fervent prayer of the faithful and atoned ones is to be found in this movement far more frequently than any other (Harrell, 1975; Synan, 1971; Wacker, 1986). Pentecostalism is further characterized by such numerous independent denominations and branches that it becomes virtually impossible to make any definitive statement about commonalities in doctrines and rituals. This calls for a heightened sensitivity with regard to denominational peculiarities: the best plan is to ask relatives or religious "brethren and sisters" about special religious beliefs of the patient and about their particular congregational affiliations, because these may differ greatly within the same denominational tradition. Nurses will probably encounter faith-healing prayer with anointing and laying on of hands, probably accompanied by "Hallelujah" and "speaking in tongues" (Popejoy, 1976); they nevertheless should safeguard their Pentecostal patients against any such activity that aggravates existing spiritual distress. Communication with patients, their families, and their peers should be established early to eliminate any friction between medically necessary procedures and patients' religious desires. Most Pentecostals observe a general prohibition of alcohol, tobacco, and other narcotic drugs. If patients are in a depressive state of mind and lonely, nurses may offer to play cassettes with favorite choruses. Children usually are not baptized except for those who have received Jesus Christ as Savior and Lord. Those who are baptized may sometimes ask for Holy Communion, in which case nurses should notify the clergy. At the point of death no special Pentecostal rites are to be observed, except in the event of unique practices in particular localities (Geradi, 1989).

Adventists

Adventists do not represent a single denomination but rather are a cluster of different groupings, among which the Seventh-day Adventists, the **Church of God** (Seventh Day), and the Worldwide Church of God remain prominent today. Their name indicates their program: like the Jews they observe Saturday, not Sunday, as the Sabbath and day of worship, which is regarded not only as scriptural but as speeding the second coming or "advent" of Christ. Any nursing plan should honor this and consequently seek to limit all activities to the bare essentials from Friday evening to Saturday evening (Numbers & Larson, 1986). However, some Adventist groups, such as the Adventist Christian Church, do not keep the seventh day (Neufeld et al., 1966; Smylie, 1990).

Adventist spirituality is characterized by a conscious notion of living in the time of the imminent advent of Christ for final judgment and the separation of the faithful from the wicked. The faithful should be prepared for this return in body, mind, and spirit: thus, they advocate a healthy lifestyle void of alcohol, tobacco, coffee, or tea and one that includes healthy exercise. Some are strict vegetarians, whereas others enjoy any kind of meat in moderation, except pork, which is regarded as religiously "unclean"; this is important to know for the dietary regimen of patients belonging to this tradition. Seventh-day Adventists, for whom the "Gospel of Health" legacy of Ellen G. White is binding, have distinctive rules about healthy living and health care to honor the body as the "Temple of the Holy Spirit" (Numbers, 1976; Schwarz, 1981). As with patients of other traditions, lifestyle questions for Adventists are questions of moral obligation and not just matters of individual preferences. Nurses should be aware that the violation of certain regulations might cause distress when one falls ill and should try to help patients abide by the religiously established regimen if the medical situation permits.

Adventists are charged to cooperate with the "laws of nature." Thus, they can be expected to comply with whatever is medically recommended or necessary for nursing. In so doing, they share in maintaining and mending the "Temple of the Holy Spirit," which means their body. Abortion and euthanasia might be acceptable, as well as organ donation (Provonsha, 1981).

Adventists in general do not approve of faith healing and oppose any type of mind cure as it is practiced by Christian Scientists or during hypnosis (Numbers & Larson, 1986). They do not administer baptism to newborns but have an infant dedication. In the rare event of patients or their families desiring Holy Communion or the ritual of anointing the sick, the officially appointed minister should be informed. Because death is seen as the natural end of earthly life, nurses do not need to look for special religious observances when Adventist patients pass away. As long as their patients are alive, nurses should provide a Bible near the bedside so that patients or their visitors can easily have access to it.

Key Points

- Christianity consists of a highly diverse group of denominations, most of them called churches. Most denominations have branched and divided, resulting in more than 30,000 different organizations.
- Important questions to ask regarding specific beliefs that might affect nursing care include observance of the religious calendar and holidays, diet, use of religious articles (e.g., prayer book, Bible, rosary), and wishes regarding visitation of clergy.
- The acknowledgment of the crucifixion and resurrection of Jesus Christ is the core of what Christians have in common across all the numerous denominations.
- Important sacraments common to many Christian churches include baptism and communion.

PERSONAL REFLECTIONS

- Have I ever provided nursing care to a person of Christian faith? If so, to which branch of Christianity did they belong? To which denomination within that branch?
- What have I done to educate myself about providing spiritually and culturally competent care to patients of various Christian denominations? What could I do to improve my knowledge in this area for the future?
- Of the various Christian beliefs and sects presented in this chapter, to which do most of patients I care for belong?
- What changes in planning nursing care would I make the next time I have a patient who is a Mennonite? Episcopal? Catholic? Methodist? Quaker? Baptist? What questions should I ask them about dietary practices? About religious observances?
- What would I do if faced with a situation in which, to support the spirituality of a patient, I had to violate a moral or ethical principle of my own? For example, if my patient refused a potentially life-saving organ transplant to obey his religious tradition, what actions would I take? How would I feel in this situation? If I were in a supervisory capacity and a family asked me to withhold an ordered treatment such as this, how would I handle this situation?
- If I were in an educational role in a teaching hospital, what strategies might I use to enhance the knowledge of my staff about religious practices among various branches of Christianity?

CASE STUDY 6.1

Samuel is the 8-year-old son of a pastor of an Assembly of God church and has just received a diagnosis of a rare, aggressive form of untreatable cancer. He is on the pediatric intensive care unit in a large teaching facility in a major U.S. city. The pastor and his wife believe that God wants to heal their son of this incurable disease but that God will wait to act until He is convinced of the strong faith of Samuel's family and their church members who are praying for him. As Samuel's condition quickly worsens, his father requests that a prayer service be held at the boy's bedside. He candidly explains to the nurse in charge that the service would involve many people crowded into the hospital room, laying hands on the boy, speaking in tongues, praying aloud, and anointing him with oil. The nurse is concerned about disturbing other patients in the pediatric ward but wishes to honor the father's request because this is an important part of their religious tradition. Samuel is too ill to voice an opinion but seems to have a deep respect for his parents and has been surrounded by caring people from his church family.

Critical Thinking
- Is there an ethical dilemma in this situation?
- What religious beliefs are at the basis of the parents' request? What are the barriers to accommodating this request?
- Would the nursing staff need to make any special interventions or precautions to arrange for such a prayer vigil in the hospital room? What factors should be considered in relationship to other patients and families on the unit?
- Is this a reasonable request? Should it be granted? Is it likely in the facility in which you are practicing that such a request would be honored? What are some implications inherent in this situation?

- Caring for the needy to ease their suffering and thereby glorify God is a hallmark of Christianity. The care nurses provide may be seen as a commitment to a greater cause than merely earning money.
- The diversity of Christian denominations makes it imperative for nurses to obtain religious information as precisely and as early as possible to devise a plan of care specific to each patient.

References

Barrett, D., Kurian, G., & Johnson, T. (Eds.). (2001). *World Christian encyclopedia* (2nd ed., 2 vols.). New York: Oxford University Press.

Barrett, D. B., & Johnson, T. M. (2002). Worldwide adherents of all religions by six continental areas, mid-2001. In *2002 Britannica book of the year* (pp. 302–303). Chicago: Encyclopaedia Britannica, Inc.

Booty, J. E. (1986). The Anglican tradition. In R. L. Numbers & D. W. Amundsen (Eds.), *Caring and curing—Health and medicine in the Western religious traditions* (pp. 240–270). New York: Macmillan.

Dodd, E. M. (1934). *Our medical task overseas.* New York: The Board of Foreign Missions of the Presbyterian Church in the U.S.A.

Douropulos, A. (1975). What is a Greek Orthodox? In L. Rosten (Ed.), *Religions in America.* New York: Simon and Schuster.

Geradi, R. (1989). Western spirituality and health care. In V. B. Carson, *Spiritual dimensions of nursing practice* (pp. 76 –112). Philadelphia: W.B. Saunders.

Harakas, St. S. (1986). The Eastern Orthodox tradition. In R. L. Numbers & D. W. Amundsen (Eds.), *Caring and curing—Health and medicine in the Western religious traditions* (pp. 146–172). New York: Macmillan.

Harakas, St. S. (1996). *Health and medicine in the Eastern Orthodox tradition.* Minneapolis: Light and Life Publishing Comp.

Harrell, D. E., Jr. (1975). *All things are possible: The healing and charismatic revivals in modern America.* Bloomington, IN: Indiana University Press.

Harrell, D. E., Jr. (1986). The Disciples of Christ—Church of Christ tradition. In R. L. Numbers & D. W. Amundsen (Eds.), *Caring and curing: Health and medicine in the Western religious traditions* (pp. 376–396). New York: Macmillan.

Holifield, E. B. (1986). *Health and medicine in the Methodist tradition.* New York: Crossroad.

Hostetler, J. A. (1974). *Hutterite society.* Baltimore: Johns Hopkins University Press.

Hudson, W. S. (1955). Denominationalism as a basis for ecumenicity: A 17th century conception. *In Church History, 24,* 32–50.

Klaassen, W. (1986). The Anabaptist tradition. In R. L. Numbers & D. W. Amundsen (Eds.), *Caring and curing—Health and medicine in the Western religious traditions* (pp. 271–287). New York: Macmillan.

Lindberg, C. (1986). The Lutheran tradition. In R. L. Numbers & D. W. Amundsen (Eds.), *Caring and curing—Health and medicine in the Western religious traditions* (pp. 32–33). New York: Macmillan.

Lippard, W. B., & Sharp, F. A. (1975). What is a Baptist? In L. Rosten (Ed.), *Religions in America.* New York: Simon and Schuster.

Marty, M. E. (1983). *Health and medicine in the Lutheran tradition: Being well.* New York: Crossroad.

McCormick, R. A. (1987). *Health and medicine in the Catholic tradition.* New York: Crossroad.

The Mennonite encyclopedia: A comprehensive reference work on the Anabaptist-Mennonite movement. (1955–1959). 4 vols. Hillsboro, KS: Mennonite Brethren Publishing House.

Neufeld, D. F., et al. (Eds.). (1966). *Seventh-day Adventist encyclopedia.* Washington DC: Review and Herald Publishing Association.

Niebuhr, R. H. (1929). *The social sources of denominationalism.* New York: H. Holt and Co.

Norwich, J. J. (1988–1995). *Byzantium* (3 vols.) [The early centuries, 1985; The apogee, 1991; The decline and fall, 1995]. London: Viking Publishing Corp.

Numbers, R. L. (1976). *Prophetess of health: A study of Ellen G. White.* New York: Harper & Row.

Numbers, R. L., & Larson, D. R. (1986). The Adventist tradition. In R. L. Numbers & D. W. Amundsen (Eds.), *Caring and curing—Health and medicine in the Western religious traditions* (pp. 447–467). New York: Macmillan.

O'Connell, M. R. (1986). The Roman Catholic tradition since 1545. In R. L. Numbers & D. W. Amundsen (Eds.), *Caring and curing—Health and medicine in the Western religious traditions* (pp. 108–145). New York: Macmillan.

Popejoy, B. (1976). *The case for divine healing.* Springfield, MO: Gospel Publishing House.

Provonsha, J. W. (1981). *Is death for real?* Mountain View, CA: Pacific Press Publishing Association.

Schwarz, R. W. (1981). *John Harvey Kellogg MD—The father of the health food industry.* Berrien Springs, MI: Andrews University Press.

Smith, D. H.(1986). *Health and medicine in the Anglican tradition.* New York: Crossroads.

Smylie, J. H. (1986). The Reformed tradition. In R. L. Numbers & D. W. Amundsen (Eds.), *Caring and curing—Health and medicine in the Western religious traditions* (pp. 204–239). New York: Macmillan.

Smylie, J. H. (1990). Adventist. In *Encyclopedia Britannica*, Vol. 1, 15th ed. (pp. 112f). Chicago: Encyclopedia Britannica Inc.

Snyder, G. F. (1995). *Health and medicine in the Anabaptist tradition: Care in community.* Valley Forge, PA: Trinity Press International.

Synan, V. (1971). *The Holiness-Pentecostal movement in the United States.* Grand Rapids, MI: Eerdmans Publ.

Tyler, A. F. (1944). *Freedom's ferment.* Minneapolis: The University of Minnesota Press.

Tyrrell, I. R. (1979). *Sobering up: From temperance to prohibition in antebellum America, 1800–1860.* Westport, CT: Greenwood Press.

Vanderpool, H. Y. (1981). The responsibilities of physicians toward dying patients. In J. Klastersky & M. J. Stuet (Eds.), *Medical complications in cancer patients* (pp. 118–120). New York: Raven Press.

Vanderpool, H. Y. (1986). The Wesleyan-Methodist tradition. In R. L. Numbers & D. W. Amundsen (Eds.), *Caring and curing—Health and medicine in the Western religious traditions* (pp. 317–353). New York: Macmillan.

Vaux, K. L. (1974). *Biomedical ethics.* New York: Harper & Row.

Vaux, K. L. (1984). *Health and medicine in the Reformed tradition.* New York: Crossroad.

Wacker, G. (1986). The Pentecostal tradition. In R. L. Numbers & D. W. Amundsen (Eds.), *Caring and curing—Health and medicine in the Western religious traditions* (pp. 514–538). New York: Macmillan.

Wanless, W. J. (1911). *The medical mission: Its place, power and appeal.* Philadelphia: Westminster Press.

Weber, T. P. (1986). The Baptist tradition. In R. L. Numbers & D. W. Amundsen (Eds.), *Caring and curing—Health and medicine in the Western religious traditions* (pp. 288–316). New York: Macmillan.

Wilkinson, J. (1980). *Health and healing: Studies in New Testament principles and practice.* Edinburgh: Handsel Press.

Woodward, K. L. (2002). Christianity's newest converts. In *2002 Britannica book of the year* (pp. 306–307). Chicago: Encyclopaedia Britannica, Inc.

7

Islam and Its Branches

Christoffer H. Grundmann and David G. Truemper

At the end of this chapter, the reader will be able to:
- Meaningfully distinguish among the beliefs of Judaism, Christianity, and Islam.
- Identify the basic tenets of Islam.
- Relate certain aspects of health behavior to the religious attitudes of those of various sects of the Muslim tradition.
- Recognize issues of spiritual and religious concern within the distinctive beliefs and practices of the Islamic faith.
- State the specific end-of-life practices that are important to those of Islamic faith.
- Gain confidence in referring patients to the appropriate religious counselors.

HISTORICAL OVERVIEW

◐ Islam—the word means "surrender" (to the will of God, or **Allah** in Arabic)—emerged as a religion in the 7th century CE on the west coast of the Arabian peninsula in what is today Saudi Arabia. Mecca, a city at the crossroads of several important caravan routes, was a flourishing marketplace with an affluent merchant population who worshipped astral deities at their central shrine, the Kaaba. In about 610 CE, Abu al-Qasim **Muhammad** ibn 'Abd Allah ibn 'Abd al-Mut talib ibn Hashim, or Muhammad (sometimes spelled "Mohammed"), began receiving revelations when staying in a certain place outside the city and continued to have revelations during a period of 20 years. Rarely were these unsought experiences visions; they mostly consisted of verbal messages of God's imminent judgment upon the people of Mecca if they did not repent to Allah, the one and only true God. Muhammad was asked to recite these messages publicly. First memorized and later written down by scribes around 650 CE, they were collected in what became the holy book of the Muslims, the "Noble **Qur'an**" (from: qara'a, meaning "to read," or "to recite"). Unlike Jesus of Nazareth, Muhammad, who died in Mecca in 633, is not known for healings or for any other type of miracles. However, it is regarded as the outstanding miracle in Islam and seen as a proof of the divine character of the Qur'an that Muhammad, who had not learned how to read and write, was the ultimate in a long line of prophets and could communicate God's undiluted will to humankind (Forward, 1997).

Muhammad and his messages were rejected at first, so much so that to escape persecution he and his small group of followers were compelled to leave Mecca in 622 for Medina, a city 250 miles north. Going into exile to surrender their lives to the will of Allah is called the **Hegira;** shortly thereafter this event made the calendar reference event of the Muslim era, counting the years after the event "AH" (After Hegira). In 632, 1 year before his death, Muhammad and the Muslim community (called **Umma**) took over Mecca and converted the Kaaba from a place of idol worship into one dedicated to the only true God, Allah (Cragg & Speight, 1980; Smith, 1981).

After Muhammad's death, Islam quickly expanded over all the Near East countries, as well as North Africa, and many rivalries developed over the authoritative leadership position of **caliph** (short for: *khalifah rasul Allah*, "successor of the Messenger of God,") of the Umma. Muslims argued over whether the caliphs should be direct descendants of the prophet or selected by virtue of their capabilities and achievements. This dispute led to the first schism in Islam between the Sunnites and the

Shiites, which occurred between 661 and 680. Today, 90% of the world's 1.2 billion Muslims are Sunnites, who regard the first four caliphs as legitimate successors of Muhammad, and 10% are Shiites, who regard Ali, the son-in-law of Muhammad, as his legitimate successor. The Shiites reside primarily in Iran, Ir , and Yemen (Barrett & Johnson, 2002, p. 302). The Sunnites (meaning *tradition*) have maintained a fair yet highly diverse coherence, but the Shiites have split into several subbranches, such as Ithna 'Ashariyah (Twelvers) or the Isma'iliyah and the Zaydiyah (Nasr, Dabashi, & Nasr, 1988; Pinault, 1992).

Although these groups adhere to different theological, legal, and political interpretations of the Qur'an and the Tradition (Sunna), the mystics (called Sufis) have added the dimension of personal piety and affectionate love for God and the prophet to the Muslim life. Emerging in the late 8th century, Sufism flourished in the Middle Ages, at the end of which various orders and brotherhoods, still in existence today, were established. The Sufis have an enormous influence on the larger population in Muslim countries through their spiritual instruction; thus, they influence the formation of Muslim society as a whole, even politically. Sufis also have been and still are responsible for and instrumental in large-scale missionary activities all over the world (Knysh, 2000).

An entirely new branch of Islam emerged in the United States during the 20th century: the **American Muslim Mission**, or **World Community of Al-Islam in the West** (members are commonly referred to as **Black Muslims**). The movement evolved out of various quasireligious U.S. African-American nationalist organizations that claimed that all black people in the United States were Moorish (and thus Muslim), and would regain their freedom from slavery after returning to Islam. This was the driving belief behind the early years of the movement, which was properly organized in 1930 by Wallace Fard Muhammad of Detroit and his Temple & University of Islam. His followers regarded him as an incarnation of Allah, and when he suddenly disappeared in 1934, he left the Nation of Islam as a legacy; his followers celebrate his birthday, February 26, as their Savior's Day (White, 2001). The movement gained considerable momentum after World War II, spurred by the nationwide rise of black consciousness and the emergence of Malcolm X (1925–1965) as its most articulate representative (Lee, 1996; Lincoln, 1961). After dissociating from the movement, Malcolm organized the rival Muslim Mosque, Inc., which he headed until his assassination in 1965. In the 1970s, the movement became the American Muslim Mission, which existed as such until 1985. It was deemed appropriate to do away with any racial or national preferences within the Umma, the worldwide community of Muslims. Today only a comparatively small splinter group retains both the name and the founding principles of the Nation of Islam. Its main mosque, Maryam, is in Chicago and has a 12-grade school called Muhammad University of Islam. The actual number of Black Muslims is 1.65 million, or about 40% of all U.S. Muslims (Barrett & Johnson, 2002, p. 303).

BASIC FEATURES AND DOCTRINES OF ISLAM

The central and fundamental message of Islam is "There is no god but God (Allah), and Muhammad is God's prophet." Every Muslim recites this basic confession, called **Sahadah**, during the formal recitation of prayers, which are said five times a day (at dawn, noon, in the afternoon, at sunset, and before sleep). This confession succinctly states what Islam is all about, namely, a radical monotheism to be observed by all humans in all walks of life and the veneration of Allah's messenger Muhammad. To associate or affiliate any other deity with Allah, or to worship someone other than God alone, is the greatest blasphemy, is regarded as idolatry, and, consequently, has to be eradicated by all means (Smith, 1981, p. 26–37). The Qur'an is the prime authority for knowing how to surrender to the will of God properly and how to be a faithful Muslim. Second to it is the Sunna ("Tradition of the Prophet"), which is collected in six compilations called **Hadiths**, and is the most important source for any advice or religious ruling. Because individuals do not primarily make the choices of how to live as a Muslim, theological authorities are listened to and consulted. In case of any uncertainty, especially with regard to family matters such as marriage, inheritance, or divorce, a fatwa, a legal statement issued by a **mufti** or a religious lawyer, is sought, which tries to reconcile the actual case with precedents in the Sunna (Smith, 1981).

Allah, as the almighty, all-merciful, and all-knowing one, cares for his servants, even when they suffer. He will be their refuge and will receive them in paradise hereafter. But for those who do not hold this belief or who mock it, Allah has prepared punishment in hell. Muslims are expected to fight such disgraceful unbelief in Allah (jihad: "struggle" or "battle" in the way of Allah) because Allah, who created them all, wants humanity to acknowledge His lordship. If they do not, Allah will decree damnation for them on Judgment Day.

A Muslim's religious life rests on five "pillars" (ark):

- The Sahadah
- Saying the ritual prayer five times daily after having cleansed oneself by washing feet, hands, and face
- Obligatory almsgiving
- Fasting in the month of **Ramadan**, meaning the renunciation of any food intake, liquid, or solid, from dawn to sunset
- If one can afford it, a once-in-a-lifetime pilgrimage to Mecca

These are conventions observed throughout the entire Umma, the worldwide Muslim community, and, as such, are very important for shaping the Muslim identity. Further specific characteristics are the circumcision of male children (and, in certain areas, also of females at a later age), the avoidance of pork and alcohol of any kind, and the prohibition of gambling and of conversion to any other religion (Esposito, 1998; Kurzman, 1998).

DOCTRINAL DISTINCTIONS AFFECTING NURSING

Providing quality nursing care to Muslim patients requires interacting with an entire family. If critical decisions have to be made, the head of the family is consulted; thus, in the case of a female patient, her husband, father, or brother must be kept informed. The nurse must keep this in mind when obtaining consent for certain procedures (such as operations or providing or removing life support) or signature of legal documents. In general, Muslim patients do not stand on their own; relatives, sometimes very distant ones, always accompany them. This tradition must be honored by the nurse: this is the Muslim way, and it makes Muslim patients feel more comfortable.

Sickness is commonly regarded as an exceptional time, so Muslims are not expected to comply with the strict religious regulations that are in effect during ordinary times. The alleviation granted is different for men and women, the latter enjoying far more, and far more frequent, lenience because of their menses, which is regarded as a time of ritual uncleanness that makes them unfit for religious observances. The lessening of religious duties affects the daily ritual prayer (called **Salat**) and fasting and diet (except for the consumption of pork); nurses should inquire which practices are important to the patient when taking the history (Rahman, 1998). This applies especially to Black Muslim patients, some of whom may not eat what may be regarded by some as traditional food of African Americans, such as collard greens and corn bread. Black Muslims also may wish to be cared for by African-American doctors and nurses and may demand a nonsmoking room or nonsmoking roommates.

Special care has to be taken in assessing and caring for women who prefer female nurses and physicians. The modesty of the Muslim woman's clothing and attitude must be respected, as should ornaments or amulets of spiritual significance which have an important influence on those who wear them (Awde, 2000). When washing or bathing the patients, these religious accessories, worn both by men and women, should not get wet and should never be removed except with the express consent of the patient.

While it can be expected in principle that Muslims, with their long and impressive history in the medical arts (Rahman, 1998; Ullmann, 1978), will normally follow medical advice, nurses may encounter some noncompliance in patients who would like to adhere strictly to this verse in the Qur'an: "And when I am ill, it is He who cures me" (26:80). This attitude must be honored by nurses, who at the same time must be careful not to unduly neglect what is medically necessary. Nurses should ensure that such patients have a copy of the Qur'an always within reach and always placed in such a way that it stands out from all other reading material or medical and nursing supplies. They should also be mindful of touching the Qur'an only with clean hands and should never put it on the floor. Nurses should offer male patients a bowl of fresh water and a clean towel and safeguard their privacy whenever they want to perform Salat, the daily ritual prayers. Women are not required to perform Salat, although some may wish to do so; should a devout Muslim woman wish to perform Salat, the nurse is advised to provide water and a bowl.

Abortion and birth control are disputed among various branches and schools of thought among Muslims. While some strictly oppose them, others take a more liberal approach. A fetus having matured beyond the 30th day after conception is regarded as a human being proper and must be handled accordingly. After delivery, the newborn child should be bathed immediately, even before the infant is handed to the father or the mother, but silently, so that parents may whisper into the child's ear the call to prayer, which should be the first words heard. Circumcision in Islam, unlike in Judaism, is not performed within the first week of the infant's life, but sometime before the boy attains puberty.

Special attention must be paid to Muslim religious observances when death is imminent. When possible, extended family members and an Imam, the prayer leader of the local mosque, should be called in to be present. After the bed is moved so that the dying person faces the direction of Mecca, the family members and Imam read the Qur'an and pray with the dying person, urging him or her to confess sins and to ask God's forgiveness in the presence of all. If no family or Imam is available, any Muslim can be asked to assist in such proper departing from the world.

Once the patient is dead, Muslim religious law requires that the corpse be washed ritually by Muslims, preferably by members of the family, and then placed facing Mecca again. When this is not possible, anyone else can do this, provided gloves are worn so as not to inflict ritual impurity on the "possession of Allah." The conception of the human body as the property of Allah makes organ donation or autopsy unacceptable to any orthodox Muslim. Instead, what belongs to Allah must be returned to Allah unmutilated and as soon as possible; for this reason, burial must take place within 24 hours after death (Athar, 1993).

PERSONAL REFLECTIONS

- Have I ever provided nursing care to a person of Islamic faith?
- What have I done to educate myself about providing spiritually and culturally competent care to Muslim patients? What could I do to improve my knowledge in this area for the future?
- How could I involve the family of the Muslim patient in the nursing care plan?
- Are there special accommodations that I would need to make if providing end-of-life care to a dying Muslim? Are there special needs for burial?
- What would I do if faced with a situation in which, to support the spirituality of a patient, I had to make exceptions to hospital rules? For example, if my patient made a request to have his death bed face east, toward Mecca, and this involved switching rooms or moving other patients, what actions would I take? How would I feel in this situation?
- If I were in a supervisory capacity and a family asked me to change assignments of my staff so that a male nurse was never assigned to care for a female Muslim patient, how would I handle the situation?
- If I were in an educational role in a teaching hospital, what strategies might I use to enhance the knowledge of my staff about religious practices among those of the Islamic faith?
  - What actions would I take if I observed prejudice among my staff in caring for persons of Islamic faith based on stereotyping because of world events?

Key Points

- The central and fundamental message of Islam is "There is no god but God (Allah), and Muhammad is God's prophet." Muslims recite this confession five times daily during the formal recitation of prayers.
- Providing quality nursing care to Muslim patients requires interacting with an entire family. Critical decisions are made by the male head of the family.
- Sickness is commonly regarded as an exceptional time, during which Muslims are not expected to comply with the usual strict religious regulations.
- Religious accessories should never be removed without the patient's express permission.
- Modesty prevails among most Muslim women, so adaptations in staffing may need to be made to allow only female nurses to care for female patients.
- Special attention should be paid to Muslim religious observances when death is imminent.

CASE STUDY 7.1

Mohammed is a middle-aged man of Muslim faith who comes from a large family that practices Muslim beliefs. Mohammed's father is dying of cancer and is a patient on the hospice ward where you work. The family has specific requests for the end-of-life care of their father. Some of these requests include activities that are considered unconventional in Western medicine but would not interfere with the father's comfort at the end of life.

Critical Thinking

- What types of religious rituals or practices would the nurse expect to see in this case?
- How can the nurse and hospice team facilitate the spiritual care of this patient and his family?
- What specific interventions could the nurse plan to spiritually support the patient and family during this time? Which religious artifacts should be at the patient's bedside?
- Are there certain distinctions within the Muslim belief system of which the nurse should be aware for Muslim patients at the end of life? How should the postmortem care be handled?
- What are the differences between the traditional hospice practices for postmortem care in the United States and those required for a peaceful death and transition in the Muslim tradition?

References

Athar, S. (1993). *Islamic perspectives in medicine: A survey of Islamic medicine; achievements and contemporary issues.* Indianapolis: American Trust Publications.

Awde, N. (2000). *Women in Islam: An anthology from the Qur'an and Had'iths.* Richmond, Surrey, England: Curzon.

Barrett, D. B., & Johnson, T. M. (2002). Worldwide adherents of all religions by six continental areas, mid-2001. In *2002 Britannica book of the year* (pp. 302–303). Chicago: Encyclopaedia Britannica, Inc.

Cragg, K. R., & Speight, M. (1980). *Islam from within: Anthology of a religion.* Belmont, CA.: Wadsworth.

Esposito, J. L. (1998). *Islam: The straight path.* New York/Oxford: Oxford University Press.

Forward, M. M. (1997). *Muhammad: A short biography.* Oxford, England/Rockport, MA: Oneworld Publications.

Knysh, A. (2000). *Islamic mysticism: A short history.* Leiden, The Netherlands/Boston: Brill.

Kurzman, C. (Ed.). (1998). *Liberal Islam: A source book.* New York: Oxford University Press.

Lee, M. F. (1996). *The Nation of Islam: An American millenarian movement.* Syracuse, NY: Syracuse University Press.

Lincoln, C. E. (1961). *The Black Muslims in America.* Boston: Beacon Press.

Nasr, S. H., Dabashi, H., & Nasr, S. V. R. (Eds.). (1988). *Shi`ism: Doctrines, thought, and spirituality.* Albany: State University of New York Press.

Pinault, D. (1992). *The Shiites: Ritual and popular piety in a Muslim community.* New York: St. Martin's Press.

Rahman, F. (1998). *Health and medicine in the Islamic tradition*. Chicago: ABC International Group.

Smith, W. C. (1981). *On understanding Islam: Selected studies*. The Hague/NewYork: Mouton.

Ullmann, M. (1978). *Islamic medicine, Islamic surveys 11*. Edinburgh: Edinburgh University Press.

White, V. L., Jr. (2001). *Inside the Nation of Islam: A historical and personal testimony by a Black Muslim*. Gainesville, FL: University Press of Florida.

8

Modern Religions and Sects of the West

Christoffer H. Grundmann and David G. Truemper

LEARNING OBJECTIVES

At the end of this chapter, the reader will be able to:
- Meaningfully distinguish between the beliefs of the modern religions and those of Judaism, Christianity, and Islam.
- Identify the basic tenets of Jehovah's Witnesses, Mormons, and Christian Scientists.
- Describe how some modern religions and sects appear to relate to Christianity but do not embrace some fundamental Christian truths.
- Relate certain aspects of health behavior to the religious attitudes of the modern religions and sects of the West.
- Recognize issues of spiritual and religious concern within the distinctive beliefs and practices of several modern religions.
- State the specific practices affecting health that are important to Jehovah's Witnesses and Christian Scientists.
- Gain confidence in referring patients to the appropriate religious counselors.

During the 19th century, several new religious movements emerged around the world: in Japan, the Muslim world, and also in the West. Some of these movements which sprung up in the West use "Church" or "Christian" in their names and regard the Bible as an important source of basic orientation. However, on closer examination, they actually deny basic tenets of the Christian faith, including the perception and understanding of the Bible, the human being, Jesus Christ, and the Trinity. Thus, they are properly called "modern religions and sects of the West." Three such movements with a large following in America today are discussed in this chapter in chronological order: the Latter-day Saints, also called Mormons; the Jehovah's Witnesses; and the Church of Christ, Scientist.

LATTER-DAY SAINTS (MORMONS)

Historical Background

Ⓜ The origins of this genuinely American religious body date to 1830, the year Joseph Smith published *The Book of Mormon* in Palmyra, New York. In it, Smith relates the history of the people of God to the people of America, indigenous as well as colonist. Referring to plates he found with the aid of an angel (and duly returned after they were translated), Smith states that a group of Hebrews migrated from ancient Palestine to America in 600 BCE. After having multiplied, the group split into the Lamanites, who forgot their faith and became the ancestors of the "heathen" Native Americans, and the Nephites, who retained their faith. Eventually their culture, characterized by great cities, was destroyed somehow in approximately 400 AD. Before this, however, Jesus appeared and taught them the "original faith." Before the Nephite culture vanished, the prophet Mormon engraved its history and religious teachings on gold plates. His son, Moroni, after making some additions, finally buried the plates in the ground, where Smith discovered them 1400 years later (*Book of Mormon*, 1830/1950).

In 1830, Smith founded the **Church of Christ** (which afterward was called the Church of Jesus Christ of Latter-day Saints) at Fayette, New York. Smith felt urged to do so by heavenly visitations telling him that all other churches were in error and that his task was to restore the true gospel. The attraction of Smith's church and teachings for many people caused much reaction from neighboring communities and denominations, who saw their members leave their churches to join Smith's. To avoid further conflicts and to find a place for undisturbed living, the "Saints" moved West via Ohio (in 1831) and Illinois (in 1839), into the desert of Utah. There, the largest group, under the leadership of Brigham Young, finally settled and founded Salt Lake City in 1847. (In 1844, Joseph Smith, at that time running for president, and his brother Hyrum were murdered [Ostling & Ostling, 1999; Shipps, 1985].)

Mormons today belong to one of five different denominations. The largest is the **Church of Jesus Christ of Latter-day Saints**, with a U.S. membership of 4.5 million and headquarters in Salt Lake City, Utah. The second largest is the **Community of Christ**, formerly called the Reorganized Church of Jesus Christ of Latter-day Saints; this denomination claims to be the genuine continuation of the original church founded by Joseph Smith, with about 150,000 U.S. members and headquarters in Independence, Missouri. The other three denominations—the **Church of Christ (Temple Lot)**, the **Church of Jesus Christ (Bickertonites)**, and the **Church of Jesus Christ of Latter-day Saints (Strangite)**—are significantly smaller and differ in several aspects of the church's teaching (Mead & Hill, 1995).

Doctrinal Distinctions

To understand Mormon teachings properly, one has to recognize the importance and authority accredited to the *Book of Mormon*. Adherents regard it as a sequel to the Bible. Adherents also regard the authority of the prophetic church leadership as teaching that is divinely inspired. Gifts such as prophecy, revelation, and speaking in tongues are an important element in church life and can establish new teachings. Mormons believe that God has evolved from man and that Christ came to earth to teach that men ought to evolve into gods by repentance, baptism (by immersion), faith, laying on of hands for receiving the Spirit's gifts, and obedience to the ordinances of the church. The important task is to do "temple work" (celebration of celestial marriages and baptisms for the dead), a term which, like many other important references in the religious life of Mormons, reflects continuity with the temple of ancient Israel, albeit without the performance of sacrifices. The supreme governing body of the church is instituted as the priesthood of **Melchizedek,** and the priesthood at the local or congregational level is known as the priesthood of Aaron, although there is no paid ministry. Every (worthy) boy becomes a deacon at 12 years of age, a teacher at 14 years, and a priest at 16 years. At 18 years of age, when they are eligible to enter into the priesthood of Melchizedek as elders, they are expected to devote as much as 18 months to missionary work, which Mormons everywhere in the world carry out at their own expense. In this way, all males become part of the church's hierarchy and part of a very close-knit organization. This is evidenced by the support Mormons show for all members in need, be it for financial, educational, or employment assistance, which the biblically ordered tithes finance.

Another important element in Mormon life is a health-conscious lifestyle free of any drugs (narcotics, alcohol, or tobacco) and free of drinks containing caffeine (tea, coffee, or cola). Likewise, Mormons regard any kind of self-inflicted mutilation of the body, such as tattooing or piercing, as nonreconcilable with their religion. At the same time, Mormons observe a vigorous work ethic, hold a high standard in moral integrity, observe a fairly rigid code of dress, and enjoy recreation and sports. This lifestyle has significantly affected the overall state of health and well-being of Mormons, which is far above that of the average U.S. population (Enstrom, 1975; Lyon & Gardner, 1984).

Because the many pre-existing spiritual beings need to be hosted in a body and can attain eternal life only when they have taken on flesh, Mormons emphasize the sanctity of family life and the importance of having many children. Thus, procreation becomes a divinely sanctioned mission and causes some discussion of how many children Mormons should have and whether sterilization might be permissible. Mormons regard marriages solemnized in their Temples as "celestial marriages," sealed for eternity. After death, families will be reunited as the families they have been on earth. The practice of some Mormons having more than one wife has been a source of debate among Christians.

Another distinct Mormon practice is the baptism of a proxy on behalf of people already dead if they happen to be 8 years of age or older. This becomes understandable in light of the importance of baptism for salvation and the Mormon tradition of adult baptism. But it is done for ancestors as well. This is why studying ancestry and keeping records of ancestry is so important in the Mormon tradition. However, the Church of Christ (Temple Lot) does not accept and does not practice baptism for the dead or celestial marriage, nor do they hold that the triune God represents three gods (Mead & Hill, 1995).

Doctrinal Distinctions Affecting Nursing

The high esteem for the body as the host of a pre-existent spirit determined to achieve life eternal is at the root of Mormon attitude toward health, healing, and illness. Bodily and mental cleanliness is of vital importance. Latter-day Saints express their ritual purity by wearing a white undergarment, which they receive as a sign of their "temple endowment," having made covenants of righteousness. Because they wear this garment day and night for the rest of life as a reminder of the sacred covenant made and a symbol of Christ-like attributes in one's mission in life, it should not be removed except in emergencies or with the patient's explicit consent. This poses a special challenge for any nursing and medical treatment.

Regarding dietary restrictions, nurses should be sure not to offer any drinks containing caffeine or alcohol. Although Mormons on the whole are not vegetarians, they prefer basic organic foods, such as fruits, grains, and herbs. When nurses must administer medicines with intoxicating side effects, they should inform patients and their families about the medication. Because family is so important, nurses should not hinder, but rather should encourage, visitations by family members, provided they do not interfere with proper medical and nursing care. When providing care for Mormons, nurses also should leave sufficient time for patients to study scriptures and prayers.

Any endowed Saint may be asked to perform spiritual administrations, such as baptism, Holy Communion, or anointing the sick, because Mormonism does not observe a distinction between laity and a specially ordained ministry. Local conventions may have different attitudes.

Birth control, preferably by natural means, is permissible for Mormons, but they strictly oppose abortion (except in the case of acute danger to the mother's life) and suicide. They also discourage artificial insemination (Bush, 1993). Occasionally, one may encounter the demand for circumcision of an infant boy in continuation of the biblical "Abrahamic Covenant," observance of which was once a teaching by Joseph Smith; currently, this practice is usually spiritualized as a "circumcision of the heart" by most Mormons.

When sick, Mormons are encouraged to seek competent medical assistance. However, when death is imminent, Latter-day Saints are taught to perceive it as a blessing and a purposeful episode in their eternal existence because they will be reunited with their body in the resurrection (Barlow, 1979). Although it is left to the discretion of family members to decide if life should be artificially prolonged, the church authority advises them not to "feel obligated to extend mortal life by means that are unreasonable" (*General Handbook of Instruction*, 1985, 11-6). Autopsy may be performed and organs donated if the deceased or the deceased's family wills so. To honor the integrity of the body, Mormons are encouraged to have the dead buried, not cremated, except in cases where the law requires cremation (Bush, 1993).

JEHOVAH'S WITNESSES

Historical Background

In the wake of the traumatic aftermath of the Civil War, Charles Taze Russell (1852–1916), a former Presbyterian haberdasher of Pittsburgh, became convinced that the Bible reveals God's precise plan of the end of the world. After acquiring rudimentary knowledge of Hebrew and Greek, "Pastor" Russell left his business in 1872 to pursue detailed Bible studies, conduct Bible classes, and publish widely. Convinced that Christ's "invisible return" had occurred in 1874, Russell proclaimed that the end of the Gentile world would come about in a fierce battle called Armageddon in 1914, after which Christ would rule God's kingdom on earth. Thus, preaching of Christ's millennial reign became Russell's vocation, as it is for all the "Witnesses" around the world today.

In 1884, the Watch Tower Bible and Tract Society was founded and soon flourished as a publishing house, mainly for Russell's own products, of which approximately 16 million copies in more than 30 languages were produced. In 1909, Russell moved the headquarters of his operations to Brooklyn, New York, where it remains today. When Russell, who is not remembered as the founder but as the "general organizer" of the movement, died, the lawyer and district judge Joseph F. Rutherford became president of the organization. An even more prolific writer than Russell, Rutherford restructured the organization; this gave rise to dissenting movements, such as the Dawn Bible Students Association, which is (ironically) located in East Rutherford, New Jersey. Rutherford also initiated international expansion in 1920, and in 1931 substituted the name **Jehovah's Witnesses** for people who were until then known as Russellites, Dawn People, or International Bible Students (Mead & Hill, 1995, 154ff; Penton, 1985).

Jehovah's Witnesses are a well-organized movement under the theocratic leadership of a governing body at the Brooklyn headquarters consisting of older and, by their judgment in accordance with scripture, "spiritually more qualified" Witnesses. What they say and rule is binding to all other Witnesses. However, there is no hierarchy; whether serving at the world headquarters, in branches, or in congregations, every Witness does the fieldwork of personally telling others about God's Kingdom, as perceived by the church's official teaching. Not only are all members expected to devote at least 8 hours per month to the work of spreading the magazines *Watchtower* and *Awake!*, but all members also have to give detailed written accounts of their activities, which are reported to headquarters for consolidated annual statistics accessible on the Internet (www.watchtower.org). Today there are more than 6 million Witnesses throughout the world, with the largest group (nearly 1 million members) in the United States.

Doctrinal Distinctions

Bible study has been and still is at the heart of the teaching of the Jehovah's Witnesses. Bearing the name of God, which they believe to be Jehovah, in their denominational designation, they use a special translation of the Bible, called "The New World Translation of the Holy Scriptures," which their headquarters authorizes. This title is programmatic because the Witnesses regard themselves now as citizens of the "New World," so their version of the Bible reflects this perception very clearly. They and their theocratic organization represent the "New World Society," namely God's Kingdom under the reign of Christ, which they bear witness to, humbly yet with high dedication, both by word of mouth and via print media (Cole, 1955).

Jehovah's Witnesses refer to what is commonly called the New Testament as the Christian Greek Scriptures, and the Old Testament as the Hebrew Scriptures. What makes the New World Translation so different is not only that it always uses "Jehovah" as God's proper name in both the Old and New Testaments, but also that it accords predominance to the books of Daniel and Revelation as God's timetables for all world affairs and as providing the definitive insight into the destiny of human beings. The translation contains many references for interpreting the scriptures accordingly and leads to a very specific perception of the history of salvation. The return of Christ is imminent, as is the final battle of Armageddon, in which Christ will victoriously fight the Anti-Christ and his powers, which are "the false teaching of the churches, tyranny of human government, and oppression by big business" (Mead & Hill, 1995, p. 157).

Thus, witnesses do not form or build churches but Kingdom Halls (without any religious symbols), and all work on the buildings is done voluntarily. They do not have an ordained ministry or hierarchy. Overseers look after the large-scale organizational issues, whereas elders and servants lead the teaching of the congregations, all without pay. Witnesses renounce the Trinity in their teaching as not being scriptural, but they nonetheless baptize new members by full immersion with a Trinitarian formula. They understand baptism as the commitment of the entire life to the sole service for Jehovah, aside from whom they serve no other masters—other masters would just be emissaries of Satan. This radical siding with the Kingdom of God leads Jehovah's Witnesses to refuse to salute the flag, vote, join military forces or, if they are compelled so to do, bear arms in war. This attitude has led them to suffer persecution and trials (Peters, 2000), but they do not want anything to do with activities associated with Satan and his powers.

Doctrinal Distinctions Affecting Nursing

Witnesses are known in medical circles for their straightforward refusal to receive blood transfusions; they similarly refuse to donate blood. This principle refers to full blood and blood products only, not to plasma expanders. This practice is defended using scripture such as Deuteronomy 15:23, Leviticus 7:26–27, and Ezekiel 33:25. Jehovah's Witnesses do not reject organ transplants in principle, provided the organ is thoroughly rinsed with a nonblood solution. These beliefs challenge the medical pro-

fession to seek alternatives, which are extensively commented upon in all the publications of the **Watchtower Society**. Because obedience to the scriptural command of
God is paramount for Witnesses, nurses may encounter Jehovah's Witness patients in
a critical situation or during an emergency requiring transfusion who are in considerable spiritual distress. Nurses should be able to inform these patients about available alternatives and ease their distress by assuring Witnesses of respect for their beliefs.

The abhorrence for mixing blood with blood has dietary repercussions as well,
although to less a degree than in the case of transfusions. Nurses should not offer
meat that has not been properly drained, or food that has blood added to it, such as
certain sausages. Appropriate meats can be readily procured through a Jewish or
Muslim vendor. Witnesses also are advised to abstain from alcohol and smoking because they harm the body.

While Witnesses oppose abortion for scriptural reasons, they leave decisions
about birth control, autopsy, and organ transplants to individual discretion. This
means that nurses do not have to consider any additional perspectives on these matters when advising Jehovah's Witnesses. The same applies to explicit religious or
spiritual assistance because Jehovah's Witnesses do not have special ministries or
rites for their sick. They celebrate Holy Communion once a year, which is consum-
mated only by those who belong to the "celestial class." Nurses should abstain from
offering to call someone in to offer Holy Communion. Nurses should see to it that
there is always a copy of the New World Translation of Holy Scriptures accessible for
the patients.

CHRISTIAN SCIENTISTS
(CHURCH OF CHRIST, SCIENTIST)

Historical Background

ⒸⓈ The term **Christian Science** denotes the particular belief of Christian Scientists,
who are members of the **Church of Christ, Scientist**. Mary Baker Eddy (1821–1910),
raised on a farm and of Congregationalist descent, founded the Church of Christ, Scientist at Boston in 1879 to accommodate the growing number of adherents to her
teachings "to reinstate primitive Christianity and its lost element of healing" (Eddy,
1936, p. 17). Her formal education being severely impaired by constant illness, Eddy
read much on her own and tried various ways of healing, including allopathic, home-
opathic, and mental techniques. After experiencing instantaneous relief from a serious condition while studying a New Testament healing story in 1866, she became
convinced that she had finally discovered the "scientific system of divine healing."
Her arduous explorations in the years that followed resulted in her book *Science and
Health with Key to the Scriptures* (Mead & Hill, 1995, p. 104; Peel, 1966, pp. 195–240).
First published in 1875 and revised for every new edition up to 1907, this book is
revered as the authoritative interpretation of the Bible and has become Holy Scrip-
ture beyond criticism for Christian Scientists. The two books (*Manual of the Mother
Church* and *Science and Health*) are regarded "as perpetual pastor of the Church of
Christ, Scientist" (Peel, 1988).

In addition to providing the teaching for Scientists, Eddy also organized the congregational life and systematically pursued the expansion of Christian Science. She

described her definite rulings for the church in the *Manual of the Mother Church*, the official church handbook, according to which a five-member board of directors at the Boston-based Mother Church is responsible for all matters regarding Scientist doctrine and teaching. Only at Boston are Christian Science teachers to be trained (the credential is Christian Science Bachelor, or C.S.B.). Only from the Mother Church is official literature to be published, and only officially appointed members of the Board of Lectureship are entitled to speak publicly on Christian Science. The purpose of this centralist organization is to ensure the untainted teachings of Christian Science, study of which is so important that Christian Scientists everywhere maintain reading rooms accessible to the public (John, 1962). The *Christian Science Monitor* is the publication that is probably most familiar to the general public.

Individual branch churches are administratively independent, but they all have officially appointed "readers," "teachers," and "practitioners," rather than clergy or a ministry of preaching. On Sundays (and Thanksgiving Day), readers read portions of the Bible, *Science and Health,* and a sermon which is prepared by a committee and published officially. On Wednesdays, Scientists also meet for a simpler gathering; the Wednesday gatherings are more appealing to many because of the healing testimonies given (*A century of Christian Science healing*, 1966).

Christian Science "practitioners" are members who engage in mental healing the Scientist way. Their names are listed in an official directory published monthly in the *Christian Science Journal*. They devote full time to this ministry after having participated in a course of study with an authorized teacher and after having demonstrated the successful healing of others. Beyond that, there are no other offices, ministries, or sacraments. Scientists speak of "baptism" and "Eucharist," but these denote mental processes. Baptism is observed as the cleansing of daily life by proper perception, and the Eucharist is a twice-yearly meditative and thus immaterial contemplation upon the "allness" of Mind that is a celebration of "at-one-ment" done in remembrance of the atonement by Christ (Gottschalk, 1973).

Doctrinal Distinctions

Chapter 12 of *Science and Health* contains a helpful glossary that unlocks much of Christian Science's teaching and shows that "science" in this context should be understood as a very particular way of thinking about life and the world (Eddy, 1971). This being the case, much attention has to be given to the fact that even common terms (not to mention the religious ones) such as life, death, mind, and matter take on different and very specific meanings; in writing, this is often indicated by capitalization of the terms, such as in "Mind," "Truth," and "Love."

Basic for Christian Scientists is the principal division between Mind as "the only Spirit, Soul, divine Principle, ... Love; ... God", and Matter, which is regarded as "mortality; ... illusion, ... the opposite of Truth; ... of Spirit; ... of God" (Eddy, 1971, p. 591). While Mind represents genuine "reality," Matter causes "illusions." "All reality is in God and His creation, harmonious and eternal. That which He creates is good ... Therefore the only reality of sin, sickness, or death is the awful fact that unrealities seem real to human, erring belief, until God strips off their disguise" (Eddy, p. 472). Disease and death are an inherent part of Matter, whereas the Spirit brings with it life eternal. Humans are freed from the deceit of their senses once they come to understand what God is all about. Attaining this knowledge is what actually heals and redeems.

As Jesus, the "highest human corporeal concept of the divine idea," healed by "rebuking and destroying error and bringing to light man's immortality" (Eddy, 1971, p. 589), so have Christian Scientists. Healing by spiritual means is their very mission, and their practitioners do not offer just an alternative to conventional scientific medicine; the reported results of their activity sometimes challenge scientific medicine, too (*A century of Christian Science healing,* 1966; Schoepflin, 1986).

Doctrinal Distinctions Affecting Nursing

Because Christian Scientists usually patronize their own practitioners or nursing homes in case of disease, they rarely make use of other medical or nursing facilities, except in cases of emergencies, fractures, or deliveries. They are reluctant to comply with public health care rulings, such as compulsory vaccination or screening. When patients are Scientists, nurses should be prepared to meet with a refusal to take any medicine because this is regarded as a breach of trust in God, the Principle and Truth. To overcome critical situations, nurses should immediately invite a Christian Science practitioner or nurse in, whose name they probably can easily obtain from the friends or relatives of the patient; if not, they may look up the official listing in the *Journal.*

Although nurses can expect a Christian Scientist not to smoke or to drink alcohol, they need not worry too much about special dietary restrictions. However, they might encounter certain reservations regarding caffeinated drinks, such as coffee or tea, and should offer alternatives. They also should see to it that patients have sufficient time for meditation and reflection, but at the same time should be aware of the overall state of distress patients suffer when experiencing the tension between official teaching and actual experience (Osler, 1910). Because Scientists do not have sacraments, rites, or a priestly ministry, sensible companionship and the patient's own meditation on the Bible and *Science and Health* are the means to be made use of in times of sickness (Peel, 1988).

PERSONAL REFLECTIONS

- Have I ever provided nursing care to a person who was a Jehovah's Witness? A Mormon? A Christian Scientist? Do I have any friends, relatives, or co-workers who follow these religions?
- What have I done to educate myself about providing spiritually and culturally competent care to patients of various modern religions? What could I do to improve my knowledge in this area for the future?
- What changes in planning nursing care would I make the next time I have a patient who is a Jehovah's Witness? Mormon? Christian Scientist? What questions should I ask them about dietary practices? About religious observances? About medical/nursing care or treatments that they may or may not be willing to participate in?

(continued)

PERSONAL REFLECTIONS (*continued*)

- What would I do if faced with a situation in which, in order to support the spirituality of a patient, I had to violate a moral or ethical principle of my own? For example, if my patient refused a potentially life-saving blood transfusion in order to obey his religious tradition, what actions would I take? How would I feel in this situation?
- If I found that a patient who was a Christian Scientist had not been taking the prescribed medications as I administered them, but the pills were later found stored in a drawer in his hospital bedside table, how would I handle the situation?
- If I were in an educational role in a teaching hospital, what strategies might I use to enhance the knowledge of my staff about religious practices among the modern religions discussed in this chapter?

Case Study 8.1

A married couple who are Jehovah's Witnesses give birth to a child with a physical problem that is easily corrected by surgery. The pediatric surgeon explains to the parents that without this surgery, the child will die, but if the operation is performed, the infant will be able to live a normal life without complications. There is a small chance the infant would need a blood transfusion during or after the operation. The father tells the surgeon that this is against their religion and they will not permit the operation to be performed. The surgeon feels that from the mother's nonverbal response, she would do anything to save her infant's life, but their religion prohibits the life-saving procedure. The physician decides to take the matter before a judge, making the infant a ward of the court so that he can operate to save the infant's life. He performs the surgery against the parent's wishes, thinking that the parents surely want their child to live and that by removing the decision from them, they are absolved from going against their religious beliefs. The child is then returned to the parents, able to physically function in a normal and healthy way.

Critical Thinking
- What is the ethical dilemma in this situation?
- What religious beliefs are at the basis of the parents' decision to refuse treatment?
- Do you agree with the physician's decision to make the child a ward of the court because the parents refuse a life-saving surgery? Are there other problems that might arise within the family because of this situation?
- What are some of the implications inherent in this situation?

Key Points

- Mormons today belong to one of five different denominations, the largest of which is The Church of Jesus Christ of Latter-day Saints, which has a U.S. membership of 4.5 million and headquarters in Salt Lake City, Utah.
- Jehovah's Witnesses are known in medical circles for their refusal to receive blood transfusions. They will accept organ transplants if certain procedures are followed.
- Christian Scientists may be reluctant to comply with medical or nursing treatment, including using medications or having surgery.

References

Barlow, B. A. (1979). *Understanding death*. Salt Lake City: Church of Jesus Christ of Latter-day Saints.

The Book of Mormon: An account written by the hand of Mormon upon plates taken from the plates of Nephi. (1830/1950). Translated by Joseph Smith, Jr. Salt Lake City, Utah: The Church of Jesus Christ of Latter-day Saints (1st ed., 1830).

Bush, L. E., Jr. (1993). *Health and medicine among the Latter-day Saints*. New York: The Crossroad Publishing Company.

A century of Christian Science healing. (1966). Boston: The Christian Science Publishing Society.

Cole, M. (1955). *Jehovah's Witnesses: The New World Society*. New York: Vantage Press.

Eddy, M. B. (1936). *Manual of the Mother Church*. Boston: First Church of Christ, Scientist.

Eddy, M. B. (1971). *Science and health with key to the scriptures*. Boston: First Church of Christ, Scientist.

Enstrom, J. (1975). Cancer mortality among Mormons. *Cancer, 36*, 825 841.

General Handbook of Instruction. (1985). Salt Lake City: Church of Jesus Christ of Latter-day Saints.

Gottschalk, S. (1973). *The emergence of Christian Science in American religious life*. Berkeley: University of California Press.

John, D. (1962). *The Christian Science way of life*. Englewood Cliffs: Prentice-Hall.

Lyon, J. L., & Gardner, J. W. (1984). Mormon health. *Journal of Collegium Aesculapium, 2*(1), 15–24.

Mead, F. S., & Hill, S. S. (1995). *Handbook of denominations in the United States*. Nashville, TN: Abingdon Press.

Osler, W, (1910). The faith that heals. *The British Medical Journal, June 18*, 1470–1472.

Ostling, R. N., & Ostling, J. K. (1999). *Mormon America: The power and the promise*. San Francisco: Harper San Francisco.

Peel, R. (1988). *Health and medicine in the Christian Science tradition*. New York: Crossroads.

Peel, R. (1966). *Mary Baker Eddy: The years of discovery*. New York: Holt, Reinhart and Winston.

Penton, M. J. (1985). *Apocalypse delayed: The story of Jehovah's Witnesses*. Toronto/Buffalo: University of Toronto Press.

Peters, S. F. (2000). *Judging Jehovah's Witnesses: Religious persecution and the dawn of the rights revolution*. Lawrence, KS: University Press of Kansas.

Schoepflin, R. B. (1986). The Christian Science tradition. In R. L. Numbers & D. W. Amundsen (Eds.), *Caring and curing—Health and medicine in the Western religious traditions* (pp. 421–446). New York/London: Macmillan.

Shipps, J. (1985). *Mormonism: The story of a new religious tradition*. Urbana, IL: University of Illinois Press.

9

Other Religions: Voodoo and Native/Indigenous American Traditions

Christoffer H. Grundmann and David G. Truemper

LEARNING OBJECTIVES

At the end of this chapter, the reader will be able to:

- Meaningfully distinguish between the beliefs of African-American or indigenous American traditions and those of Judaism, Christianity, Islam, and modern religions.
- Recognize the basic beliefs and practices of Voodoo.
- Identify the basic tenets of Native American religious traditions.
- Relate certain aspects of health behavior to the religious attitudes of Native Americans.
- Recognize issues of spiritual and religious concern within the distinctive beliefs and practices of several major Native American tribes.
- State those specific practices affecting health that are important to Native Americans.

VOODOO

Historical Background

🔵 **Voodoo** is the name for the "spirit" species in the language of the **Fon** people from Benin, West Africa. The Voodoo cult originated in Africa and was first introduced to the United States by slaves, then later by immigrants from the Caribbean islands, especially Haiti, where the cult assimilated certain elements of Roman Catholicism and has a stronghold still (Laguerre, 1989). Suppressed by the officially established churches for a long time, Voodoo thrived in secrecy and is found today mainly in southern states, especially Louisiana (New Orleans), neighboring states, and wherever Haitian immigrants have settled (Tallant, 1990).

Doctrinal Distinctions

Voodoo, like any cult similarly expressed in detailed ritual, perceives of spirits as the all-decisive forces in life for both good and bad. Every individual has his or her **met tet** (master of the mind) as guardian. To better their lots, influence the outcome of a critical situation in life, or turn bad fate into good, adherents seek to communicate with and influence these spirits. To do so, they need the help of people who are knowledgeable of the highly diverse spirit world, the inhabitants of which are called **loa**, which means "mystery" in the language of the Yoruba, another West African people (Brown, 1989). The loas have different names in different traditions and clans; sometimes these names are tainted by the names of Christian saints (that is, names are called upon that sound like names from the Christian tradition, but they are understood entirely differently). The many loas, which are by no means all benign, are divided into two main groups, the Rhada loas and the Petro loas. The Rhada loas are always wise and benign, represent the historically older spiritual authorities from Africa, and demand a somewhat serene rite. The Petro loas represent authorities of more recent and not necessarily African origin, are harsher and not necessarily benign, and demand more agitated and violent rituals.

Knowing the exact name of a particular loa and where to find it in the spirit world is vitally important for calling upon it and addressing it properly. Those who assist in this difficult and demanding task are called **houngan** (male priest) or **mambo** (priestess). They do so by means of elaborate ceremonies involving animal sacrifice, music, drumming, and dance. Participants in a ceremony attempt to get themselves into a trance state or help a medium do so in front of a lavishly decorated altar in the temple, thereby inviting the respective loa to come and take possession of all that is displayed on the altar. The loa comes because the basic principle of spirit world cults is the reciprocity of human action and spirit behavior: as humans depend on the help and guidance of spirits for securing work or staying healthy, the spirits depend on humans for food and due acknowledgment.

As long as the spirits can be appeased and kept in a good mood, life will flourish, but neglect of these duties will inflict harm. However, sometimes bad things happen to people despite all efforts to observe the cult properly. Ill fate or diseases are interpreted as something not merely incidental. It is not just "fate." It is explained as the workings of **caplatas**, "witches" who engage in "left-handed Voodoo" or "black magic." Caplatas can effectively curse people on demand, a procedure in which the famous needle-pricked Voodoo dolls have been commonly used, the dolls representing the unaware victims (Olmos & Paravisini-Gebert, 1997).

Doctrinal Distinctions Affecting Nursing

Voodoo is mainly practiced by a particular group of African Americans who are very much aware of and concerned about their identity as Africans; therefore, when possible, African-American nurses should be assigned to care for patients who practice Voodoo in order to ease communication. Whoever provides care for patients who believe in Voodoo will probably notice a pragmatic attitude both toward scientific medicine and ritual treatment, because to these patients there is no either/or (Kraut, 1990): the more agencies that are employed, the more promising the outcome. This attitude should not be viewed as mistrust on the part of the patient with regard to conventional medicine, but rather as compensation for what conventional medicine cannot provide; care should be taken not to disparage the patient's beliefs and practices. Strange paraphernalia on the table or amulets worn by the patient should be respected, and permission should be sought before these objects are moved or removed (DeSantis, 1989).

Dietary regulations may be prescribed by certain cults and should be inquired into as soon as the history is taken. Sometimes, to soothe the spirits, it may be necessary to call in a houngan or mambo; these priests and priestesses not only officiate in temple rituals but also provide counseling, serve as healers, and shield against witchcraft and sorcery. For the Voodoo patient, spirits are very particular and definite realities; they are nothing to be played with or joked about, and they must be respected as potential powerful sources of patient unrest and agony. The nurse's understanding of and respect for the patient's beliefs may determine the outcome of the treatment.

When a Voodoo patient dies, the nurse should see to it that family or cult members have the chance to perform the proper ritual to avoid having the deceased turning into a zombie, which would be regarded as very inauspicious (Davis, 1983; Raboteu, 1986). According to Voodoo belief, one should never rush the dead; therefore, the nurse should be wary of moving the body immediately out of the sickroom and into the mortuary.

NATIVE AMERICAN RELIGIONS

Historical Overview

❶ The native peoples of North America include Indians, Aleuts, and Eskimos (Inuits). American Indians are the descendants of Asian nomadic hunters who came to the continent about 20,000 to 35,000 years ago. Eskimos and Aleuts, who have Asian features, are believed to have migrated to North America from northeastern Asia more recently, some 5,000 years ago; they make up the native population of the Arctic and sub-Arctic regions. Native Americans developed different traditions after settling in different areas—for example, the meat-eating and fur-wearing hunting societies of the West, the Great Plains, and eastern North America; the agricultural and horticultural societies of the Southwest; and the Pueblo societies in the deserts of the far Southwest.

When European colonists reached the American shores in large numbers in the 17th century, they interacted with the natives in very diverse ways. The Catholic Spaniards tried to Christianize the Native Americans of the South and relocate them to designated areas, as they did in Latin America as well. The French established trade relations with the Native Americans. The British, politically farsighted, prohibited unauthorized confiscation of Native American land and in 1763 appropriated the entire area west of the Appalachians to Native Americans. When the British North America Act established Canada in 1867, it endowed Canada with exclusive legislative rights regarding the Native Americans and their lands.

In 1830, Native Americans in the United States experienced a change in attitude in the white settlers when President Andrew Jackson signed the Indian Removal Act. This act enforced the relocation of tribes westward, to what were then out-of-the-way places, especially in the northwestern territories, which were not so desirable for the colonists. But the legal securities the Native Americans were given by this act soon were nullified in wars and often were violated, especially after gold was discovered in California in 1848. Trade with Native Americans was prohibited in 1871. In 1887, when Native Americans had migrated to their more than 100 newly assigned reservations, the General Allotment Act, although intended to help assimilation, actually brought about the immediate loss of 62% of newly acquired Native American territory. On top of this deplorable situation, many tribes faced extinction by infectious diseases (especially smallpox), a situation that gave rise to the perception of the Native American as "the vanishing American" (Osborn, 2000).

But Native Americans did not vanish. In addition to their courageous self-defense in battles, they developed indigenous means of spiritual survival and identity. A unique yet tragic expression of spirituality was the Ghost Dance religion, which arose in the reservations of the northern Plains at the end of the 19th century (McGregor, 1972; Sayer, 1997). The typical songs and ceremonies of this religion promised the Native Americans a return to the old way of life and reunion with their departed kinsmen. This era came to an abrupt end at Wounded Knee Creek, South Dakota, on December 29, 1890, when the prominent leader, Sitting Bull, and more than 200 men, women, and children were shot dead by troops of the 7th cavalry (Brown, 1972).

The 20th century saw a remarkable shift in the official attitude toward Native Americans, the first major breakthrough being the Indian Reorganization Act of 1934, which tried to reverse many of the rulings of the Allotment Act and give due respect to tribal autonomy, custom, and religion. The intention of this act was reinforced in later decades with a noticeable emphasis on civil rights. It has encouraged the formation of indigenous Native American organizations and has led to a heightened awareness of Native American identity. However, in 1973, Wounded Knee again became the focus of Native American protest when members of the American Indian Movement occupied the village for more than 2 months to draw renewed attention to the needs of Native American peoples in the United States. They left this historic site only after having been assured negotiation of their grievances (Gonzalez & Cook-Lynn, 1999). Today, reservations are entitled to operate gambling casinos to raise revenue.

As a result of the destruction of their traditional way of life, many Native Americans are unemployed, with alcoholism and diabetes being the current leading health problems for this population (Rhoades, Mason, Eddy, Smith, & Burns, 1988).

Doctrinal Distinctions

In North American, several tribes of Native Americans have accepted Christianity, whereas others have not or have done so only to a certain degree. Many have mixed their indigenous culture and tradition with Christian elements over the years, some of them very consciously. This is the case with the **Native American Church,** which was formed in 1918 by groups of the prosecuted Peyote religion in order to get government recognition. A unique practice of this church is the use of the hallucinogenic juice of the Peyote cactus, which is ritually consumed by devotees to enable spirit communication. Coupled with this spirit communication is a high ethical demand on the life of those who are on the "Peyote road," as the life of the devotees is called. They must shun alcohol, be committed to care for their families and their brothers of the tribe, and support themselves through steady work (La Barre, 1989; Marriott & Rachlin, 1971).

Only a very general outline of some of the basic structures of the Native American belief systems is possible, because they differ quite substantially: those held by the Native Americans of the Plains differ from those of the Native Americans of the Northwest Coast, and those of the Southwest tribes differ from those of the Southeast tribes. However, they do have certain elements in common, namely the belief in the powers of the spirit world and the institution of the medicine man or shaman (Bonvillain, 1996).

All beings, including animals, have a spirit that can be communicated with and that should never be provoked. Depending on the tradition, the spirits are called **digi, boha, maxpe,** or **manitous,** some of which have replaced the older *orenda* of the Iroquois or the *wakan* of the Sioux. Humans have two "life spirits" or souls: the free soul, which leaves the body when a person is asleep and traverses into the spirit world, an indication of which is a person's dreams; and the body soul. Once the body soul goes on an errand (during a dream, for instance), the individual is left highly vulnerable and prone to serious diseases, which are then regarded as "partial loss" of the body soul. These diseases can be properly dealt with only by a "soul catcher," a shaman or medicine man whose task is to catch the soul and return it before it leaves completely— for the "happy hunting grounds," as in the case of Native Americans of the Plains, or the "gloomy underworld" in the north, as in the case of the Navajo.

Leading a prosperous life requires not only living according to the ethical codes of the tribe but also pleasing the manitous or spirits. Supplicants may beg the spirits to bestow favors for the furthering of life, the individual's as well as the communal life; when something goes wrong, these spirits have their share in it. Native American religions also know the reality of witches and the feared black magic exercised by "skinwalkers" (Kluckhohn, 1967).

Another feature common to all Native American Indian societies is the institution of the medicine man or shaman; women as well as men can hold this office. Medicine men are "called by the spirits," which means they have the ability to communicate successfully with the spirit world. Before being called by the spirits, medicine men usually have overcome a severe illness, which is interpreted as having visited the spirit world, and sometimes have served a lengthy apprenticeship with an acknowledged and well-recognized medicine man. At the end of a protracted training period and at a time designated by the mentor, an elaborate ceremony is performed that publicly confirms the spiritual capabilities of the adept. The symbols of medicine men's spiritual powers find expression in their attire and are contained in the paraphernalia of the medicine bag carried by each of them thereafter.

The main task of medicine men is to diagnose and cure (severe) illnesses, but they also are expected to know where things not yet seen by others may be located and found, such as game, enemies, or lost property. Medicine men can "see" these things because the spirits they are in communication with see them. Common to all Native American peoples is the belief that disease is caused by the intrusion of a foreign substance into the body, which the medicine man is expected to extract from the patient by sucking or pulling it out. But it is not just the sucking or pulling that is important: the special sequence of narratives that are chanted in the process of the treatment is believed to make the process efficacious.

To enhance the power of the narratives of the medicine men, certain societies in the Southwest (especially the Navajo) employ elaborately designed sand paintings. These are colorfully designed holy places that depict the guardian spirits and all other spirits, which are regarded as potencies for dealing with particular diseases. Once the sand painting is properly completed, the spirits portrayed inhabit it immediately. The patient is then requested to sit down in the center of that painted space while the medicine man chants the appropriate song and dialogues with the patient. After the ceremony, the painting is destroyed by the patient, who applies the colored sand to his or her entire body (Newcomb & Klan, 1964; Newcomb & Richard, 1975).

The dominant role accorded to the medicine man or "medicine societies" in Native American cultures derives from the importance of medicine in the life of the people, with "medicine" meaning any substance considered powerful to ward off evil and safeguard well-being. Because every being—human, animal, plant, water, air, soil, sky, the dead—is inhabited by a particular spirit not necessarily perceived as a personal being, the art of good living consists in reconciling the various demands of the spirits and living in harmony with them. To Native American peoples, all of nature is a sacred totality, meaning that nothing seen and experienced is just a thing or a happening as such; all belongs to the sphere of religion somehow. This leads to a certain restraint from modern society's active manipulation of life by interfering medically or technically without any reference to the sacred powers at the roots of life. Their beliefs and practices not only make Native Americans ecologically sensitive, but also led them to develop a highly sophisticated medical approach to life as well, an approach which differs from tribe to tribe. All things medical have a strong religious connotation in Native American society, and this definitely has a bearing on the nursing care of Native American patients (Hultkrantz, 1989, 1997).

Doctrinal Distinctions Affecting Nursing

Nursing care of Native Americans normally takes place on a reservation, either in the dwelling place of the sick individual or in the reservation's health care center, all of which since 1955 have been managed by the Indian Health Service (IHS). Rarely does nursing care take place in a hospital, an institution alien to Native American culture. Proximity to family and the tribal brothers and sisters is important and should be cherished because "the caring of the sick is a prominent feature of Indian social care" (Hultkrantz, 1997, p. 166).

As long as diseases are diagnosed as diseases of object intrusion, medical intervention does not cause too much of a problem: the intruding object has to be removed anyway, so surgery is easily accepted. But when it turns out to be a really serious sickness with the (partial) loss of body-soul, and not just a malfunctioning of the bodily system, patients will avail themselves of a dual approach to get well again. In addition to the medical treatment, patients are very anxious that their soul be properly and completely recaptured by the specialist; thus, indigenous medicine men should be invited in to chant their songs to ease patients' spiritual distress and to help them to cope. It is important for believers that the old tales are being told because it is these stories that provide plausible explanation and thus hold the answers to the "Why?" of the current situation.

It is also important that people are present to reassure patients of their belonging and to encourage them with words of comfort. Such comfort will hardly ever involve an expectant hope in an eternal life or a heavenly paradise because concepts such as these are not very much developed in Native American spirituality. What matters is fitness for actual life, for which some cultures practice a special Blessingway ceremony. If life is impeded by disease or disability, Native Americans have a hard time bearing it. Much of their tradition holds that to die healthy and strong at a young age is to be preferred over invalidism; this caused some of their strongest members in the 19th century to prefer suicide to living with the consequences of smallpox (Hultkrantz, 1997, p. 166). Despite this, in most cases when disease strikes, it is borne with remarkable equanimity by the patients. When death is imminent, many Native Americans who were around during the patient's illness may try to avoid any contact with the deceased because the corpse is regarded as something contagious of that part of the spirit world with which one had better not have contact. Some believe that the body-soul, when departing, needs 4 days to reach the land of the dead, a period during which the corpse is not to be buried.

When nursing assistance is sought in childbirth, nurses should be aware that many different ritual observances apply in the various Native American traditions. Childbirth is viewed as something very natural and as highly significant for the individual, as well as for the entire clan, because new life is coming about. The birth of twins traditionally poses a serious problem because of the duality of souls coming into life; twins are not regarded as a good omen, and in the past this has led to the practice of killing one twin. Although attitudes have changed, nurses should be alert to the spiritual distress that the delivery of twins might arouse. Once the child has been born and has shown signs of normal life, the naming ceremonies, which are regarded as vital for the well-being of the baby, may begin. Names are not just given as labels, but contain power; giving the children names of important ancestors or dominant spirits endows the new life with these powers. Nurses should see to it that the performance of the proper rites is not hindered.

PERSONAL REFLECTIONS

- Have I ever provided nursing care to a person who believed in Voodoo?
- How familiar am I with the history of Native Americans? How would this knowledge potentially enhance the nursing care I could provide?
- What have I done to educate myself about providing spiritually and culturally competent care to Native Americans? What could I do to improve my knowledge in this area for the future?
- How could I involve the family of the Native American patient in the nursing care plan?
- What are the most common health problems among Native Americans? Where is most health care provided?
- What would I do if faced with a situation in which to support the spirituality of a patient, I had to violate a moral or ethical principle of my own? For example, if my patient wished to use a Voodoo doll to cast a spell on an enemy to give retribution for his part in the patient's injury, what actions would I take? How would I feel in this situation?
- When caring for Native Americans, what will likely be the greatest barrier for a non-Native American nurse in gaining access to the patient population? What are some strategies a nurse could use to gain entry or acceptance into this group?

Key Points

- Voodoo perceives spirits as the all-decisive forces in life for good and for bad. Sometimes it is necessary to call a houngan or mambo in to sooth the spirits. They not only officiate in temple rituals but also provide counseling, serve as healers, and shield against witchcraft.
- Paraphernalia belonging to the patient or amulets worn should not be moved or removed without permission.
- Beliefs and practices among Native Americans vary widely according to tribe, but certain elements are common, such as the belief in the powers of the spirit world and the institution of the medicine man or shaman.
- Nursing care of Native Americans rarely occurs in a hospital but more likely on the reservation or in the home. Caring for the sick is important in Native American society and involves the family.
- Alcoholism and diabetes are major health problems among Native Americans.

CASE STUDY 9.1

Amy is a young Anglo-American nurse who feels called to work with Native Americans. She accepts a government job working on a reservation in Arizona but finds that the people do not readily come to receive needed health care from the clinic there. One of Amy's biggest barriers to helping the families living on the reservation is that they see her as an outsider and do not seem to trust traditional Western medicine. Amy has identified that many of the children are not receiving adequate care and lack immunizations, and that there is a severe problem with teenage alcoholism and related issues. In addition, a high rate of diabetes has been found among the young adult population, and the life expectancy for many of the area tribes is less than 56 years.

Critical Thinking

- What barriers can be identified in Amy's situation? What strengths can she build upon?
- Are there ways in which Amy could be accepted as a health care provider among the tribes on the reservation? Why might the people not wish to come to a clinic?
- Whom should Amy consult with to learn more about the different tribes on the reservation?
- What are the common health problems she has identified? How should Amy begin to plan when proposing a comprehensive health care program on the reservation?
- What types of funding may be available to assist with her goals of improving health for these people?

References

Bonvillain, N. (1996). *Native American religion*. New York: Chelsea House Publishers.

Brown, D. A. (1972). *Bury my heart at Wounded Knee: An Indian history of the American West*. New York: Bantam Books.

Brown, K. M. (1989). Afro-Caribbean spirituality: A Haitian case study. In L. E. Sullivan (Ed.), *Healing and restoring—Health and medicine in the world's religious traditions* (pp. 255–285). New York/London: Macmillan Publishing.

Davis, E. W. (1983). Ethnobiology of the Haitian zombies. *Journal of Ethnopharmacology, 9*(1), 85–105

DeSantis, L. (1989). Health care orientation of Cuban and Haitian immigrant mothers: Implications for health care professionals. *Medical Anthropology, 12*(1), 69–89.

Gonzalez, M., & Cook-Lynn, E. (1999). *The politics of hallowed ground: Wounded Knee and the struggle for Indian sovereignty*. Urbana: University of Illinois Press.

Hultkrantz, A. (1989). Health, religion, and medicine in native North American traditions. In L. E. Sullivan (Ed.), *Healing and restoring—Health and medicine in the world's religious traditions* (pp. 327–358). New York/London: Macmillan Publishing.

Hultkrantz, A. (1997). *Shamanic healing and ritual drama—Health and medicine in native North American religious traditions*. New York: Crossroad Publishing Company.

Kluckhohn, C. (1967). *Navajo witchcraft*. Boston: Beacon Press.

Kraut, A. M. (1990). Healers and strangers: Immigrant attitudes toward the physician in America—A relationship in historical perspective. *The Journal of the American Medical Association, 263*, 1807.

La Barre, W. (1989). *The Peyote cult*. Norman: University of Oklahoma Press.

Laguerre, M. S. (1989). *Voodoo and politics in Haiti*. New York: St. Martin's Press.

Marriott, A. L., & Rachlin, C. K. (1971). *Peyote*. New York: Crowell.

McGregor, J. H. (1972). *The Wounded Knee massacre: From the viewpoint of the Sioux*. Rapid City, SD: Fenwyn Press Books (1st ed. 1940).

Newcomb, F. J., & Klan, H. (1964). *Navajo medicine man and sandpainter*. Norman, OK: University of Oklahoma Press.

Newcomb, F. J., & Richard, G. A. (1975). *Sandpaintings of the Navajo shooting chant*. New York: J. Augustin (original 1937). Reprinted New York: Dover.

Olmos, M. F., & Paravisini-Gebert, L. (Eds.). (1997). *Sacred possessions—Vodou, Santería, Obeah, and the Caribbean*. New Brunswick, NJ: Rutgers University Press.

Osborn, W. M. (2000). *The Wild frontier: Atrocities during the American-Indian War from Jamestown Colony to Wounded Knee*. New York: Random House.

Raboteu, A. J. (1986). The Afro-American traditions. In R. L. Numbers & D. W. Amundsen (Eds.), *Caring and curing—Health and medicine in the Western religious traditions* (pp. 539–562). New York/London: Macmillan Publishing.

Rhoades, E. R., Mason, R. D., Eddy, P., Smith, E. M., & Burns, T. R. (1988). The Indian Health Service approach to alcoholism among American Indians and Alaska natives. *Public Health Reports, 103*(6), 621–627.

Sayer, J. W. (1997). *Ghost dancing the law: The Wounded Knee trials*. Cambridge, MA: Harvard University Press.

Tallant, R. (1990). *Voodoo in New Orleans*. Gretna, LA: Pelican Publishing Co.

10

South Asian Traditions

Theodore M. Ludwig

LEARNING OBJECTIVES

At the end of this chapter, the reader will be able to:

- Describe the basic beliefs and practices of South Asians, including Hindus, Jains, and Sikhs.
- Discuss the main principles, diagnostic techniques, and treatments of Ayurvedic medicine.
- Describe some concerns about spiritual care and health felt by Hindus, Jains, and Sikhs.
- Recognize the implications for providing nursing care for people of South Asian traditions.

Adi Granth (Guru Granth Sahib)   karma
atman   meditation
Ayurveda medicine   nonviolence (ahimsa)
dharma   samsara
Guru Nanak   three doshas
Jainism   yoga

Evolving from earlier traditions, Hinduism, Buddhism, and Jainism developed together in India from about the 6th century BCE (before common era) onward. Buddhism eventually disappeared from India, after spreading to other parts of Asia. Jainism has remained a fairly small tradition in India, and Sikhism did not begin until the 16th century CE (common era). Apart from the large Muslim populations of India, Pakistan, and Bangladesh, and the Buddhist majorities of Sri Lanka and Bhutan, Hinduism has long been the dominant religion of South Asia, observed by nearly 80% of India's population of 1 billion and nearly 90% of that of Nepal. During the past century, immigration also has created a significant diaspora of Hindus, Jains, and Sikhs in the Western world.

HINDU RELIGIOUS AND CULTURAL TRADITIONS

③ Hindus trace their ancestry to the ancient Aryans, a pastoral Indo-European people who apparently migrated to South Asia sometime after 2000 BCE. The pre-Aryans of the Indus Valley created a sophisticated civilization with large cities and extensive agriculture; some of their religious ideas and practices, as well as those of other pre-Aryan peoples in India, may have influenced the development of Hinduism and other South Asian religious traditions. The Aryans composed Sanskrit scriptures, which they called Vedas (*veda* means "knowledge"). The Vedas were organized into four collections: *Rig Veda* (hymns to the Gods), *Sama Veda* (verses sung during the sacrifice), *Yajur Veda* (formulas spoken by the priests), and *Atharva Veda* (incantations, including medical formulations). Throughout the centuries, additional texts were added to these original Vedas, in particular the philosophical scriptures known as the Upanishads. All these early Sanskrit scriptures eventually became known as Veda, the eternal truth. All modern Hindus still highly revere these scriptures as possessing great wisdom and power. Many other scriptures also were composed in ancient India, such as the **dharma** sutras, the great Epics (including the *Bhagavad-Gita*), and the Puranas. Although these scriptures generally do not have the high status of the Veda, they are well known and influential among Hindus, laying out concretely the various facets of the Hindu way of life and belief.

Hinduism has had many phases of development, as documented in the history of these extensive sacred texts, and some would argue that it is still developing today. The religion of the early Vedas focused on fire sacrifice to the various Gods and Goddesses, accompanied by the chanting of the powerful words of ancient hymns, to obtain success, long life, and many children. A class ("caste") system developed, with the priests (Brahmins) as the highest class, followed by warriors, workers, and servants. The Vedic sacrificial rituals and chants were considered central for maintaining order and life, and today Hindus still believe that it is important for Brahmin priests regularly to perform some of these ancient rituals.

In addition to these Vedic ritual practices, many other religious perspectives and practices developed in classical Hinduism. The Upanishads show a spiritual search for understanding that gave expression to fundamental Hindu ideas of the One Reality (Brahman), **karma**, rebirth, and the cycles of **samsara**, together with the practice of **meditation** and the goal of liberation (moksha) from the cycles of rebirth. The dharma sutras laid out fundamental Hindu ideas of order and social structure, suggesting appropriate actions and duties for everyone based on class, gender, and stage of life. The great Epics, *Mahabharata* and *Ramayana*, through stories of heroes and Gods, provided models for the whole Hindu way of life, including involvement in society through following one's dharma (or calling), spiritual fulfillment through worshiping the Gods, and the alternate path of withdrawal through meditation and **yoga**. The Hindu tradition continued to develop in the medieval period, with the rise of philosophical schools, further discoveries of cosmic spiritual forces through esoteric Tantric practices, strong surges of theistic devotion to the great Gods, and the impact of Islamic ideas and spirituality.

In modern times, Hindus have responded to Western influences in India and have carried their traditions into the Western world. For Hindus living in the Western diaspora, maintaining a sense of Hindu identity in the midst of Western secular education, interfaith marriage, and the lack of a Hindu social order is challenging. Traditional distinctions of class, caste, and sectarian adherence tend to become less important among Hindus in the West, and they are attracted to a more inclusive kind of Hindu orientation.

Hindu World Views

Although Hindu philosophers have adopted a number of differing perspectives on the world and ultimate reality, a very influential view is that developed in the Upanishads and elaborated by the great philosopher Shankara, generally known as Nondualism (Advaita). This tradition asserts that all of reality is One, even though humans may perceive it as many. Called "Brahman," the One Reality is the absolute spirit, the source of all, which pervades all and is in fact not differentiated from all. For those who truly know and understand, all of this world is really the one Brahman.

Hindus recognize different ways of conceiving the relation between the Brahman and the world as humans experience it:

- The Brahman is the All, and there is nothing else.
- The Brahman is real, and the multiplex world is illusion.
- My true and eternal self (**atman**) is Brahman, not this changing, perishing self.

Shankara made a helpful distinction between two ways of talking about Brahman: *Brahman nirguna* (Brahman without qualities), and *Brahman saguna* (Brahman with qualities). Brahman nirguna is the perception, first, of the highest truth, that all is Brahman, with no distinctions, and second, that all other perceptions are illusion (*maya*). But the lower way of perceiving Brahman saguna is also true, namely, Brahman experienced as the Soul of the world, as God (Ishvara), as the Real at the heart of all.

An alternate perspective on reality is offered by the Samkhya philosophical school, a vision that has been influential in yogic practice and in Ayurvedic medicine. Samkhya posits two eternal realities: *purusha*, which is pure spiritual consciousness, and *prakriti*, which is pure materiality. The universe evolves from prakriti, including the whole person with mind and senses, whereas purusha is formless, pure transcendent consciousness, the eternal soul. Purusha becomes entangled with prakriti because of ignorance and desire on the part of the embodied mind. The goal of yogic practice is to discipline the mind–body complex to disentangle purusha consciousness from the material self and mind and bring about liberation. These spiritual and physical disciplines also bring about mind–body health and wholeness.

Some Hindu holy men and women (samnyasins) have achieved the highest spiritual perfection and contemplate Brahman as the one reality, reaching a level of self-realization that sees no difference between self and Brahman. This can be experienced to a degree in certain forms of meditation and yoga, and it forms an important part of Hindu spiritual practice. But for many Hindus, the more concrete way of experiencing the divine source is through bhakti yoga (yoga of devotion), in which a great God or Goddess is worshiped as the personal supreme reality. Hinduism allows for many Gods—330 million of them, according to tradition—because the divine source can be seen in all living things. But most Hindus follow their family tradition and devote themselves to one of several great Gods/Goddesses, together with their consorts and associated Gods.

The two great Gods for most Hindus are Vishnu and Shiva, and Goddesses associated with them also are widely worshiped. Vishnu is the creator and preserver of the world. Vishnu can also be worshiped through his consort Lakshmi, Goddess of wealth and beauty, and especially through his avataras (incarnations), such as Krishna and Rama. The other great God is Shiva, whose cosmic dance continually creates and destroys the world, and who embodies both male and female generative powers, as symbolized in the lingam and yoni (male and female organs). Shiva is the supreme yogin who keeps the world operating through the power of his meditation. Shiva's female aspect (Shakti) is often highlighted in worship, in the form of Parvati his wife, or Durga the great warrior Goddess, or even Kali, the fiercely destructive mother Goddess. Oftentimes, their devotees raise these female forms of the great Goddess to supreme status.

Traditional Hindu views of the world suggest a process of gigantic time cycles in which the world evolves and devolves like waves on the sea. Hindu scriptures give different pictures of the origin of the world, but one well-known version comes from the *Vishnu Purana*. In it, Vishnu is the supreme lord, containing the entire potential universe in his own nature and resting on his cosmic serpent Sesha. His wife, Lakshmi, tickles his feet, and engaging in play, Vishnu evolves the whole universe from himself. He then becomes the preserver, supporting the world through gigantic time cycles until it is exhausted, at which time he destroys the world in a great conflagration and sleeps on the great serpent, until he once again is stirred to create the world for another cosmic cycle.

Yet even within these changing worlds, there is an eternal order, *dharma*, the right way for everything. The world is real, and it functions by dharma. Even the great Vishnu (according to *Bhagavad-Gita* 3.22–24) has his dharma to fulfill: upholding the whole world and all its functioning. All aspects of the world, including humans, fit into that order and have dharma to fulfill.

In thinking of the nature and role of humans, Hindus believe a distinction must be made between the *real self* and the *empirical self* that we experience living in this phenomenal world. The empirical self seems to be the real self, for it is made up of the physical body as well as the subtle body of vital breaths, organs of action, and organs of knowledge, mind, and intellect. But Hindu wisdom says the real self is something other: the *atman*, which is the eternal and formless soul, in essence none other than the Brahman or pure cosmic consciousness. In a famous dialogue in the Upanishads, the wise father Uddalaka instructs his son Svetaketu, telling him to place salt in some water in a basin and then taste it from different ends, finding that the whole water is pervaded by salt. Thus it is with Brahman, which pervades all reality: "That is Reality. That is Atman. That you are, Svetaketu" (*Chandogya Upanishad* 6.13.1–3). The true self for each human being is the atman, which is really the supreme Brahman. The spiritual goal for Hindus is fully to realize the atman and thus reach complete unity with Brahman, the experience of moksha, liberation from the sufferings of the rebirth cycle.

This fundamental Hindu teaching does not mean that the lower, concrete realities of self are unimportant. The physical, mental, psychological, and social aspects of life make up the arena in which one's dharma is lived out. Hinduism teaches that the atman is embodied according to the working of the law of karma: the actions the atman performs in one lifetime, depending on their moral quality, determine the conditions for the next embodiment of the atman. This law of karma works neutrally and brings about the results of one's actions through rebirth after rebirth. In addition, according to Hindu belief, because there are countless living beings, each embodying atman, there are many levels of rebirth, from those in the hells to plants, animals, humans, and Gods. Each rebirth depends on the quality of karma built up during the previous lifetimes.

Thus, in traditional Hindu thought, concerns for physical well-being and spiritual well-being coincide. Living the right kind of life leads to higher levels in the rebirth cycle, with corresponding advancement in well-being and spiritual fulfillment. In the same way, living the wrong kind of life leads to lower levels in the cycle, with increased physical and spiritual deficiencies. The quality of karma determines the state of rebirth, including the makeup of mind and body, health, susceptibility to disease, and spiritual abilities (Leslie, 1999).

According to the Upanishads, the basic problem that mires the atman in repeated existences in samsara is ignorance of the true nature of the atman. The true self, atman, is really the Brahman (supreme consciousness), but we humans in our ignorance tend to think that our phenomenal self, consisting of body, mind, and feelings, is our real self. Out of such ignorance, attachment and desire arise, leading to action (karma) done out of these selfish desires, and the accumulation of karma done out of desire continues the cycle of unhappiness, suffering, redeath, and rebirth. The solution is fundamentally a spiritual one: knowledge of the Brahman, detachment from selfish desire, and dedication to fulfilling dharma. Such is the path of spiritual advancement toward moksha, as well as physical health and well-being.

Hindu Spiritual Paths

Hinduism recognizes that different people have different spiritual capacities because of their particular place in the rebirth cycle, and their correspondingly unique makeup of body and mind. The *Bhagavad-Gita* (14:5–18) teaches that there are three universal *gunas* or qualities that pervade all creation: *sattva* (light, spirit, clarity), *rajas* (movement, passion), and *tamas* (inertia, darkness, dullness). Each person, because of past karma, is born with a particular configuration of the gunas and, thus, with different mental and spiritual capabilities. Many different spiritual practices are available in Hinduism, appropriate to each spiritual level, involving almost every conceivable type of religious pursuit. Following the model set forth in the *Bhagavad-Gita*, Hindu thinkers have suggested that these various spiritual practices can be grouped into three basic paths (*margas* or *yogas*):

- The path of knowledge (*jñana-yoga*)
- The path of action (*karma-yoga*)
- The path of devotion (*bhakti-yoga*)

These three broad paths intersect at many points, and Hindus may typically follow practices associated with two or all three, but each path has a special focus and structure.

Those who are more spiritually advanced strive to follow the path of knowledge (jñana-yoga), with disciplines of study, withdrawal, and meditation to help advance toward moksha. Although all Hindus can engage in these practices, the ideal is to reach the point of withdrawing from attachments in family and society and devote oneself fully to these spiritual disciplines. Some might retreat to an ashram to live under the guidance of a guru and engage in study and meditation. Or some might follow the path of yoga as taught by Patañjali, with its emphasis on mind–body unity in ethical, bodily, and mental discipline. For the spiritually highly advanced, becoming a samnyasin (renouncer) means totally cutting ties with family and society and devoting oneself full-time to austerities and meditation.

But for the vast majority of Hindus, the path of action (karma-yoga) provides a means of spiritual advancement while fulfilling one's role in family and society. Because karma caused by selfish actions is understood to cause problems in this life and lower rebirth in the next, Hindus are taught by the *Bhagavad-Gita* to abandon selfish desire and simply fulfill their dharma, that is, their role in life according to their birth, whether priest, warrior, worker, or servant, whether man or woman. Performing one's actions out of duty (according to one's dharma), rather than doing actions out of desire, builds up good karma and leads to happiness in this life and a higher rebirth in the next. Hindus believe that fulfilling one's proper role in life, as determined by caste and gender, is a spiritual path that brings blessing and wholeness for the individual and for the community.

A third path is available for spiritual and material wholeness—the path of devotion to one's God (bhakti-yoga). The *Bhagavad-Gita*, while teaching the path of knowledge and the path of action, presents the path of worshiping God as the highest path, and one open to all classes or castes, men and women equally. By focusing all one's mind and spirit, desires, needs, thoughts, and passions on one's God, karma and suffering can be surmounted through divine power. The *Bhagavad-Gita* counsels everyone to worship the great God Vishnu in the form of Krishna, Vishnu's avatar (incarnation). As the divine source of all, Vishnu can lift one up beyond samsara and bring salvation. Other Hindus devote themselves to the great God Shiva through songs, austerities, and yogic meditation, finding saving power for liberation from karma and rebirth through his cosmic power. Some Hindus are moved to ecstasy through the divine grace of Lakshmi or Parvati or another form of the great Goddess, while strong-minded Hindus focus their worship on Kali, a destructive form of the great Goddess, for empowerment and salvation. The Gods are not jealous and exclusive, so many Hindus participate in devotion to various Gods, even while maintaining special devotion to the God traditionally worshiped by their family. The path of bhakti is full of colorful rituals, festivals, music, dance, pilgrimage, and much more, forming an important part of the spiritual identity of many Hindus.

The Hindu life cycle follows a dynamic rhythm, defined by special ritual times called *samskaras*, sacraments of passage (Desai, 1989, pp. 24–34). There are many such rituals, but almost all Hindus observe a few major ones. Birth rituals include the important naming rite about 10 days after birth, as well as the first haircut at about 3 years. An important step for boys of the three upper classes is initiation (*upanayana*) into the student stage of life; the boy's head is shaved, a sacred cord is placed over his left shoulder, and he is taught the words of sacred Vedas. Marriage (*vivaha*) is a key family event, arranged between two families and celebrated with many rituals over several days. The last samskara, the death ritual (*antyesti*), traditionally includes proceeding with the body to the cremation grounds and placing the body on a pyre of wood, with the eldest son setting it aflame while repeating an ancient Vedic prayer. The bones are gathered and placed in a river, and final rituals (*shraddhas*) involve offering cakes of rice and water, symbolically constructing a next-worldly body for the deceased in the realm of the ancestors.

Thus, for Hindus, a wholesome, healthy life is one that embodies Dharma in all its ramifications: to live in the proper order of class and caste, family role, and stage of life; to honor the Vedic scriptures and the wisdom of the sages; and to perform the daily rituals, worship the Gods, and participate in the festivals. The so-called Four Aims of Life sum up the Hindu ideal: to seek success, pleasure, dharma, and moksha. Depending on one's particular age, stage of life, and spiritual progress, the emphasis changes. For example, for a householder, success and pleasure are important values, along with doing one's dharma. For an aged person, or one spiritually advanced, movement toward moksha becomes the more important value.

OTHER SOUTH ASIAN RELIGIOUS TRADITIONS

Two other religious traditions that have grown up in South Asia are Jainism and Sikhism. There are fewer adherents to these religions than Hindus, but they also are representative of South Asian culture and are present in significant numbers in the Western world.

The Jain Religious Tradition

While Jainism never became a large movement numerically—there are perhaps 4 million **Jains** today—it has been a significant part of the culture of India. Jains believe that in each vast world cycle a series of Jinas ("conquerors") arise to reach enlightenment and guide others to liberation. The first Jina in our current world age established civilization; the 24th and last Jina for our age was Mahavira, who was born in India about 599 BCE. He was a householder but renounced the world when he was 30 years old and followed a path of extreme asceticism, going unclad, fasting often, and practicing **ahimsa (nonviolence)** toward every living thing. After 12 years, he reached the highest enlightenment (*kevela*), became the Jina, and taught disciples, monks, nuns, and lay persons, until he was fully liberated with his death at 72 years. His life and teachings have been the model for the Jain community ever since.

Jains do not believe in a creator God or supreme being. Rather, the world process operates on its own through endless world cycles of evolution and degeneration. The universe is eternal, and its constituents are space, motion, rest, time, and matter, as well as infinite individual souls (jiva). All these souls (except those who have reached liberation and dwell in the pure state in the highest realm of the universe) are embodied in matter because of karma, and continue in the rebirth cycle (samsara) almost endlessly because of continuing desire and karma. There are four realms of rebirth: Gods, humans, hell-beings, and animals or plants. The animal–plant category is almost infinite, including even microscopic beings with only the sense of touch, whose body is air, water, fire, or earth. Jains teach that every individual soul has already been reborn millions and millions of times, in all possible forms. The human rebirth form is particularly important because this form is most favorable for spiritual progress toward liberation.

Despite this vision of a vast number of rebirths, Jains do not believe that the soul is hopelessly trapped in the rebirth cycle. Even in its defiled state, the soul retains certain capabilities that can change the effect of karma and begin movement toward liberation, even though it often falls back again. The time will come when the soul is in a relatively pure state and encounters the teachings of a Jina, a transforming event that completely redirects the soul toward liberation so that, no matter how many lifetimes it takes, it never falls back. The soul is said to progress through 14 stages of purification until it reaches final liberation. After reaching the fourth stage, the stage of true insight, the soul is irreversibly on the path to liberation; at this stage it becomes possible to follow the religious path, whether as a monk or nun, or as a dedicated lay person (Jaini, 1979).

To be a Jain monk or nun means to observe a whole series of restraints and other disciplines on a path of complete renunciation. Monks and nuns take five Great Vows: to refrain from

1. Injuring life
2. False speech
3. Taking what is not given
4. Unchastity
5. Possession

These restraints are observed in a very strict and complete fashion. For example, monks and nuns extend the restraint of not injuring life to all living things, even one-sense beings. Thus, they cannot bathe, walk in the rain, dig in the earth, light or extinguish fires, or fan themselves because all such activities would injure delicate one-sense beings who have earth, water, fire, or air as their bodies. Monks and nuns follow many other disciplines, and rigorous meditation techniques are used to attain deeper insight.

Lay persons follow a similar ascetic path but at an appropriately less vigorous level, taking 12 "partial" vows or restraints. Lay persons also participate in rituals such as worshiping the Jinas, keeping the holy days, participating in festivals, and going on pilgrimages to holy places. Jains have a full round of rituals of the passages of life, beginning with a ritual for the protection of the expectant mother and embryo, and ending with the death rituals of cremation and throwing the ashes in a river.

Jains have maintained their identity in India and more recently have spread throughout the world. One reason for their continued vitality is the close association of the monks and nuns with lay persons. The Jain vision of the good, wholesome life is strongly shaped by their underlying idea of karma, which attaches to the soul through deeds of desire and violence. The first of the five Great Restraints is very important: not doing injury to living beings (*ahimsa*). Willful violence toward living organisms causes karma in abundance, so practicing nonviolence is a hallmark of the Jain way of life. Lay persons are permitted to harm one-sense organisms (such as vegetation) for the obvious reason of providing food for society, but they are strictly enjoined from harming animals and thus practice vegetarianism. Jains also avoid occupations that entail violence to living beings, such as leather-working, military service, and farming. Teaching that nonviolence and the other restraints are to be fulfilled in positive ways that benefit society, Jains are well-respected in occupations such as educators, physicians, business, and societal leaders.

The Sikh Religious Tradition

Today Sikhs number about 22 million, 80% of whom live in India; they form the majority of the population in the Punjab region in northwest India. Compared with Hinduism, Jainism, and Buddhism, the Sikh religious tradition arose relatively recently in India, founded by **Guru Nanak** in the 17th century. Nanak was born near Lahore into a Hindu family, but he also had contact with Muslims, who by then were very populous in India. The devotional atmosphere was very strong in both Hinduism and Islam at this time, and Nanak composed and sang hymns together with a Muslim friend. When he was 30 years old, Nanak had a transforming religious experience, being carried up to God's presence and given a divine call. When he reappeared he proclaimed, "There is neither Hindu nor Muslim, so whose path shall I follow? I shall follow God's path." Nanak now was the guru, who gives voice to the word of God, the true Guru. He pursued his divine calling by traveling about India for many years, teaching and singing evangelistic hymns, gathering disciples ("Sikhs") and thus founding the Sikh community.

After Guru Nanak's death, nine more gurus arose to lead the Sikh community. The hymns that Guru Nanak composed, as well as hymns composed by the gurus after Nanak and also by several non-Sikhs, were eventually gathered and published as the sacred scriptures, the **Adi Granth** (Original Collection), also called **Guru Granth Sahib** (Guru Sacred Collection). Amritsar in the Punjab became a religious center, where the well-known Golden Temple was built. The tenth guru, Gobind Singh (1666–1708), founded the military society called *Khalsa* in 1699, originally for the protection of Sikhs in those tumultuous times, but eventually it became the central Sikh community. Before his death, Guru Gobind decreed that no more human gurus would arise; rather, from that point on the Holy Book, the *Adi Granth* itself, would be the Guru, the vehicle for the presence of God's word in the world.

Sikh teachings revolve around God as the sole reality who is beyond all form, and yet God's self-manifestation is the whole creation. God is also personal, revealed to the human heart through God's word in all creation and especially through God's name, *Nam*, the dimension of God's presence that can be known and loved. God creates the universe and dissolves it time and again in divine play. Humans are part of the creation emanating from God, like sparks from the fire. The soul is immortal and takes bodily form according to the will of the creator; it is the basic link with God as the receptacle of God's love. When the body dies, the soul appears before God and, depending on its karma, is sent to be reborn in another body, whether animal, human, or in heaven or hell. The ultimate goal of the Sikh religious life is to attain final nirvana, transcending heaven and hell and the rebirth cycle in blissful union with God.

The human problem, Guru Nanak taught, is separation from God because of ignorance and self-centeredness. This is the cause of all suffering, whether physical, mental, social, or spiritual. Because of this self-centeredness, the soul is trapped in evil and has to endure countless rebirths in the samsara cycle. But through the Guru, the path to God is revealed, for God's word reverberates through the Guru, and by meditating on God's word and God's name, disciples are given God's grace and favor. Guru Nanak rejected the traditional Hindu and Muslim rituals and practices, and taught that the true path is an inward preparation of the heart to receive and experience God. Practical disciplines for preparing the heart include singing God's praises (*kirtan*) and meditating on God's name, repeating it over and over (*Nam simaran*) so that the divine sound fills one's whole being. With respect to health, the ritual of repeating God's name is believed by Sikhs to bring physical wholeness and even to cure diseases (Singh, 1999).

Sikh worship is focused on the *Adi Granth*, the Sikh sacred scripture, through which the word of God is experienced concretely. Devout Sikhs keep the *Adi Granth* in a special room of the house and read from it with great respect. Worship also means visiting the gurdwara, the temple where the Sikh community gathers for communal worship. The central object is the *Adi Granth*, placed on a cot and draped in embroidered silks with a royal awning above, before which Sikhs bow before sitting on the floor. Both men and women read from the holy book, and trained musicians lead the faithful in devotional music. *Karah prasad*, a sacred food made of flour, sugar, and clarified butter, is served to everyone present. Guru Nanak rejected the caste system and the lower status of women, and this equality is demonstrated concretely in the community kitchen (*langar*) associated with most gurdwaras, where people of all sorts sit together and partake of the same food without any distinction between the high and the low.

Although Guru Nanak did not approve of excessive ritual, Sikhs do have commonly observed festivals, such as the commemoration of Guru Nanak's birthday and the martyrdom of the fifth Guru Arjun. Rituals observing life passages include reciting the first five verses of the morning prayer in the ears of a newborn child, naming the child, and celebrating when a boy has his first turban ceremoniously tied on. When Sikh boys and girls come of age, they may be formally initiated into the order of the khalsa. Men who are initiated may for the rest of their lives wear the five symbols of the khalsa: uncut hair (kept under a turban), a comb, a dagger, a wrist guard, and short pants. Men entering the khalsa often take the surname Singh (lion), and women take the name Kaur (princess). A Sikh marriage takes place in the presence of the *Guru Granth Sahib*, with the couple solemnly circumambulating the holy book in a counterclockwise direction while the wedding hymn is sung. When death occurs, the family accompanies the body to the crematorium singing hymns, with no wailing; a close family relative lights the pyre, and mourners may return to the family home to sing hymns and begin a complete reading of the *Guru Granth Sahib*.

Sikhs believe that the love of God leads to a good ethical life, which brings happiness, grace, and self-realization. Sikhs are not to withdraw from life to follow asceticism but are to involve themselves fully in family and society while displaying the fundamental virtues: wisdom, truthfulness, justice, self-control, contentment, and courage. All should be productive in society in right livelihood, helping the needy, avoiding slander and enmity, and practicing altruism toward all, for in serving humanity one is serving the guru and serving God. Thus, Sikh hospitals, educational institutions, and social relief agencies flourish in India today.

SOUTH ASIAN PRACTICES OF HEALTH AND MEDICINE

Practices of health and healing have been abundant among the peoples of South Asia. Many of the traditions are spiritual in nature, involving meditation, yoga, and spiritually powerful healers. More-specific medical practices also have a long history; in particular, several organized systems of medicine have developed in India, namely, the Siddha, Unani, and especially the Ayurvedic systems.

Healing and Health for Spiritual Ends: Meditation and Yoga

The many practices of meditation and yoga developed in the South Asian religious traditions are intended as means for spiritual advancement, as we have seen. At the same time, experience has shown that many of these practices contribute to physical, mental, social, and psychological health as well. This is appropriate because sickness and health are understood holistically. Mental stress can contribute to sickness, as can physical stress, and healing involves both mind and body. Practices of meditation and yoga typically calm, focus, or enhance mental functioning, and often the mental exercises are linked with bodily exercises, such as a special sitting position, breathing exercises, walking, chanting, or singing.

Meditation, in its various forms, calms the mind and brings deeper insight and awareness. Two major types of meditation are widely used among the Eastern peoples. One is *concentration* or fixed meditation, which focuses on an internal or external object. The other is known as *mindfulness*, in which the meditator simply observes alertly everything that passes through the mind. To give one example: the progression of meditation suggested in the *Mandukya Upanishad* is a four-stage movement from outer reality to inner enlightenment. This meditation is linked to the mantra *AUM (Om)*, which symbolizes Brahman, the ultimate sacred reality. The meditation begins with the letter *A*, representing the normal waking state, with mind and senses turned outward and full of activity. As meditation turns inward, the *U* stage represents the "dream-like" stage, with the mind still active but now totally internal, detached from outer objects. Next, the *M* stage is like "deep sleep" with no mental activity, but only a massive consciousness, calm, and peaceful. The fourth stage is represented by the silence that precedes and follows the mantra *AUM*; it is the cessation of sense and mental activity and the experiencing of the nondual source of all, union with Brahman, which brings bliss and wholeness. Studies have shown how practices of meditation are effective in reducing stress and promoting mental and physical health (Griffiths, 2002).

The word *yoga* as used in the South Asian traditions can refer to many types of spiritual/mental/physical disciplines, including bhakti-yoga (worshiping God), karma-yoga (the spiritual discipline of right action), and mantra-yoga (chanting sacred sounds). A most influential system of yoga is the classical yoga developed by Patañjali in his *Yoga-sutras*. This system of yoga includes eight steps and encompasses a holistic body-mind practice: restraint in life, observance of moral purity, bodily postures, breath control, withdrawal of senses, concentrating the mind, meditation, and experiencing a higher trance-like state. Following these extensive yogic disciplines involves a holistic regimen that aims at spiritual liberation but also brings mental and physical wholeness (Fields, 2001; Iyengar, 2001). Box 10.1 describes the eight limbs of classical yoga.

Hindus, Buddhists, Jains, Sikhs, and others find some or all of these spiritual practices conducive to health: meditation, yoga, bodily movements, breathing exercises, prayer, and chanting. Some of these practices also have become adopted for healing and health by peoples of the Western world.

Ayurveda System of Traditional Medicine

A wide variety of healing practices exists throughout South Asia, as herbalists, bone-setters, yogins, tantrists, homeopaths, and many others practice their traditional healing arts. Of particular importance are several integrated, holistic systems of medicine that since ancient times have been associated with written medical treatises and

---

BOX 10.1 Eight Limbs of Yoga

Classical Yoga, as set forth in the *Yoga-sutras* of Patañjali, is directed toward discriminative knowledge, which distinguishes between a person's physical–mental existence (prakriti) and his or her true nature as cosmic consciousness (purusha), and leads to liberation. Suffering is experienced because of afflictions of mind and body that arise from ignorance of one's true nature. Yoga cultivates the psychophysical person in order to reach discriminative knowledge and thus liberation and wholeness.

The eight limbs of Patañjali's Yoga can be grouped into three areas: ethical values, physical practices, and cultivation of consciousness.

ETHICAL VALUES
1. Moral self-restraints (yama): nonviolence, truthfulness, nonstealing, sensual restraint, nonacquisitiveness
2. Moral commitments (niyama): purity, contentment, self-discipline, self-education, dedication to God

PHYSICAL PRACTICES
1. Postures (asanas): steadiness, endurance, equilibrium, relaxation of effort, meditation on infinite
2. Regulation of vital energy through breath (pranayama): controlling the energy of the mind–body system by breath exercises
3. Withdrawal of the senses (pratyahara): eliminating mental distraction from sensory sources

CULTIVATION OF CONSCIOUSNESS
1. Concentration (dharana): one-pointed mental concentration on a single object
2. Meditation (dhyana): sustained and unwavering attention to the object
3. Meditative trance (samadhi): complete absorption of mind in object, leading to higher states and liberation of purusha from prakriti

texts. These traditional systems are, of course, related to the religious traditions, but their primary purpose is healing and maintaining health. The most influential of these systems is Ayurveda, described briefly below, but the Siddha and Unani systems also have considerable followings. These systems have become quite popular in modern times with the upsurge of interest in India's national heritage. The government of India has set up a special Department of Indian Systems of Medicine and Homoeopathy within the Ministry of Health and Family Welfare to promote and regulate these traditional systems of medicine (Ministry of Health & Family Welfare, Government of India, 2002a).

Among the Tamils of south India, the Siddha system of medicine is still widely used, with an extensive medical literature in the Tamil language. Siddha medicine is closely related to Ayurveda in its view of the body, diagnostic techniques, and therapies (Ministry of Health and Family Welfare, Government of India, 2002b; Narayanaswami, 1983). It looks especially to the healing accomplishments of 18 perfected saints called Siddhas, and makes considerable use of drugs derived from metals and minerals, as well as herbs.

Some Muslims of South Asia continue to practice the Unani system of traditional medicine. They believe that Unani originated from the ancient Greeks, was passed on through Persian and Arab peoples, and was brought to India by Muslims in the medieval period and practiced during the Mughal dynasty. Unani medicine is based on maintaining equilibrium among the various aspects of the body, made up of four elements, different temperaments, simple and compound organs, and four humors. Diagnostic techniques include examination of the pulse, urine, and stool; treatments include exercise, massage, Turkish bath, douches, diets, and herbal drugs (Ministry of Health & Family Welfare, Government of India, 2002c).

Ayurveda means "knowledge of life," and its roots are in the Vedic knowledge of ancient India, associated especially with the *Atharva Veda*, which contains formulations for treatment of disease. It developed as an auxiliary science with important treatises and practices. Three particularly important ancient texts define some of the basic principles and techniques of Ayurveda: the *Caraka Samhita*, the *Sushruta Samhita*, and the *Ashtanga Hardayam Samhita*. Although Western biomedicine has become important in India in modern times, with government support Ayurveda has experienced a significant revival, and India now has approximately as many recognized Ayurveda practitioners as physicians of Western medicine. South Asians living in the Western world often take interest in Ayurveda, and this system has also become well-known among non-Asian Westerners who are interested in alternative health practices.

Ayurveda is based on the traditional Hindu Samkhya world view, which holds that all things arise from the co-presence of cosmic consciousness (purusha) and primordial materiality (prakriti). Everything in the world (prakriti) operates through the interaction of the three universal gunas or qualities: *sattva, rajas*, and *tamas*. Sattva is white and bright, bringing clarity of perception; rajas is red, causing passion, emotion, sensation, and movement; tamas is dark and causes inertia, heaviness, and confusion. All characteristics of the world and of humans derive from these three qualities and their interactions. Human temperaments and mental characteristics are classified according to which of these three gunas predominates. For example, people with sattvic qualities are loving, pure, followers of truth and righteousness, alert, creative, full of luster, and intelligent. People with rajasic qualities are egoistic, ambitious, controlling, perfectionists, restless, jealous, fearful of failure, and loving to those who help them. People with tamasic qualities are lazy, depressed, less intelligent, greedy, irritable, and love food and sleep.

With respect to the body, according to the Ayurvedic texts, all forms of matter are composed of the five basic elements (space, air, fire, water, and earth), each produced by a particular combination of the gunas. What is present in the cosmos (macrocosm) is present in the body (microcosm), so all of these five elements are present in the human body (Fields, 2001). Synaptic and cellular space in the body permits the flow of intelligence between cells. Air is *prana*, the vital life force that communicates and governs all sensory stimuli, motor responses, and other movements within the body. Fire (*agni*) regulates body temperature, is responsible for digestion, absorption, and assimilation of food, and is active within each organ and even within each cell. Water exists as the bodily fluids, plasma and saliva, carrying energy from one cell to the other and from one system to the other. Earth is present in all solid structures and tissues and cells.

Although the body itself is made up of the five elements, the functioning of the body is governed by the **three doshas** or biological energy forces: *vata* (from space and air), *pitta* (from fire and water), and *kapha* (from earth) (Frawley & Ranade, 2001; Lad, 1999; Zysk, 1996). These three energy forces are also present in every cell, tissue, and organ and differ in their combinations in each person. Ayurveda distinguishes seven basic body types: monotypes, with vata, pitta, or kapha prevalent; dual types, vita-pitta, pitta-kapha, or kapha-vata; and the equal type, with the three doshas in equal proportions. But even within these seven body types, each individual has a unique combination of the three doshas.

Vata is the energy of movement. Its qualities are dry, light, cold, mobile, active, astringent, and dispersing, and all of these qualities can be found in people in whom vata is dominant. For example, a person in whom vata is dominant would have dry skin and hair; would tend toward constipation; would have a light body frame, cold hands and poor circulation; would be very active and perceptive; and would have emotions of anxiety and insecurity. People with unbalanced vata are susceptible to diseases involving air, such as emphysema, pneumonia, and arthritis, or nervous system disorders and mental confusion.

Pitta is the energy of digestion or metabolism. Its qualities are hot, sharp, light, liquid, sour, oily, spreading, and having a strong smell and bitter taste. Thus, a person with much pitta has a strong appetite, warm skin, perspires easily, has sharp features and mind, oily hair that gets grey early, moderate body frame, an aggressive and dominating personality, is critical of others, and is a perfectionist. People with unbalanced pitta tend to have diseases involving the fire principle, such as fevers, inflammatory diseases, jaundice, skin rashes, ulcers, colitis, and sore throats.

Kapha is the energy that forms the body's structure. Its qualities are heavy, slow, cool, oily, liquid, dense, thick, static, cloudy, sweet, and salty. A person in whom kapha dominates has heavy bone, muscles, and fat, easily puts on weight, has slow metabolism, cool and clammy skin, thick wavy hair, a slow but steady memory, walks slowly and does not like exercise, is loving and compassionate, and has a slow mind and a sweet tooth. People with unbalanced kapha tend to have diseases connected with the water principle, such as influenza, sinus congestion, diabetes, excess weight, and headaches.

In addition to the three doshas, the body is made up of tissues (*dhatus*) and waste products (*malas*). Seven tissues, as the structure of the body, are responsible for nourishment: plasma, blood cells, muscle, adipose, bone, bone marrow, and reproductive tissue. The wastes are the nonretainable substances (urine, feces, and sweat), which need to be released to cleanse the body.

The Ayurvedic concept of health is a well-balanced state of this total body matrix that includes the three energy forces, seven tissues, and waste products, as well as the mental temperament and the functioning of the five elements in the process of nourishment. This is a holistic notion of health involving physical, mental, social, emotional, and spiritual well-being. Intrinsic or extrinsic disturbances in this natural equilibrium can bring imbalances that, if not corrected, build up toxins (*ama*) and lead to various diseases. Such disturbances include dietary misuse, undesirable habits, improper exercise, wrong use of sense organs, incompatible actions of body and mind, or imbalanced emotions. For example, fear and anxiety are associated with vata, and if these emotions are repressed, the kidneys tend to be disturbed; anger and hate, connected with pitta, can unbalance the liver; and greed and possessiveness, linked with kapha, can cause disturbance in the heart and spleen. External causes, such as seasonal abnormalities, hereditary pathologies, external trauma, or supernatural causes, may also have an effect. All such factors can increase or deplete one or more of the doshas to a level that is not a healthful balance for that particular individual. Each body type also has a tendency toward certain disorders, depending on such factors as age and season of the year. For example, vata disorders can be traced to the colon and are aggravated in autumn and winter, whereas pitta disorders begin in the small intestine, often in summer, and kapha disorders occur in the stomach with aggravation in winter and spring.

In the Ayurvedic view, the progression of disease begins with the accumulation of the aggravated dosha in its location: kapha in the stomach, pitta in the small intestine, and vata in the colon. Such accumulation is not unusual (it happens seasonally, for example), and therapy is fairly simple at this point. But in the second stage, the dosha begins to provoke the surrounding organs, and by the third stage the dosha begins to circulate through the body. Next, the aggravated dosha settles in a weak area of the bodily tissue and begins to dominate and cause toxins, and the cardinal symptoms and signs of the disease become manifest, leading to structural changes and complications involving other tissues and systems (Frawley & Ranade, 2001; Lad, 1999).

Ayurvedic physicians employ a variety of diagnostic techniques involving the whole person and environment: questioning about life history, observing parts of the body, listening, and palpating. Great emphasis is placed on pulse diagnosis, which is felt by three fingers (vata, pitta, and kapha pulses) and provides much information to the physician about the body type and the health of the internal organs. Also important is tongue diagnosis, which investigates characteristic patterns in different areas of the tongue that reveal pathological conditions of the internal organs. In addition, urine and feces are analyzed, and skin, nails, lips, eyes, voice, and other parts of the body are observed (Frawley & Ranade, 2001).

The goal of treatments prescribed by Ayurvedic physicians is to help the person to restore the healthy balance of the whole body matrix, as is natural and unique to each person. Depending on the diagnosis, a variety of treatments are used (Frawley & Ranade, 2001). Some treatments aim at *palliation* (alleviating the disease), by balancing the doshas, kindling the gastric fire, and burning toxins. These treatments involve many types of herbal formulations, as well as fasting, restricting intake of liquids, yogic stretching, lying in the sun, and breathing exercises. Another major type of treatment involves *cleansing* excess doshas and toxins from the body through the *pan-*

chakarma (five actions): enemas, purgation, therapeutic vomiting, nasal medicinal insufflation, and blood cleansing. To prepare for *panchakarma,* oil message and sweat therapy are given for several days, and then the appropriate cleansing treatment is applied through such means as herbal formulas, salt water, and castor oil. Once the doshas are in balance again, the physician prescribes specific therapies to promote strength and vitality through diet, minerals, and exercise. Additional therapies deal with mental hygiene and spiritual health through use of mantras, meditation, and rituals (Lad, 1999).

Ayurveda medicine appeals to many South Asians (and others) as an alternative system of medicine that is rooted in their religious world view, takes account of health in its full context, and considers physical, mental, psychological, emotional, social, and spiritual factors. It allows for differences of mental temperament and physical types, and factors in such variants as lifestyle, season, and age to provide personalized diagnosis and treatment. The techniques of diagnosis and the treatments are based on centuries of experimentation in India and place great value on nutrition, herbal medicine, exercise, meditation, and general lifestyle. Many practitioners think that, although Western allopathic medicine should be used in cases of acute disease, Ayurvedic medicine is helpful for maintaining health; dealing with chronic conditions such as rheumatoid arthritis, stroke paralysis, or multiple sclerosis; and avoiding the kinds of disorder that lead to acute diseases. Some also think that Ayurvedic medicine can effectively deal with the side effects often caused by the administration of powerful biomedical drugs used in Western medicine and that Ayurvedic principles can help physicians decide on the appropriate biomedical drugs to prescribe for people, taking into consideration whether the person is a vata, pitta, or kapha type.

HEALTH AND SPIRITUAL CONCERNS FOR SOUTH ASIANS

Appropriate health care for South Asians includes attention to their spiritual needs, particularly because their world view links physical, mental, social, and spiritual well-being very closely. For example, the person's sense of identity and well-being is linked closely with his or her place in family relationships and the traditional social system. Medical diagnosis and treatment are often matters for decision not just by the patient but also the family. Nurses should ensure that family members are present during visits by physicians or other health care providers when important decisions are being made.

    ❸ For Hindus in particular, concerns about pollution are prominent: pollution through blood, sickness, death, improper kitchen and food preparation, and stagnant water. Nurses should include asking Hindus about their preferences regarding diet and bathing in assessments. Keeping rooms clean and removing dirty linens from the room promptly support Hindu concerns. High-caste Hindu men consider the sacred cord worn over one shoulder an important spiritual symbol that should be treated with great care.

Jains need proper vegetarian foods and assurance that violence to living beings is not done on their behalf. In addition to asking about food preferences, nurses should assess whether Jains will take medications or use products that have been tested on animals.

Even when hospitalized, Sikhs may want to retain the symbols of their khalsa identity, such as uncut hair, bracelet, and symbolic dagger. If these need to be removed for some reason, nurses should do so with care and sensitivity; for example, it is said that some Sikhs would rather die than submit to having their hair cut because of surgery (Nesbitt, 1997; Singh, 1999). Nurses should never remove any personal item without the consent of the patient or family. Nurses in emergency and surgical departments should avoid shaving body parts when providing care.

Nurses should present Western treatments in light of Eastern concepts. For instance, when patients are receiving physical therapy, it might be helpful to explain procedures in terms of the vata, the energy of movement. Patients familiar with Ayurvedic and Unani practices should be comfortable providing urine and stool samples because these substances are frequently assessed in these Eastern traditions.

Given the key role that karma plays in their thinking, patients may feel conflict between their acceptance of disease as a result of karma and the need to actively fight the disease (Leslie, 1999). In the case of dying patients, these religious traditions emphasize the importance of calmness and detachment so that additional karma is not built up for future effects. Among Jain monks and nuns, self-willed death by fasting with the approach of old age and disease is a well-known tradition, and some Jains and Hindus look to this as a spiritual ideal in terminal illnesses when treatment becomes ineffective. In the context of modern Western medicine, of course, this raises issues about whether caregivers can assist patients in such practices of self-willed dying (Young, 1989). Nurses need to examine their feelings regarding these practices and determine if their personal values will interfere with providing spiritually appropriate care.

The spiritual needs of South Asians in health care include opportunities for spiritual practices that bring calm, balance, and wholeness, such as forms of meditation, prayers, reading of scriptures or devotional material, music, and offerings to Gods. For many, opportunity for Ayurvedic diagnosis and treatment, as a supplement to their Western medical treatments, helps them feel more secure and at peace. By providing a calm and caring presence, nurses can facilitate the use of spiritual practices that support patient needs.

PERSONAL REFLECTIONS

- How could you see yourself relating to a person who lives by one of the South Asian religions?
- Are you comfortable accepting the importance of their beliefs and practices and encouraging them to strengthen them?
- Do you feel that you have enough understanding of each of these religious traditions to be able to provide appropriate spiritual care?
- What features of the South Asian religions do you think make the most sense?
- Are you uncomfortable with any of the teachings and practices of the South Asian religions?
- Do you feel that the holistic notions of health and healing present in Ayurveda medicine could be helpful also in Western medicine?
- Are you comfortable supporting patients who want Ayurvedic treatments while maintaining their Western medical regimen?
- Do you find personal spiritual or health benefits from practices such as yoga and meditation?

CASE STUDY 10.1

Mrs. Singh is visiting from India with her relatives in the United States. During her month-long visit, Mrs. Singh becomes quite ill with severe abdominal pain and vomiting. Her relatives take her to the emergency room, and she receives a diagnosis of partial bowel obstruction. She is moved to a medical-surgical floor, where she undergoes medical treatment and observation. A consultation with a surgeon is ordered. While in the nurse's care, Mrs. Singh expresses extreme distress regarding this recent episode. She reluctantly expresses that she had been having similar bouts for quite some time and that her suffering may be the result of her grief over the loss of one of her adult sons about 3 months earlier. She states that she is extremely religious and must deal with this in her own way.

Critical Thinking
- What questions should the nurse ask to further explore Mrs. Singh's feelings?
- Which of the South Asian religions discussed in this chapter might she practice?
- How should the nurse prepare her for the possibility that surgery might be needed or proposed?
- Whom could the nurse ask questions about how best to approach this situation?
- How can the nurse demonstrate cultural and spiritual sensitivity toward this patient?
- What challenges might this patient face with regard to surgical treatment?
- What types of treatments might Mrs. Singh have tried at home before seeking care for this recent episode?

Key Points
- Eastern religions and cultures emphasize a holistic understanding of health that includes body, mind, spirit, family, and nature.
- Hindus, Jains, and Sikhs understand the eternal soul to be embodied according to the law of karma in the rebirth cycle of samsara, progressing through spiritual disciplines toward wholeness and liberation.
- Ayurvedic medicine is based on the Hindu world view that the cosmic forces of three gunas, five elements, and three doshas operate within the human body, and that sicknesses caused by imbalances of the three doshas can be remedied by treatments of herbal medicines, breathing exercises, and spiritual disciplines.
- Providing holistic care to people influenced by the South Asian traditions requires understanding their religious and medical traditions as well as responding to their particular spiritual concerns.

References
Desai, P. N. (1989). *Health and medicine in the Hindu tradition: Continuity and cohesion.* New York: Crossroad.

Fields, G. (2001). *Religious therapeutics: Body and health in yoga, Ayurveda, and tantra.* Albany: State University of New York Press.

Frawley, D., & Ranade, S. (2001). *Ayurveda, nature's medicine*. Twin Lakes, WI: Lotus Press.

Griffiths, P. J. (2002). Psychoneuroimmunology and Eastern religious traditions. In H. G. Koenig and H. J. Cohen (Eds.), *The link between religion and health: Psychoneuroimmunology and the faith factor* (pp. 250–261). New York: Oxford University Press.

Iyengar, B. K. S. (2001). *Yoga: The path to holistic health*. London: Dorling Kindersley Publishing.

Jaini, P. S. (1979). *The Jaina path of purification*. Berkeley: University of California Press.

Lad, D. V. (1999). Ayurvedic medicine. In W. B. Jonas & J. S. Levin (Eds.), *Essentials of complementary and alternative medicine* (pp. 200–215). Philadelphia: Lippincott Williams & Wilkins.

Leslie, J. (1999). The implications of the physical body: Health, suffering and karma in Hindu thought. In J. R. Hinnells & R. Porter (Eds.), *Religion, health and suffering* (pp. 23–45). London: Kegan Paul International.

Ministry of Health & Family Welfare, Government of India. The Department of Indian Systems of Medicine and Homoeopathy. (2002a). *Gateway for information on Indian systems of medicine & homoeopathy*. Available at: http://indianmedicine.nic.in/sitemap.htm.

Ministry of Health and Family Welfare, Government of India. Department of Indian Systems of Medicine and Homoeopathy. (2002b). *Siddha*. Available at: http://indianmedicine.nic.in/html/siddha/siddha.htm.

Ministry of Health and Family Welfare, Government of India. The Department of Indian Systems of Medicine and Homoeopathy. (2002c). *Unani*. Available at: http://indianmedicine.nic.in/html/unani/unani.htm.

Narayanaswami, V. (1983). Ayurveda and Siddha systems of medicine: A comparative study. In S. V. Subramanian and V. R. Madhavan (Eds.), *Heritage of the tamils: Siddha medicine* (pp. 568–576). Madras: International Institute of Tamil Studies.

Nesbitt, E. (1997). The body in Sikh tradition. In S. Coakley (Ed.), *Religion and the body* (pp. 289–305). Cambridge: Cambridge University Press.

Singh, P. (1999). Sikh perspectives on health and suffering: A focus on Sikh theodicy. In J. R. Hinnells & R. Porter (Eds.), *Religion, health and suffering* (pp. 111–138). London: Kegan Paul International.

Young, K. (1989). Euthanasia: Traditional Hindu views and the contemporary debate. In H. Coward, J. Lipner, & K. Young (Eds.), *Hindu ethics: Purity, abortion, and euthanasia* (pp. 71–130). Albany: State University of New York Press.

Zysk, K. (1996). Traditional Ayurveda. In M. S. Micozzi (Ed.), *Fundamentals of complementary and alternative medicine* (pp. 233–242). New York: Churchill Livingstone.

Recommended Readings

Brannigan, M. C. (2000). *Striking a balance: A primer in traditional Asian values*. New York: Seven Bridges Press.

Eck, D. L. (2002). *A new religious America: How a Christian country has become the world's most religiously diverse nation*. New York: Harper.

Hinnells, J. R., & Porter, R. (Eds.). (1999). *Religion, health and suffering*. London: Kegan Paul International.

Lipner, J. (1994). *Hindus: Their religious beliefs and practices*. London: Routledge.

Resources

The Ayurvedic Institute
11311 Menaul Blvd. NE, Albuquerque, NM 87112
Phone: (505) 291-9698
http://www.ayurveda.com

Department of Indian Systems of Medicine and Homoeopathy
Ministry of Health & Family Welfare, Government of India
http://indianmedicine.nic.in/sitemap.htm
Gateway for information on Indian systems of medicine and homoeopathy.

The Hindu Universe
Hindu Students Council, P.O. Box 9185, Boston, MA 02114-0041
Phone: (617) 698-1106
Fax: (617) 444-8725
http://www.hindunet.com

National Center for Complementary and Alternative Medicine (NCCAM)
National Institutes for Health, Department of Health and Human Services, Bethesda, MD 20892
http://nccam.nih.gov/

The Pluralism Project
Harvard University, 201 Vanserg Hall, 25 Francis Avenue, Cambridge, MA 02138
Phone: (617) 496-2481
Fax: (617) 496-2428
http://www.pluralism.org/index.php
The Pluralism Project was developed by Diana L. Eck at Harvard University to study and document the growing religious diversity of the United States, with a special view to its new immigrant religious communities.

Wabash Center Guide to Internet Resources for Teaching and Learning in Theology and Religion: World Religions
Wabash Center, 301 W. Wabash Avenue, Crawfordsville, IN 47933
Phone: (765) 361-6047; (800) 655-7117
Fax: (765) 361-6051
Hinduism, http://www.wabashcenter.wabash.edu/Internet/hinduism.htm
Sikhism, http://www.wabashcenter.wabash.edu/Internet/sikhism.htm
The Wabash Center for Teaching and Learning in Theology and Religion seeks to strengthen and enhance education in North American theological schools, colleges and universities.

11

*B*uddhist Traditions

Theodore M. Ludwig

LEARNING OBJECTIVES

At the end of this chapter, the reader will be able to:
- Describe the basic beliefs and practices of Buddhists.
- Identify the Four Noble Truths and other central teachings of Buddhism.
- Discriminate among Theravada, Mahayana, and Vajrayana Buddhism, including the locales where each type is most popular.
- Describe some typical concerns about spiritual care and health felt by Buddhists.
- Recognize the implications for providing nursing care to people of Buddhist traditions.

The fundamental truth about reality, the Buddha taught, is the truth of *pratitya samutpada*, dependent co-arising. "When that exists, this comes to be; on the arising of that, this arises. When that does not exist, this does not come to be; on the cessation of that, this ceases" (*Majjhima Nikaya* 1.262–264). This truth expresses the interconnectedness of everything. A supreme being does not cause things, nor do things happen randomly. Rather, everything results from something prior in an interrelated process. That means that every condition contributes to the next and is itself conditioned by other determining conditions.

From this central truth arises the third mark of existence, that all aspects of reality, including humans, have no atman (anatta), no self-standing and permanently existing self or soul. In contrast to Hindu teaching about the real self, the eternal atman, the Buddha taught that the character of all reality is conditioned and impermanent, including everything that makes up a person. He taught that a person is made up of five aggregates or clusters: bodily matter, sensations, perceptions, mental formations, and bits of consciousness. These five aggregates are constantly changing, brought together in a lifetime by karma from previous lifetimes, dissipating again when that karma runs out and the person dies. The karmic formations built in that lifetime cause another birth and another lifetime, and the cycle continues (Box 11.1).

The Buddha's teachings about impermanence and no-self were intended as therapeutic teaching. Because ignorance about the true nature of reality leads to attachment and suffering, realizing that there is no permanent reality or self to cling to will bring the cessation of attachment and thus the cessation of suffering. That realization, when it is total and complete, is nirvana, which means "blowing out" the flame of desire and attachment, and thus experiencing the permanent state of peace, joy, and equanimity. The Buddha and many disciples through the ages since achieved this, and still today the attainment of nirvana is understood to be the spiritual goal of the Buddhist path.

**BOX 11.1   From Suffering to Wholeness:
              Elements of the Buddhist Way**

THE REALITY: THE THREE MARKS OF EXISTENCE
Dukkha: Suffering, anxiety, discontent, dying
Anicca: Impermanence, conditionedness, changing, arising, and ceasing
Anatta: No-self, nonsubstantiability, non–self-existing

DIAGNOSIS AND THERAPY: THE FOUR NOBLE TRUTHS
1. *Suffering:* All existence is permeated with suffering.
2. *The Arising of Suffering:* Suffering is caused by clinging.
3. *The Stopping of Suffering:* The cessation of clinging brings the cessation of suffering.
4. *The Way* which leads to the stopping of suffering consists of:

Right views	Right livelihood
Right resolve	Right effort
Right speech	Right mindfulness
Right conduct	Right concentration

Although nirvana is the end of the path, in the characteristic Buddhist thinking about samsara, the never-ending cycles of life, nirvana may be many lifetimes away. Thus, the Buddhist path has practices appropriate for people at every stage along the way, which bring spiritual benefits and enhancement of life.

The Buddhist Monastic Community

For monks and nuns who have reached higher levels of spiritual perfection, the practices are more intense and are designed to root out all attachments and bring one closer to nirvana. The Buddha set up monastic orders for both men and women, setting down Ten Precepts and more than 200 rules for the mendicant lifestyle. The Ten Precepts are to refrain from (1) taking life, (2) taking what is not given, (3) sexual activity, (4) lying, (5) drugs and liquor, (6) eating after noon, (7) watching shows, singing, and dancing, (8) using adornments, perfumes, or ointments, (9) sleeping in a broad high bed, and (10) handling gold or silver. The additional rules lay out a disciplined life involving, among other things, total celibacy, no possessions, cultivation of compassion and loving kindness for all beings, dependence on others for support (begging), and the practice of meditation—all designed gradually to eliminate the sense of selfish attachment and bring the quality of nirvana into one's life. The ultimate goal of the monastic life is to attain completely the state of nirvana. One who has attained this state, called an *arhant*, has rooted out all clinging and thus has stopped all outflows of karma. When the arhant's lifetime ends, there is no rebirth, only that permanent state of nirvana, beyond the cycle of birth and death.

In Theravada Buddhist lands today, the role of the samgha (the monastic community) continues to be important for the benefit of the whole society. Because of the vicissitudes of history, the community of fully ordained nuns, the *bhikkhuni* samgha, has disappeared from all Theravada Buddhist lands (although it still exists in Mahayana Buddhism). Although many women still follow the religious path, they cannot become fully ordained (which requires the presence of fully ordained nuns), and thus are regarded as novices or as dedicated laywomen. This means that even though they perform many valuable functions of teaching and service, they do not enjoy the same spiritual status in society as the order of monks, the *bhikkhu* samgha. Buddhists believe that the presence of the samgha brings many spiritual benefits to the whole society, through teaching and guiding lay persons, and chanting scriptures for various occasions. Above all, they are fields of merit in the community: monks and nuns serve as models, and by supporting them, giving them food, and meeting other needs, the lay people also build up merit themselves.

The Buddhist Laity

Despite its emphasis on detachment and the higher spiritual life of monks and nuns who have withdrawn from society, Buddhism does accord value to the much larger segment in society who cannot be completely detached from the world, namely, the lay people. Lay people are encouraged to follow the basic ethical precepts and engage in devotion and meditation. Lay persons follow the Five Precepts: namely, to refrain from taking life, taking what is not given, wrong sexual relations, lying, and drugs and liquor. These precepts provide an outline of ethical life designed to lead away from self-centered acts to acts of compassion and loving kindness. Lay people renew their commitment to the Buddhist path through daily rituals and devotions, or by going to the temple on the fortnightly holy day, or by participating in festivals. They build up merit by giving food, robes, and other provisions to the monastic community.

Through such activities, lay people make spiritual progress, bringing a quality of peace and wholeness to life, and possibly leading to a future lifetime at a higher spiritual status. Most Buddhists are familiar with the traditional teaching of different realms of rebirth, depending on the quality of karma acquired in this lifetime. There are six such realms of rebirth: in the hells, as animals, as wandering ghosts, as humans, as demigods, or as gods. All of these realms are part of the continuing samsara cycle, and are thus conditioned and impermanent. Buddhists consider the human realm to be a fortuitous birth because conditions are most favorable in the human realm for making spiritual progress and eventually reaching nirvana, which is outside the samsara cycle.

ADDITIONAL MAHAYANA AND VAJRAYANA BUDDHIST TEACHINGS

The basics of Buddhism in the Theravada perspective have been described as they are understood even today by Buddhists of South Asia and Southeast Asia. To a large extent, all Buddhists accept this fundamental perspective, but some important additions and expansions developed in the Mahayana and Vajrayana traditions. A brief look at them will be helpful in understanding the spiritual outlook and needs of Buddhists today in the East Asian communities: Chinese, Koreans, Japanese, Mongolians, Vietnamese, and Tibetans. East Asian peoples are also influenced, of course, by their indigenous, pre-Buddhist religious traditions, in particular, Confucianism, Daoism, and (in Japan) Shinto. These indigenous Chinese and Japanese traditions are discussed in Chapter 12.

Mahayana Buddhism

The term "Mahayana" means "larger vehicle," and this tradition of Buddhism developed broader, expanded teachings and practices. For example, Mahayana Buddhists felt that Theravadins put too much emphasis on monks and nuns who reach nirvana (arhants), developing a kind of elitist spiritual class. The Mahayanists taught that lay persons could participate more fully and even reach nirvana. While there still are monks and nuns in Mahayana communities, there tends to be less distinction made between the monastics and the lay people.

Further, the Mahayanists felt that the teaching of the Buddha was contained not only in the *Tripitaka* scriptures, but also in many additional sutras (scriptures) that the Buddha taught secretly, to be revealed publicly several centuries later, sutras such as the *Lotus Sutra, Garland Sutra, Perfection of Wisdom Sutra, Nirvana Sutra*, the **Pure Land** sutras, and many more—all of which also are "Word of the Buddha." So Mahayana Buddhists today, even lay people, may study some of these sutras and use them in devotions.

Two of the most characteristic and important Mahayana teachings concern the nature of the Buddha and the ideal of the **bodhisattva**. For Theravadins, the Buddha is Siddhartha Gautama, the human being who reached enlightenment and became the teacher of the Dharma; while Buddha images are venerated, the Buddha is not worshiped or prayed to. Mahayana Buddhists take a greatly expanded view of Buddha, teaching that there are three dimensions of Buddha-hood: the universal Buddha nature, human forms of Buddha, and heavenly Buddhas. The fundamental dimension is the universal Buddha nature, the eternal inner essence of all reality. We all share in this universal Buddha nature: it is the true Self for us to realize and experience, as opposed to our illusory and passing self. Awakening to the universal Buddha nature, which is equivalent to achieving enlightenment, brings the experience of nirvana right within the world of samsara. In fact, Mahayana Buddhists say that samsara is the same as nirvana in the sense that the universal Buddha nature is the true quality of all aspects of life in this world.

The universal Buddha nature can be experienced in two additional dimensions, at the human level and at the heavenly level. Siddhartha Gautama was a human form of Buddha to guide humans in our world era to enlightenment. The *Lotus Sutra* says there have been countless numbers of such Buddhas, in all worlds and ages, using various means to teach and guide living beings to enlightenment. Further, there are many "Enjoyment Bodies" of Buddha, cosmic Buddhas who out of their great storehouse of merit have created Buddha realms. These Buddhas can teach and save vast numbers of living beings, imparting wisdom, merit, and salvation. Some of these heavenly Buddhas are widely worshiped in the Mahayana Buddhist world, almost as savior beings. For example, Amitabha (Amida Buddha), a Buddha of great compassion who took 48 vows to save all beings who cannot save themselves, is the object of worship in the Pure Land Buddhist school. Worshipers chant Amida's name with single-minded faith and devotion, based on the promise of the Pure Land sutras that Amida Buddha will grant them rebirth in his heavenly Buddha realm, the Pure Land. These cosmic Buddhas can grant physical well-being as well as spiritual help. For example, the Buddha called Master of Healing, Bhaishajya-guru, provides help in all aspects of the medical arts, promising health and longevity for those who worship him.

Another important Mahayana emphasis is on the *bodhisattva* (one who is becoming a Buddha) as the ideal goal of the Buddhist path. A bodhisattva is one who reaches nirvana but out of great compassion vows to remain in the samsara cycles of birth and death to help all other living beings. Bodhisattvas willingly are reborn in all of the realms of rebirth, to provide spiritual and physical help to beings suffering in these realms. In particular, cosmic bodhisattvas living in the Buddha realms are available to help all who call upon them in distress of any kind. One such bodhisattva worshiped all over the Mahayana world is Avalokiteshvara, praised in the Lotus Sutra as an omnipresent savior deity, rescuing those who invoke him from all sicknesses and distresses. In East Asian Buddhism, Avalokiteshvara is often represented in feminine form as a goddess of compassion. The Chinese translate her name as Guanyin, whereas in Japan she is known as Kannon; in Korea, as Kwanse'um; and in Vietnam, as Quan-am. She has a special following among women, who desire her help during pregnancy, and among the elderly, who pray for a peaceful old age free from senility.

One characteristic of Mahayana Buddhism, with its large number of sutras and diversity of teachings, is the development of special schools or lineages of masters who put their emphasis on one of the central themes of Mahayana. Thus, in understanding Mahayana Buddhists it is of some significance to know which particular school or sect to which they belong. Two classical, broad Chinese schools are Tiantai (Japanese Tendai) and Huayan (Japanese Kegon). Tiantai is a scholarly school that synthesizes all scriptures and forms of Buddhism in a progressive unfolding, with the Lotus Sutra recognized as the culmination of the truth for all. Huayan promotes the deep philosophic wisdom of the Garland Sutra, teaching the complete interpenetration of all reality with the Buddha nature.

Out of Buddhist interaction with the Chinese religious traditions, two more schools developed that stressed simple practice and direct benefit: Pure Land Buddhism and Chan (Zen) Buddhism. These two schools show two sides of the Mahayana path, with its emphasis on the universal Buddha nature. Pure Land Buddhists believe that the world is in an evil age and that salvation is possible only by believing in Amida Buddha and calling on his name for the gift of rebirth in the Pure Land paradise. Knowing that help comes through the "other power" of Amida Buddha, humans can live with assurance of salvation. In the midst of trouble, suffering, and death, faith in Amida Buddha keeps one from despair and maintains peace and contentment, a foretaste of the bliss of the Pure Land.

On the other hand, adherents of Chan (Zen) Buddhism emphasize a "self-power" approach through meditation. Because everyone possesses the Buddha nature, the direct way to enlightenment is simply to practice meditation, emptying the mind and "seeing directly" the Buddha nature. The source of human confusion is the mind, filled as it is with attachments and desires. Zen masters teach their disciples to practice insight meditation, simply observing mind and body with detachment, letting thoughts go until the mind is emptied, so that the true nature of reality can be seen directly. Such experiences of *satori* (awakening) help one to live ordinary daily life with detachment and thus freedom and wholeness.

A third simple and direct school developed in Japan was founded by the charismatic master Nichiren. Nichiren Buddhists believe that the whole Buddha reality is present in the Lotus Sutra, so that by chanting the title of the Lotus Sutra, this very life can be infused with the Buddha realm, bringing health, happiness, and well-being.

Vajrayana Buddhism

One more Buddhist school that has taken on special significance, especially in the Tibetan sphere of influence, is Vajrayana, the thunderbolt vehicle. This can be considered a further development of Mahayana, although some scholars would characterize it as the third division in Buddhism, along with Theravada and Mahayana. Drawing from the idea of the universal Buddha nature and the identification of samsara and nirvana, Vajrayana developed elaborate rituals and practices of meditation that lead to the experience of being a Buddha in this very body. For example, the whole world can be considered the cosmic body of the great Sun Buddha, Mahavairochana, and thus the world process consists of the thoughts, actions, and sounds of the Sun Buddha. Humans share these "three mysteries," so ritual activity focused on thought (meditating on mandalas), speech (chanting mantras), and action (performing mudras) can bring the experience of oneness with the great Sun Buddha. In Tibet, Vajrayana practitioners have developed esoteric methods of meditation involving, among others, visualization of Buddhas, gods, and goddesses for empowerment and transformation; invocations and transformations of demonic evil forces into positive means of spiritual progress; and ritual activities that use human passion and sexual symbolism as means for spiritual transformation. Buddhism in Tibet incorporates many aspects of the indigenous Bon shamanistic religion of Tibet into the overall Vajrayana Buddhist framework.

After the Chinese takeover of Tibet in the 1950s, many Tibetan lamas went into exile from Tibet to places such as Nepal and India, and many have immigrated to the Western world, spreading and popularizing the practice of Vajrayana Buddhism. One of the best-known Buddhists in the world today is the Dalai Lama, who escaped from Tibet in 1959 and has tirelessly traveled throughout the globe, advocating peace and reconciliation among all peoples. The Dalai Lama, believed to the reincarnation of the previous Dalai Lama, as well as an incarnation of the bodhisattva Avalokiteshvara, teaches and practices the Vajrayana path.

All of these schools and forms of Buddhism are well represented in the Western world today, so considerations of spiritual care in healing practices will include influences from Buddhism. Listing different types of Buddhists present in the Western world is formidable: Theravada Buddhists with ethnic differences from Thailand, Burma, Cambodia, Laos, and Sri Lanka; a great variety of East Asian Mahayana Buddhists from the Pure Land, Zen (Chan), Nichiren, Tendai, Kegon, and Shingon schools; and Tibetan Vajrayana Buddhists with colorful rituals and elaborate teachings. Currently, one might say that there are two types of Buddhist communities in the West: Asian ethnic communities, representing all the groups listed here, that tend to stay within their own ethnic and sectarian groups, and significant numbers of non-Asian Westerners, who have joined Buddhist religious organizations or at least participate in some Buddhist activities. These non-Asian Buddhist groups have tended to follow the meditation traditions of Theravada, Zen, and Vajrayana in particular, while not stressing the ethnic–cultural aspects of the particular tradition of Buddhism.

HEALING AND MEDICAL PRACTICES IN BUDDHISM

Ever since Siddhartha Gautama taught the Noble Eightfold Path as the way to the cessation of suffering, Buddhists have considered their spiritual practices conducive to a healthful mental and physical life. The central Buddhist practice of meditation, including calming the mind and emptying the mind, promotes wellness by reducing stress and engaging the mind positively in the healing process (Olendzki, 2000). Other spiritual and ritual practices for diagnosing and healing diseases were also cultivated among Buddhists, such as astrology and divination, recitation of sutras and healing formulas, use of amulets, and exorcism (Samuel, 1999; Skorupski, 1999).

❸ ◐ With respect to medical practices in Buddhist cultures, the diversity and multi-ethnic character of Buddhism prevented a single traditional system from developing for all Buddhists. In India, Buddhists contributed to the development of Ayurvedic medicine, so traditional medicine is influenced by Ayurveda in some Buddhist lands, such as Tibet, Sri Lanka, and parts of Southeast Asia. In East Asia, Buddhists have long lived with, and helped to shape, traditional Chinese medicine and its variant forms in Korea, Japan, and elsewhere. Further, in all Buddhist lands, each ethnic community has had traditional shamanistic healing practitioners, who usually combine Buddhist practices with indigenous folk religious practices. Buddhism as a religious path does not negate the usefulness of the traditional indigenous practices, whether supernatural or natural, that are considered to bring benefits for living a healthful life in this world.

The Buddhists of Tibet, with their unique pattern of influences from the indigenous Bon religion as well as from India and China, developed a system of medicine,
complete with written texts, that is gradually becoming more known with the diaspora of Tibetans in the Western world. An important feature of Tibetan medicine,
similar to Ayurveda, is the theory that every form of existence is conditioned and depends on the three elements or energies: space or movement, digestive energy, and
material. Tibetan medicine holds that the nature of every phenomenon is determined
by the interaction and balance of these three elements (Badmaev, 1999). In human life,
health is a state of well-functioning balance between these elements, whereas disease
results from disruption of this balance. Tibetan medicine understands this balanced
health not only in physical terms; it also believes that emotional and spiritual health
are intimately connected with the harmonious interaction of the three elements.

In diagnosing disease, an important factor is determining the person's basic psychosomatic type, depending on the natural balance of the three energies. The physician examines the whole appearance and mental–emotional state of the patient, also
using a complex pulse reading as well as examination of the urine. Tibetan medicine
treats illness with diet, herbs, massage, yogic breathing exercises, and moxa treatments (burning a moxa herb above the skin to apply heat). Because every cell, tissue,
organ, or system of the body is composed of a particular balance of the three elements, and this balance changes with such factors as the seasons and times of day, Tibetan medicine attempts to adjust the delivery of nutrients with specific foods, herbs,
and minerals. Because of the functioning of the central nervous system, emotional
and mental digestion is equally important for the proper flow of energy through all
of the body's energy channels.

Tibetan medicine takes account of spiritual factors in disease and healing based
on Vajrayana Buddhist principles. Spiritually empowered medicinal substances can
be obtained from monasteries and lamas. The ideal state of health is a feeling of compassion, with the mind devoid of ignorance, attachment, anger, jealousy, and pride,
so rituals and spiritual disciplines are important to facilitate the healthy functioning
of the whole mind–body complex (Badmaev, 1999; Samuel, 1999).

HEALTH AND SPIRITUAL CONCERNS FOR BUDDHISTS

As we have seen, health concerns and spiritual concerns are closely connected for
Buddhists. Suffering itself has spiritual benefits, for it is the recognition of suffering
that impels one to seek liberation by following the Buddhist path. Detachment from
desire and clinging brings peace and liberation from suffering, but that does not
mean that one will avoid sickness and dying. The idea of karma often leads Buddhists to take a resigned attitude toward sickness and dying. Nurses should realize
that sickness may not be seen by patients who are Buddhist as something that must
be cured.

Buddhists consider a calm, peaceful mind to be important at death because it
minimizes the karma that propels the rebirth cycle onward. Thus, Buddhist meditation and other religious rituals are considered important to help one face dying with
calmness and detachment. Caregivers need to understand that, ideally, Buddhists
want to avoid analgesics and sedatives as they approach the end of life so that their

mind can be filled with wholesome thoughts, aided perhaps by Buddhist rituals and scriptures (Ratanakul, 2002). Nurses need to collaborate with patients who are Buddhist before administering any medication that might affect the patient's level of awareness and ascertain what are acceptable alternative treatments for care, particularly palliative care at the end of life.

Many Buddhists today seek to develop ways of applying Buddhist principles to questions of health care and spiritual guidance for sickness and dying. Medical practices of concern to Buddhists include such issues as abortion, euthanasia, organ transplantation, and definitions of brain death. Harming or taking life is contrary to the first Precept, so Buddhist teachings stand against abortion and euthanasia (Tedesco, 1999). Yet some contemporary Buddhists believe that Buddhism, with its teachings of both nonviolence and compassion, may be able to offer a thoughtful "middle way" between the extremes of today's abortion debate (Keown, 1999). In cases of euthanasia, not only is killing involved, but the natural working out of karma in the dying process is thwarted (Ratanakul, 2002). Western definitions of brain death are based on the assumption that the brain is the only determinant of life, whereas in Buddhist thought, life is interdependent with many factors and conditions. Because of their opposition to the criterion of brain death, Buddhists also have concerns about organ donations from still-living bodies. At the same time, some Buddhists have come to think that pledging to donate one's own organs is a bodhisattva-like act done out of compassion; they refer to a story about how the Buddha, in a previous lifetime, gave his own living body to be eaten by a starving tigress (Ratanakul, 2002; Umehara, 1994).

PERSONAL REFLECTIONS

- How do you see yourself relating to a person who lives by one of the Buddhist traditions?
- Are you comfortable accepting the importance of their beliefs and practices and encouraging them to strengthen them?
- Do you feel you have enough understanding of each of these religious traditions to be able to provide appropriate spiritual care?
- Which features of the Buddhist religions do you find to make the most sense?
- Are you uncomfortable with any of the teachings and practices of the Buddhist religions?
- How do you see yourself providing spiritual care to someone who believes that his or her sickness is determined by karma and that death will lead to rebirth in another state of life?
- Do you believe your own spiritual health and awareness are important factors in enabling you to provide spiritual care for people of Buddhist religions?
- Are you comfortable with the need to learn, communicate, think critically, and be willing to change your own perspectives in caring for people of Eastern religions and cultures?

CASE STUDY 11.1

The nurse is caring for a 45-year-old male patient who has recently converted to the Buddhist religion. He has received a diagnosis of amyotrophic lateral sclerosis (ALS). The nurse recognizes that this terminal disease eventually will rob the patient of his motor function while leaving his sensory function intact. During teaching about the prognosis and course of the disease, the patient tells the nurse that he believes the suffering he may endure from ALS has been allowed to make him a more whole being, to purify him, and that he will use meditation to combat the difficult times ahead as he loses voluntary control of physical function. He expresses happiness that his cognition and sensation will remain intact until the time of his death.

Critical Thinking

- What are appropriate courses of action the nurse can take to provide spiritual care to this patient?
- Are there additional referrals the nurse could or should make?
- What additional information should the nurse have to provide competent spiritual care for this man?
- How is the nurse's assessment of the patient's understanding of the Buddhist religion illuminated by the information provided in this chapter?
- List several potential nursing diagnoses related to spirituality that may need to be addressed in this situation.

Key Points

- Eastern religions and cultures emphasize a holistic understanding of health, including body, mind, spirit, family, and nature.
- Buddhists understand suffering to be caused by attachment and thus practice spiritual disciplines of meditation and compassion to stop attachment and attain peace and wholeness.
- Mahayana Buddhists of East Asia consider all life to be grounded in the universal Buddha nature, which can be experienced through meditation or through the help of bodhisattvas and heavenly Buddhas.
- Providing holistic care to people influenced by the Buddhist traditions requires understanding their religious and medical traditions as well as responding to their particular spiritual concerns.

References

Badmaev, V. (1999). Tibetan medicine. In W. B. Jonas & J. S. Levin (Eds.), *Essentials of complementary and alternative medicine* (pp. 252–274). Philadelphia: Lippincott Williams & Wilkins.

Keown, D. (1999). Buddhism and abortion: Is there a 'middle way'? In D. Keown (Ed.), *Buddhism and abortion* (pp. 199–218). Honolulu: University of Hawaii Press.

Olendzki, A. (2000). Meditation, healing, and stress reduction. In C. S. Queen (Ed.), *Engaged Buddhism in the West* (pp. 307–327). Boston: Wisdom Publications.

Ratanakul, P. (2002). A Buddhist perspective on death and dying. In T. M. Ludwig & H. Mwakabana (Eds.), *Explorations in love and wisdom: Christians and Buddhists in conversation* (pp. 107–114). Geneva: The Lutheran World Federation.

Samuel, G. (1999). Religion, health, and suffering among contemporary Tibetans. In J. R. Hinnells & Roy Porter (Eds.), *Religion, health and suffering* (pp. 85–110). London: Kegan Paul International.

Skorupski, T. (1999). Health and suffering in Buddhism: Doctrinal and existential considerations. In J. R. Hinnells & R. Porter (Eds.), *Religion, health and suffering* (pp. 139–165). London: Kegan Paul International.

Tedesco, F. (1999). Abortion in Korea. In D. Keown (Ed.), *Buddhism and abortion* (pp. 121–155). Honolulu: University of Hawaii Press.

Umehara, T. (1994). Descartes, brain death and organ transplants: A Japanese view. *New Perspectives Quarterly, 11*(1), 25–29.

Recommended Readings

Brannigan, M. C. (2000). *Striking a balance: A primer in traditional Asian values.* New York: Seven Bridges Press.

Eck, D. L. (2002). *A new religious America: How a Christian country has become the world's most religiously diverse nation.* New York: Harper.

Hinnells, J. R., & Porter, R. (Eds.). (1999). *Religion, health and suffering.* London: Kegan Paul International.

Mitchell, D. W. (2002). *Buddhism: Introducing the Buddhist experience.* New York: Oxford University Press.

Resources

Buddhanet
Buddha Dharma Education Association Incorporated, P.O. Box K1020 Haymarket, Sydney NSW 2000 Australia
http://www.buddhanet.net/
Buddhist information and education network.

National Center for Complementary and Alternative Medicine (NCCAM)
National Institutes of Health
Department of Health and Human Services, Bethesda, MD 20892
http://nccam.nih.gov/
The official site for the National Center of Complementary and Alternative Medicine; connects consumers with the most current and reliable information on CAM.

The Pluralism Project
Harvard University, 201 Vanserg Hall, 25 Francis Avenue, Cambridge, MA 02138
Phone: (617) 496-2481
Fax: (617) 496-2428
http://www.pluralism.org/index.php
The Pluralism Project was developed by Diana L. Eck at Harvard University to study and document the growing religious diversity of the United States, with a special view to its new immigrant religious communities.

Wabash Center Guide to Internet Resources for Teaching and Learning in Theology and Religion: World Religions
Wabash Center, 301 W. Wabash Avenue, Crawfordsville, IN 47933
Phone: (765) 361-6047; (800) 655-7117
Fax: (765) 361-6051
Buddhism, http://www.wabashcenter.wabash.edu/Internet/buddhism.htm
The Wabash Center for Teaching and Learning in Theology and Religion seeks to strengthen and enhance education in North American theological schools, colleges and universities.

*E*ast Asian Traditions

Theodore M. Ludwig

At the end of this chapter, the reader will be able to:
- Discuss the basic beliefs and practices of East Asians, including Chinese, Japanese, and Korean people.
- Describe the traditional worldview of the Chinese, explaining the interaction of the macrocosm and the microcosm in terms of the various operational forces.
- Compare and contrast the Confucian and the Daoist religious traditions, showing how they complement each other in China's religious environment.
- Describe the religious world view of Japanese people and state how a number of religious traditions are integrated in Japanese culture.
- Recognize the diversity of Korean religious and spiritual beliefs.
- Discuss the main principles, diagnostic techniques, and treatments used in traditional Chinese medicine.
- List and discuss some of the typical concerns about spiritual care and health of Chinese, Japanese, and Korean people.
- Recognize the implications for providing nursing care for individuals from East Asian traditions.

acupuncture   qi
divination   traditional Chinese medicine
five agents   yang
moxibustion   yin

⑤ The peoples of East Asia—Chinese, Tibetans, Japanese, Koreans, Mongolians, and Vietnamese—have always esteemed their traditional religions and cultures. Chinese culture, which had reached a high and sophisticated point 2000 years ago, has tended to be dominant in the whole region. Yet each people of East Asia developed their own distinct culture and religious practices, with which they accepted and transformed the continual influences from Chinese culture that reached them. These ancient traditions are still represented in modern forms in these countries: Shinto in Japan, Bon in Tibet, Mudang shamanism in Korea, and traditional Mongolian shamanism. Throughout East Asia, the major Chinese traditions of Confucianism and Daoism have long provided common beliefs and practices for maintaining the spiritual balance necessary for health and well-being. Furthermore, Mahayana Buddhism in its different forms has been integrated as a common feature of all East Asian cultures and has further shaped the overall religious and cultural perspective of these peoples.

Today, many of the peoples of East Asia have become quite Westernized and participate fully in modern technological culture, yet their longstanding traditional cultures and religions continue to play significant roles. In China, the Communist movement fiercely attacked traditional culture and religion, especially during the Cultural Revolution, with the result that religious and spiritual practices have been greatly diminished among Chinese living in the People's Republic of China. However, since the end of the Cultural Revolution, there has been a significant growth in the Chinese people's appreciation for their traditional culture, including their religious and medical traditions. Among Chinese people living in Taiwan, Hong Kong, Singapore, and elsewhere, including the West, traditional religion and culture still play a fairly significant role.

CHINESE RELIGIOUS AND SPIRITUAL TRADITIONS

An overall key concept of Chinese religious traditions is harmony or balance. For a good, wholesome life in this world, it is important to understand and maintain harmony with all the spiritual forces, including the forces operating in the natural process of the cosmos; the various gods, goddesses, and spiritual beings of the cosmos and community; and the ancestral souls that influence the ongoing life of the family.

Traditional Chinese World View
The Chinese have always viewed the world as a self-generating and self-sustaining divine reality. Although they believe in gods and goddesses, no outside creator and

governor of the world exists; all the creative powers operate within the world. Through centuries of experience and experimentation, the Chinese developed a view of the cosmos as a unified, dynamically functioning organism that operates according to set patterns. Texts that speculate on the origins of the world suggest an original state of chaos or potentiality, out of which is generated the multifaceted world, with all its functioning forces. A text from the *Dao de jing* identifies the original state as *Dao* (Way), from which the world is generated and continues to function:

> Dao produces the One.
> The One produces the two.
> The two produce the three.
> And the three produce the ten thousand things.
> The ten thousand things carry **yin** and embrace **yang**,
> And by blending vital energy (**qi**) they attain harmony
>
> —*Dao de jing, ch. 42*

This cosmological perspective sees Dao as the source and root of all things, an undifferentiated reality, replete with creative material and energy (qi, also written ch'i or chi), which gives rise to a separation between finer and brighter elements (yang, heaven) and coarser and darker elements (yin, earth). From the interaction of these polar forces, yin and yang, all things arise and function. Yin qualities are coarse, dark, mysterious, feminine, wet, cold, passive, and yielding. Yang qualities are fine, bright, clear, masculine, dry, hot, active, and structuring. Thus water, moon, north, and winter have more dominant yin qualities, whereas fire, sun, south, and summer have more yang qualities. In the microcosm of the human body, food, and life functions, there is also a proper balance of yin and yang forces for health and well-being.

This is a dynamic view of natural forces because the balance of yin and yang constantly is changing in cyclic patterns of growth and decline. Such changes include the seasons, of course, and also changes of temperature, weather, moon and stars, planting and harvest, government, bodily functions and processes, and stages of life. The interaction of yin and yang in all these processes needs to be understood and kept in harmony.

The Chinese have deepened their view of these life processes by connecting yin and yang with the **five agents** (elements) or operational forces. The five agents are wood, fire, earth, metal, and water, and this set of forces is linked with many aspects of reality, such as seasons, weather, cardinal directions, and planets. These are dynamic operational agents that move in cyclical changes; each agent has its time to rise, flourish, decline, and be taken over by the next agent. The Chinese extended this ecological balance by connecting the yin–yang polarity and these five operating agents not only with all the processes of nature but also with all physical, mental, emotional, psychological, political, and sociological human processes. Thus, the traditional Chinese world view allows people to understand and attempt to balance their lives with these natural forces, whether for bodily health, family happiness, material prosperity, or social harmony.

In addition to the need for balance with these natural forces, the traditional Chinese world view assumes that health and well-being are dependent on harmony with a wide variety of gods, spirits, ancestors, the human community, and the family. The traditional Chinese pantheon has an array of popular gods and goddesses, functioning rather like celestial bureaucrats, from the Jade Emperor to the city Gods of Moats and Walls to the local Earth God, Tudi-gong. The ancient Shang rulers worshiped a high god called Shangdi, "Lord Above," who provided rain and fortune with the help of many other gods and goddesses associated with natural forces. Later, the Zhou ruling family worshiped the high god Tian, "Heaven," emphasizing the moral order upheld by this deity. Daoist priests invoke the "Three Pure Ones" of the unchanging prior heavens, together with the powerful gods and goddesses of the posterior heavens.

The supernatural realm is also inhabited by many spirits, both gods and demons, who were once humans. Foremost in importance among these are the family ancestors, still present and powerful in spiritual form. In traditional Chinese thought, the human being is constituted of two souls, the yang soul (*hun*) from heaven and the yin soul (*po*) from earth. After death, through the elaborate funeral rituals, the family puts the yin soul to rest in the tomb, where it continues to be present as an earthy spirit (*gui*), whereas the yang soul is enshrined on the family altar as a heavenly spirit *(shen)*. The family continues to worship and serve the ancestral spirits, so that happiness, harmony, and blessing will continue from the ancestors. Occasionally gui spirits are neglected and abandoned by the family, and the resentful gui becomes a homeless ghost, wandering about and causing evil happenings, sickness, and death. On the other hand, some shen spirits have become powerful over wide regions and are worshiped by many as high gods. For example, the goddess Mazu originally was a fisherman's daughter who died young, performed miraculous deeds, and over the course of centuries was elevated to the status of Queen of Heaven and worshiped all over China.

So that the human community, family, and individual can stay in harmony with this rich array of spiritual forces (yin–yang and the five agents, gods and goddesses, spirits and demons, ancestors) traditional Chinese people have available longstanding wisdom and ritual techniques for understanding these forces. From ancient times the Chinese have made use of many methods of **divination**, techniques for reading signs to interpret the operation of these forces. Already in the Shang era, to provide advice to the Shang rulers, diviners heated bones and shells, then plunged them in water, reading and interpreting the cracks that appeared. Their inscriptions on these oracle bones and shells are the first instances of the Chinese pictographs that eventually developed into the Chinese written characters. The classic system of divination, embodied in the *Yijing* (Classic of Changes), approaches a divinatory question by ritually constructing a hexagram of broken (yin) and unbroken (yang) lines. Once the six lines are determined, the *Yijing* is consulted, for it contains judgments and commentaries on each of the 64 hexagrams, helping people to understand how the universal forces are operating in that particular context and how to stay in harmony with them.

Another traditional custom that involves divination is the practice of *fengshui* (wind and water), which is the art of reading the balance of yin and yang and the other forces at a particular place, to determine the best location and shape of an ancestral grave or a house. Inhabitants of a house with bad fengshui are at risk of poor health, poverty, and early death. The fengshui expert determines where the yin and yang "breaths" are pulsating, finds the outlines of the azure dragon (yang) and the white tiger (yin) in the landscape, and devises the best way to retain the vital energy (qi) in maximum harmony and vitality, which contributes to the health and welfare of the inhabitants.

Other methods of divination are available in traditional Chinese communities to communicate with gods, spirits, and ancestors. For example, one may consult a spirit diviner who can communicate with the spirits through trances, spirit writing, or chair divination. One simple method of divination is to present oneself before the temple altar, perform acts of worship, and throw two divination blocks on the floor. Each block has a rounded and a flat side, signifying yin or yang; an affirmative answer to a question is provided when yin and yang are in balance (one yin and one yang block).

Thus, in the traditional Chinese way of thinking, an individual person's health and well-being are to be found in a large range of relationships with family, community, ancestors, gods and spirits, forces of yin and yang, and the five agents. Rituals and techniques for maintaining these relationships in a harmonious way have been passed on from early times and are still used by many today. Alongside these traditional practices, and to some extent growing out of them, impressive intellectual, philosophic, and religious traditions have also developed in China, producing important sacred texts, teachings, and practices for living a good, wholesome life. The two most lasting and influential of these traditions are Confucianism and Daoism. Many Chinese follow Confucian and Daoist teachings along with the traditional popular views and practices, as well as Buddhist teachings (see Chapter 11).

The Confucian Tradition

The little that is known about the sage Confucius (Kongzi) suggests that he lived in the sixth or fifth century BCE (before the common era) in a time of upheaval and anarchy. He was well educated in the classic texts and taught a way of life that was designed to transform society and bring harmony and well-being. Although he failed to persuade rulers to follow his way, he gathered a group of disciples who passed on his teachings until finally, in the early Han period (ca. 120 BCE), the emperor established the Confucian teaching as standard for government civil service examinations. Thus, Confucianism has had an enormous influence on the culture and thought of the Chinese people and the other peoples of East Asia through the centuries until the present day.

Confucius did not create a new religion but rather developed and taught a way of life based on traditional Chinese values and wisdom. According to tradition, he edited the "Five Classics" supposedly written by sages in the earlier Zhou period, the *Classic of Rites, Classic of History, Classic of Poetry, Classic of Changes,* and *Spring and Autumn Annals.* His own teachings, in the form of brief sayings, were passed on as the *Analects of Confucius.* Another important Confucian text comes from a later disciple, Mengzi (Mencius), who elaborated at greater length on the Confucian principles. A series of important neo-Confucian thinkers in later eras elaborated and shaped the Confucian path still further.

The way of life taught in these Confucian texts and traditions is based on the vision that humans can, through education and discipline, be nourished and transformed so that they develop into "people of humaneness" (*ren*). This process would start with rulers, leaders, and teachers and move out through family, community, state, and world, for peace, health, and well-being for all. The one who cultivates humaneness will become a Noble Person, a sage who can then help others to cultivate humaneness. As Confucius said, "A person of humaneness, wishing to establish his own character, also establishes the character of others. Wishing to be noble himself, he helps others to be noble." (*Analects* 6:28).

At first glance, the humanism taught in Confucianism does not seem particularly "religious," and Confucius himself downplayed the importance of gods and spirits. For example, when asked about worshiping spirits and gods, he said, "We do not yet know how to serve humans, so how can we know how to serve the gods?" (*Analects* 11:11). But his humanism is a religious humanism in that it is oriented to the higher spiritual order of things, expressed in the notion of the "Will of Heaven," which to Confucius is the universal moral order by which everything should be measured (Ching, 1993). He was convinced that his way coincided with the will of Heaven, and that, therefore, it would bring harmony and wholeness in human society. He said, "Without knowing the Will of Heaven, one cannot become an exemplary person" (*Analects* 20:3).

This path presupposes the view that humans by nature can be nourished and transformed to become people of humaneness. It is true that there was extended discussion about human nature among various teachers in ancient China, and some Confucian teachers, such as Xunzi, argued that by nature humans are greedy and prone to do evil to others. But even Xunzi agreed that humans can, through training and discipline, be educated to become good. The dominant Confucian perspective was expressed firmly by Mengzi (Mencius): all humans by nature have the beginning impulses for goodness. If, he argues, a person sees a child about to fall into a well, the first impulse is not some self-serving thought but pure compassion for the child, based on innate humaneness (*Mencius* 2.A.6). This shows that humans are humane and righteous by nature, and that if that in-born goodness is cultivated and nourished, humans will become people of humaneness.

The reason that people are violent and evil, according to this view, is that, because of anarchy in society and the lack of virtuous leaders and teachers, human goodness is not cultivated and nourished, and it withers away like a garden that is untended, continually hacked at, and stomped on. Therefore people are selfish and hurtful, family values break down, community wholeness is destroyed, and the whole society lives in unrest, war, and violence.

The Confucian solution is a way of education and transformation based on the deliberate cultivation of traditional wisdom and values, starting with leaders and teachers and extending to all. The main elements in this Confucian path are studying the classic writings, cultivating ritual behavior and attitudes, and practicing propriety in social relationships. These are formative disciplines to educate and nourish humaneness in oneself and, by extension, in family, community, and society.

The religious humanism taught by Confucius affirms the self-transformative character of study and learning. The Five Classics contain the wisdom of the earlier sage/kings, who listened to the Will of Heaven and expressed it in these classic texts, and through studying them, one's character is tuned to the Will of Heaven. The course of study laid out in Confucianism is a classic liberal arts program, encompassing historical studies (*Classic of History*), natural scientific studies (*Classic of Changes*), social and political studies (*Spring and Summer Annals*), religious studies (*Classic of Rites*), fine arts and literature (*Classic of Poetry*), and performing arts (*Classic of Music*, no longer extant). A famous saying from Confucius attests to the value of the lifelong discipline of learning:

> At fifteen I was set on study, at thirty I had established my character, at forty I had no uncertainty, at fifty I knew the Will of Heaven, at sixty I was in constant accord with things, and at seventy I could follow my heart's desires without overstepping what is right. *Analects 2:4*

Later neo-Confucian thinkers such as Zhu Xi (1130–1200) further extended the idea of study to the investigation of all things. These thinkers developed the view that a unified, universal principle (*li*), the Great Ultimate, underlies all reality, is always linked to material force (*qi*), and thus is manifest in the countless things. Humans have the universal principle as their original nature, actualized in material force, which clouds and obscures this principle. So it is important for humans to penetrate through to principle by investigation of things and by meditation, thus identifying with that unifying nature of all things. A further approach was taught in the Mind School of neo-Confucianism, by thinkers such as Wang Yangming (1472–1529), who identified principle and mind. Because the mind innately contains all principles, the way to self-cultivation is not through study of external things but through the cultivation and extension of the innate knowledge of the mind, through inner moral and spiritual cultivation. Thus, overall the Confucian path strongly emphasizes intellectual and spiritual cultivation through study of the ancient wisdom, investigation of the principles of self and world, and meditation on the innate principles of the mind.

Confucius' curriculum involved personal and social disciplines as well as study. A key term in his teaching is *li*, which means "ritual" in its narrower sense and "reverent action" or "propriety" in its broader sense. It is difficult for Westerners to understand the importance of ritual behavior in Chinese traditional society, from rituals of sacrifice and prayer to rituals of greeting guests and kowtowing to parents and ancestors. Linking ritual action with their cosmological views, some ancient thinkers suggested that the whole universe, nature as well as human society, operates and is kept in order by ritual. Through ritual, heaven and earth are harmonious, sun and moon are bright, and the four seasons are ordered. Ritual keeps ancestors in honor, elevates rulers and teachers, balances love and hatred as well as joy and anger, and keeps society in order (*Xunzi*, ch. 19). The heart of ritual, for the Confucians, was the practice of sacrifice and worship offered to the ancestors; this was the source of well-being for individual, family, and community. Confucius made it clear that the most important factor was not the effect of ritual on the ancestors, but the heart and spirit of the descendant whose character is transformed through the ritual of dedication to the ancestors. Through ritual, one's innate goodness is nourished and conforms more to the pattern of heaven, earth, and ancestors.

Confucianism teaches that one can become a person of humaneness especially by practicing the rules of "propriety" (*li*, the same word as ritual). The fundamental idea is to display a similar attitude of reverence and respect shown in ritual to the ancestors in all human relationships, with appropriate adjustments for the type of relationship. The focus is on relationships in family and society. The Confucian tradition talks about the "rectification of names," that is, transforming oneself so as to practice one's proper role in family and society. Confucius said, "Let the prince be the prince, the minister be minister, the father father, and the son son" (*Analects* 12:11). Many people do not live according to their proper role: they usurp the authority of the elders, fail to respect the rulers, and undermine proper family roles. To transform ourselves into our potential human goodness, Confucius taught, we need to discipline ourselves to live as a father, a son, a sister, a ruler, a subject. The Confucian tradition suggests that there are five basic human relationships: parent–child, husband–wife, older sibling–younger sibling, ruler–subject, and older friend–younger friend. Although this is a hierarchical structure, each relationship is reciprocal, so that the proper type of propriety is practiced by all in their different roles. Because this accords with the will of Heaven, humane goodness is nourished and family and society live in harmony and wholeness.

Over the course of two millennia, the Confucian tradition has seen many changes and developments, both because of China's turbulent history and its interactions within other cultures of East Asia. As is natural in China, a state cult of Confucius developed, with temples, priests, and festivals. In addition to providing an ethos and set of values for the people, Confucianism was wedded with government, education, literature and art, and traditional religious practices. Today it is difficult to identify Confucianism as a "religion" of the Chinese and specify its components. Yet traditional Chinese are still steeped in the Confucian worldview. Rituals and festivals directed toward ancestors or community gods and family rituals such as marriage, funerals, and New Year celebrations are often associated with Confucianism in the minds of the people. Their cultural values, family relationships, sense of what is right and good, and definitions of health and wholeness are permeated with Confucian ideas.

The Daoist Tradition

Daoism forms a balance with Confucianism in the religious streams of China. Confucianism represents the yang pole: positive, active, structuring, hierarchical, and masculine. Daoism is the necessary balance, the yin pole: negative, passive, yielding, unshaped, feminine. Never as dominant or as structured as Confucianism in China, Daoism has long been esteemed by the Chinese people as the alternative tradition. Actually, "Daoism" encompasses a great variety of religious territory in Chinese history, from the early philosophic texts (the *Dao de jing* and the *Zhuangzi*), to the Daoist alchemists and meditation masters seeking immortality, to Daoist priestly orders with scriptures, liturgies, monasteries, and many gods. In addition, many of the popular religious practices of divination, spirit mediums, and exorcism are often labeled as Daoist religion, as are qigong and taiji exercises. Although large numbers of the Chinese today would not label themselves Daoists, their cultural and spiritual perspectives have been influenced by this long and variegated tradition.

Daoism arises from the ancient Chinese naturalistic world view, but its founding as a religious tradition is shrouded in the mists of history. Tradition looks to Laozi, supposedly born around 604 BCE, as the founder, although scholars suspect that the legends of his life are collective representations of sages who withdrew from society and practiced harmonizing with nature. Laozi, according to legend, eventually withdrew to the western mountains to become an immortal, but before he left he wrote the 5000 characters of the *Dao de jing*, "Classic of the Dao and its Power," to explain his way. This text, very influential in China and the Western world, suggests a way of life tuned in to the operation of the mysterious Dao, the "path" that all things follow. A later disciple, Zhuangzi, contributed an additional text that elaborates a Daoist perspective through many stories and examples, as well as philosophic statements. These texts are sometimes considered the philosophic basis of the Daoist way, but closely related are more specifically religious developments involving ritual masters, alchemy, meditative and yogic techniques, scriptures, priesthoods, great gods and goddesses, and liturgies.

In contrast with the Confucian focus on structure in family and society, Daoists seek spiritual fulfillment in union with Dao, which is somehow connected with the process of nature itself, as the sacred source of all. Dao, which literally means "way," cannot really be defined. The *Dao de jing* opens with the perplexing statement, "The Dao that can be spoken is not the eternal Dao; the Name that can be named is not the eternal Name." All concepts and language differentiate and manage reality, but Dao is prior to division and analysis. Rather than defining Dao, the *Dao de jing* suggests images and metaphors for understanding it. Dao is the mother of the world, the valley, the child, the empty bowl that is never exhausted, the uncarved block. Prior to heaven and earth, it is the undifferentiated source from which all things arise and to which all things return. Not knowing Dao leads to disaster; to be in total harmony with Dao is to be eternal like Dao.

Because harmony with Dao is the root of happiness and well-being, in this view, it is most important to understand how Dao operates—not through force, structure, activity, or propriety, but through "no-action" (*wu-wei*), that is, through yielding and passivity. This turn toward yin values is perhaps most characteristic of the Daoist perspective and is based on observation of how nature itself operates. Of all the yielding and weak things in the world, water is the most so, but nothing is superior in attacking what is hard and strong; the weakest things in the world overcome the hardest things (*Dao de jing*, chs. 78; 43). The yielding flow of water will eventually wear down even the mightiest mountains. Dao always abides in no-action, yet there is nothing that is not done; it flows everywhere and all things depend on it for life, yet it does not master or possess them (*Dao de jing*, chs. 37; 34). So the wise person, like Dao, abides in no-action and yielding—that is, cultivates a way of life in which everything is done in harmony with the flow of Dao.

Based on this naturalistic perspective, Daoists believe that human problems in life arise from artificiality and unnaturalness. Humans are always trying to structure and manage reality, going against nature to make things the way humans think they should be. Zhuangzi jokingly suggests that such attempts are like trying to lengthen the duck's legs or shorten the crane's legs to make them the way they "should" be, which of course winds up causing suffering and pain (*Zhuangzi*, ch. 8). The early Daoists were critical of Confucianists, for they felt that artificiality and coercion were promoted, especially by social institutions such as laws, education, ceremonies, and rules of morality and propriety. Going against the stream of nature itself, judging right and wrong, planning strategies, forcing people into roles, and trying to change what is naturally given causes evil, misery, war, sickness, and early death.

This same basic notion flows over into the more widespread religious Daoist view of our human problems: humans get out of balance with the cosmic forces that support and sustain them. These forces can be understood as the great gods of the stellar constellations who manage the operation of yin and yang and the five agents. In more popular understanding, these forces include the gods and goddesses that operate in the state and the local community and also the ancestral spirits that oversee the family and dispense weal or woe in accordance with the family's harmony with them. In all of these ways, Daoists sense that humans bring problems on themselves by being out of harmony with Dao and the cosmic forces.

Thus, the path offered in Daoism consists of ideas, disciplines, and practices designed to lead to harmony with Dao and all the spiritual forces that operate in our universe. According to the early Daoist thinkers, the way to harmony involves practicing "no-action," meditation, and withdrawal from society's constraints. Practicing no-action prescribes a way of life in which nothing is done against the natural course, no actions are forced, no mental concepts are imposed on the Dao, and even judgments about good and bad or desirable and undesirable are avoided. This calls for disciplines and practices of nonstriving, noncontrol, and nonstructure: simply letting the natural take its course. Early Daoists would often withdraw from society and live as hermits in the mountains, living simply and cultivating harmony with the natural processes. Central to this way is the practice of meditation as an emptying out of the mind, letting go plans, strategies, and structures so that the natural flow of Dao might fill the whole being. Zhuangzi talks of a "fasting of the mind" or "listening with the spirit" that brings harmony with Dao (*Zhuangzi*, ch. 4). Zhuangzi shows how this harmony can be experienced in the normal, everyday activities of life, such as butchering an ox, carving a bell stand, or enduring a disfiguring sickness or even the death of a spouse.

Many modern people, Chinese and otherwise, are fascinated with this Daoist perspective on life. In particular, the practice of no-action and yielding has been cultivated in some of the arts, such as landscape painting, poetry, and dance, and it provides the foundation for some of the bodily exercises and martial arts that operate with softness, yielding, stillness, and silence. These practices of meditation and movement are influential in healing therapies and wellness techniques today.

Yet there is more to the Daoist path than a philosophy of life and techniques of movement and meditation; a wide range of religious practices is also associated with Daoism. Daoism today is one of the five recognized religions in the People's Republic of China, and there are many Daoist temples and priests in Taiwan, Hong Kong, and all the other Chinese communities. The masters and priests of the Daoist sects and communities start from the basic Daoist perspective and offer religious practices that relate concretely to the human concerns of health, well-being of family and community, material happiness, and even immortality. The Daoist priests and experts generally follow the religious path for their own spiritual transformation and power so that they can share their expertise and power with the community. Thus, the religious path of Daoism operates both on the level of the priest or expert and on the level of the ordinary people in the community.

Daoist priests typically go through long periods of training in the scriptures and rituals and receive an ordination rank, depending on how extensive is their command of the spirit world. Because the local temple and even the human body are microcosms of the great universe, the sacred forces of the cosmos can be called down to inhabit the temple or human body. Through long study and practice, the Daoist priest memorizes the spirit registers and becomes adept at the rituals, able to summon the great powers into this realm and into his own body to bring renewal and transformation. In ancient times, Daoist practices included alchemy, creating a kind of gold dust fluid to drink to nourish the inner forces and prolong life. More important today are various practices of bodily exercise and meditation designed to nourish the internal life forces. Daoists feel that the key elements in the body are breath or energy (*qi*), spirit (*shen*), and spermatic essence (*jing*), present throughout the body but especially concentrated in the three Cinnabar fields, that is, the head, the heart, and just below the navel. These are the special fields of the Three Pure Ones, the great stellar gods that inhabit the body. Yin and yang are also at work: as life goes on, yang forces are used up, and yin increases, leading to an imbalance, until finally spirit, breath, and seminal essence are dissipated in death. The practices of the Daoist adept are designed to reverse this process, renewing the heavenly yang forces and thus restoring vitality. Among these practices are inner meditations in which the One Dao is focused on, and a visualization technique through which the Three Pure Ones are summoned into the three fields of the body to bring renewal. In addition, Daoist priests use breathing techniques, gymnastics, and dietetics to purge the body of impurities, clear the channels of circulation through the body, and nourish the primal breaths.

Because the Daoist priests and adepts can practice this path, ordinary people look to them for their services in the great festivals of community renewal, in critical life events, such as marriages and funerals, and in times of sickness and other need. The priests can restore the balance of sacred forces by exorcising the evil spirits and calling down the great gods to restore harmony and renew life forces. But ordinary people also can take their own steps on the Daoist path through such actions as going to the local temple to worship the gods there who have demonstrated their power and importance for the community, throwing divination blocks to receive guidance, and participating in qigong exercises. In ordinary religious life, boundaries are very flexible between Daoist religious practices and popular practices linked to Buddhism, Confucianism, ancestor worship, and folk religions. The life needs of a Chinese family or community are met through spiritual care that comes from all of these traditions.

JAPANESE RELIGIOUS AND SPIRITUAL TRADITIONS

Today, Japanese people are very modern and secularized, yet there still is a unique Japanese identity, influenced, in part, by the long religious heritage of Japan. As an island people, the Japanese developed distinct religious practices (later called Shinto) that shaped their culture. When Chinese influences started entering in about the sixth century CE (common era), the Japanese accepted Buddhism, Confucianism, and Daoism, integrating them into their Shinto-based culture. They likewise adopted the Chinese traditional principles of medicine and treatment, which became standard in Japan even until modern times (Lock, 1980; Ohnuki-Tierney, 1984; Sakade, 1989). The Japanese characteristic has been to accept new influences but never to throw anything away. Later, Western culture and Christianity reached Japan, and again the Japanese accepted much but reshaped it in a distinctly Japanese way. Today, a typical Japanese person is outwardly secular and westernized, but still participates in Shinto and Buddhist religious activities, follows Confucian values and perspectives, pays attention to Daoist ideas of calendar and geomancy, takes interest in Christian ideas and perhaps has a Christian-style wedding, enjoys the folk religious traditions of his or her own locality, and uses traditional Chinese medicine along with Western medicine.

The Shinto Tradition

Ancient pre-Buddhist Japanese religion was a fertility religion related to rice growing and focused on myriads of nature spirits called *kami*. Myths from ancient Japan suggest a tripartite world, consisting of the plain of high heaven, the earth, and the world of darkness (death). The sun kami, Amaterasu, was a major kami who was worshiped especially by the imperial clan, with myths telling how the emperor is a direct descendent of Amaterasu. But each local community also had important kami, which they worshiped in their own ways. With the coming of Chinese civilization in the sixth century, the Japanese accepted Buddhism and other Chinese traditions but continued to practice their native religious traditions of kami. Eventually these native traditions were called "Shinto," a Chinese word meaning "way of the kami." Today tens of thousands of Shinto shrines are scattered throughout Japan in every community, and most Japanese participate in at least some of the festivals and other activities associated with these shrines, perhaps also keeping a small shrine in their own house.

The Shinto perspective is simple but has permeated Japanese culture to the core. The whole world is full of kami, with no sharp lines drawn between gods, humans, and the natural world. Anything experienced as specially powerful, unusual, awesome, terrifying, or beautiful can be thought of as kami; Mt. Fuji, a thunderstorm, a beautiful waterfall, disease, a fox, a powerful warrior, sexual power, ancestors, and a mirror all can represent the presence of kami. Stories tell how the whole world was created by Izanagi and Izanami, two primordial kami who descended from the plain of high heaven. Through sexual intercourse and giving birth, these kami engendered the myriads of kami who constitute the whole world, so that the very nature of the world is kami. Humans also share with all of nature in being "children of kami."

Because the kami are pure, good, and beautiful in nature, the whole world, including human nature, is originally pure, good, and beautiful. Thus, the Japanese have always cultivated a sense of sharing in the beauty and goodness of the world through artistic practices and appreciation of nature, which are viewed as means of communing and cooperating with the kami. There are, of course, evil things, suffering, and death in the world. According to Shinto mythology, all such things arise from pollution that enters the world from the underworld. Pollution includes human moral wrongs and sins but also natural disasters and bodily functions, such as bleeding, menstruation, sickness, and death. Pollutions of various kinds break down the harmony with the kami and bring about all kinds of evils to the individual and the community. Thus, the main Shinto rituals have to do with purification: cleansing away the pollution and restoring harmony with the pure, life-giving kami.

Worshiping the kami can be done simply and in many ways. Traditional Japanese families have a kami shrine (*kamidana*) in their home for daily worship. A worshiper also can stop by the local shrine at any time. Because the kami are pure, the first step in worship is purifying oneself, usually through washing the hands and rinsing the mouth. The worshiper pulls the shrine bell rope, and with bowing, clapping of hands, offerings, and prayers, communion with the kami is experienced. Often, the local shrines have festivals in which the whole community participates. These festivals are understood to "entertain" the kami and serve to purify and restore the community. At festivals, the priests purify the whole gathered people by waving purification wands over them, present offerings of food and other gifts, and solemnly chant ancient prayers to the kami. Following this, worship of the kami also involves festival celebrations of various kinds. These celebrations include special shrine dances and music, as well as presentations of art, such as flower arranging or calligraphy. Various sports, such as horseback riding, archery, and wrestling, may also help to entertain the kami and the people. Symbols of the kami may be placed in a palanquin (a portable shrine carried by worshipers) and taken through the streets of the neighborhood, the kami coming to purify and bless the people.

Shinto ideas and rituals are closely linked with the family and, especially, the passages of life. Birth itself is polluting because of the blood, so the mother is purified and the infant is brought to the shrine to be dedicated to the family kami. On special days, such as birthdays or the Seven-Five-Three Festival (for girls 7 and 3 and boys 5 years of age), children are dressed in fine clothes and presented at the shrines.

New Year's Day has become a big festival in modern Japan, with most people visiting the shrines to purify the coming year and bring home new shrine amulets. Traditional Japanese weddings are performed with Shinto rituals, with the new couple and their parents sanctifying the union by exchanging a cup of o-sake before the kami. Students often visit shrines to seek help from the kami in passing examinations for college. Adult's Day, a modern festival for people reaching 20 years of age, draws many young women and men to the shrines dressed in their finest. Priests may purify new homes and business buildings before they are occupied. In all these ways, Shinto remains important and intertwined in the lives of many Japanese.

Japanese Buddhist Tradition

Shinto has to do with that which promotes life, such as marriage and the birth of a child, but when death comes, the family calls in Buddhist priests. Death is polluting, in the Shinto view, but Buddhism has long provided an understanding of death and rituals for handling it. The Japanese saying, "Born Shinto, die Buddhist," characterizes the complementary function of these two religious traditions in Japanese culture. Buddhism teaches the kind of detachment from life that prepares for death and assists in attaining a better rebirth. The Japanese family is very concerned about their ancestors, and Buddhism offers a means for them to provide a meaningful funeral for the dead one, to pray for the ancestors on memorial days after death, and to provide merit for them in the afterlife.

◐ ⑤ Japanese Buddhism also offers spiritual help in other crises of life. The healing Buddha, Yakushi (Bhaishajya-guru), can be invoked in times of sickness, as a supplement to medical help. The Bodhisattva Jizo is protector of travelers, so his statue often stands at crossroads. Because Jizo is also the protector of children, families with sick or deceased children worship small statues of Jizo and pray for the welfare of the souls of their children. Modern medical technology has facilitated the availability of abortions for Japanese women, and their Buddhist faith draws women who have had abortions to certain Buddhist temples, where they can have Buddhist priests conduct rituals for the repose of the souls of their aborted children (mizuko, water-child) (Harrison, 1999). Many worship Kannon (Bodhisattva Avalokiteshvara) for healing in sickness and help in pregnancy. It is particularly popular among aging Japanese to implore Kannon as the goddess who can prevent senility and grant a timely, speedy death so that they will not become a burden on their children in old age.

◐ ⑤ For engaging in regular spiritual practice in their lives, many Japanese look to one of the schools of Buddhism. They may turn to the Pure Land school and worship Amida Buddha for the gift of rebirth in the Pure Land Buddha realm. Some choose one of the sects in the Nichiren tradition and chant the title of the Lotus Sutra for spiritual and material well-being, and some follow the Zen path of meditation for mental strength and spiritual awareness.

Many so-called new religions have arisen in Japan, beginning in the 19th century and increasing rapidly after World War II. Some estimates suggest that one-third of the Japanese people have had some relationship with one or another of these movements. The success of these new religions seems related to the fact that they meet people's spiritual and physical needs in very concrete ways: offering healing practices, counseling, and providing direct experiences of divine power, fellowship, and an array of earthly benefits. These movements generally have been founded by charismatic leaders (often women) who often draw from several of the Japanese religions, even Christianity, to offer a new revelation and practice. Some of these movements have become quite large and mainstream, such as Tenrikyo and Soka Gakkai, and have even drawn Western followers into their fold.

Like other aspects of Japanese culture, healing and medical practices have been adopted from a variety of sources. Today this pluralism of Japanese medicine still is apparent, as Japanese typically seek help from religious (Shinto and Buddhist) sources, **traditional Chinese medicine** (*kanpo*), and Western biomedicine (Ohnuki-Tierney, 1984).

KOREAN RELIGIOUS AND SPIRITUAL TRADITIONS

Religion in Korea has been heavily influenced by Chinese traditions. Values and attitudes relating to family life and society are deeply Confucian, and the perspective on the natural world and the human life process is related to the traditional Daoist ideas. The Chinese traditional medical system likewise has exerted much influence over Korean ideas of health and healing (Shin, 2001).

 At the same time, other religious traditions also play a role for the people. Most Koreans are Buddhist, so Buddhist ideas play a large role in their understanding of life and death (Tedesco, 1999) (see Chapter 11). The percentage of Christians in South Korea is higher than in the other countries of East Asia, making up nearly half of the population. The indigenous religion, worshiping the gods and the ancestors in the traditional ways, still attracts many people (Kendall, 1987). And some new religious movements have attracted attention, such as the Unification Church of Rev. Sun Myung Moon, a quasi-Christian movement that emphasizes conservative family values and suggests Rev. Moon as a new type of messiah.

TRADITIONAL CHINESE MEDICINE

The main lines of Chinese medicine were shaped over centuries as scholar physicians drew on traditional knowledge and practice developed in the religious traditions: the operation of yin and yang and the five agents, alchemy, techniques of meditation and bodily movement, methods for controlling breaths and circulation systems of the body, and dietary practices. Important medical and pharmacologic texts were produced, some claiming great antiquity. For example, one of the earliest and most often cited compilations of Chinese medical knowledge, the *Huangdi Neijing* (*The Yellow Emperor's Classic of Internal Medicine*), traditionally is ascribed to the legendary emperor of the third millennium BCE, who brought benefits of civilization to the Chinese people. This medical text and others were known by time of the Han era (220 BCE–200 CE), and tradition venerates a series of sages of medicine over the next centuries who experimented and augmented medical knowledge and practice. A fairly consistent system of traditional medicine developed by the time of the Sung era (960–1280), complete with medical schools and extensive medical texts.

In modern times, those who attempted to modernize China along Western lines and establish Western medicine in China tended to disregard traditional Chinese medicine, but in the second half of the 20th century, a great revival of interest in the Chinese traditions of medicine took place among the Chinese and even among Westerners. Today the traditional system is supported and taught at Chinese medical schools together with Western medicine. Traditional Chinese medicine now has training schools and licensed practitioners, and it also has gained respect and recognition in the West. Some Western physicians remain skeptical about the scientific basis of the traditional system, with its cosmological assumptions and methods of diagnosis, but practices that have shown empirical results, such as the use of acupuncture for analgesic purposes, are widely recognized.

Ⓢ As in traditional Chinese religion, the central notion in medicine is balance or harmony, within the microcosm as within the macrocosm. Key to this balance is the healthy state of qi, vital energy, which flows in the universe and in the human body. This vital energy includes not only physical energy but also mental and spiritual energy. Imbalances cause qi to dwindle and become weak, or to be obstructed and congested, resulting in loss of wellness and eventual sickness. Proper balance maintains vigor and well-being in the body, mind, and spirit. Qi, like everything in the universe, functions through the dynamic interaction of yin and yang and the phases of the five agents. Yin is the passive and constitutive principle, with the qualities of earth, moon, nighttime, darkness, winter, femininity, cold, wet, internal, small, and weak, whereas yang is the active principle, with the qualities of heaven, sun, daylight, brightness, summer, masculinity, hot, dry, external, big and strong. Yin is the more steady state: concrete, solid, completed. Yang tends to be the stronger factor in transitions: beginnings, moving, and changing.

Yin and yang have particular qualities that are understood to pertain to sickness and health in human life and, particularly, in the bodily functions. For example, yin tends to be associated with the time between noon and midnight; whatever acts on or moves toward the interior; stable essence (*jing*); stable fluids; energy exhaustion; anything that is murky or opaque, soft, or savory; and the transformation phases of the metal and water agents. On the other hand, yang tends to be associated with the time between midnight and noon; whatever is on the surface or moving toward the surface; the back; active qi energy; heavenly spirit (*shen*); active fluids; energy abundance; anything that is clear, hard, and tasteless; and the transformation phases of the wood and fire agents. But yin and yang are dynamic forces, so phenomena that have yang qualities also are influenced by yin, and vice versa, as natural changes take place. Thus, natural, healthy balance in body and spirit is not a static state but one in which the natural rhythms of yin and yang with respect to season, time, organ, circulation, and mood are maintained in optimal harmony.

Practitioners of Chinese medicine connect the yin–yang principles with the continuum of five elements or agents (*wu xing*): wood, fire, earth, metal, and water. These are not substances, as the word "elements" might mistakenly suggest; rather, they are transformational agents or phases. For example, the movement of the five agents in the cycle of yang and yin may begin with the yang phase, with potential activity (wood) that leads to full activity (fire). After a transitional shift (earth) to the yin phase comes potential settling (metal), which leads to actual settling (water), which again produces potential activity (wood). This sequence of agents, in which one agent produces the next, is called the "productive sequence." But this sequence is simultaneously balanced by another sequence, in which these active phases are controlled by their constructive counterparts. In this "conquest sequence," wood is conquered by metal, metal is conquered by fire, fire is conquered by water, water is conquered by earth, and earth is conquered by wood. Thus, we see that the interplay of these agents is rather complex. For example, while wood is producing fire, metal is conquering wood; and while metal is producing water, fire is subduing metal. In addition, while earth is conquering water, metal is producing water; and while fire is subduing metal, earth is producing metal.

In traditional Chinese medicine, the fundamental perspective is that the operation of yin and yang through these two sequences (creating and subduing) of the five agents is the basis of health and vitality. When the interplay of all these forces is normal and natural, healthy life is experienced. But when these processes are disrupted by some cause, the normal flow of energy becomes weak and deficient in some areas, and becomes stopped up and congested in other areas. The result is that the sequences of the five agents break down, and sickness results.

In understanding the relation between the various outward observable phenomena and the inner vital functions of the body, Chinese medicine operates with a particular view of anatomy that sees the human body as a constellation of energy (qi) in which the vital functions are concentrated in a group of "organs" or functional fields. Associated with these organs are a number of meridians or pathways for the flow of energy. The organs or functional fields relate to the fundamental vital functions, of course, but they are also classified in relation to yin and yang, the five agents, cosmic and natural phenomena, bodily regions and meridians, and physical and sensory projections. The solid organs (liver, heart, spleen, lungs, and kidneys) are associated with yin in that they create energy and are storage organs. The hollow organs (gall bladder, small intestine, stomach, large intestine, and bladder) are associated with yang in that they are passage organs and distribute energy. Each of the storage organs (yin) is linked with one of the passage organs (yang) that complements its function.

Chinese medicine looks on these organs more as functional fields than as precise physical entities, and they are linked to the operation of the five agents (Table 12.1). Thus, the liver and the gall bladder together are linked with the agent wood (potential activity). The liver is the controller of the other organs and the reservoir of constructive energy, storage of the individual personality qualities and demeanor, and

TABLE 12.1   Correspondences of the Five Agents or Phases

	Wood	Fire	Earth	Metal	Water
Season	Spring	Summer	Late summer	Autumn	Winter
Direction	East	South	Center	West	North
Time of Day	Dawn	Forenoon	Afternoon	Early evening	Night
Weather	Wind	Heat	Damp	Dryness	Cold
Color	Green	Scarlet	Yellow	White	Black
Yin Organ	Liver	Heart	Spleen	Lungs	Kidney
Yang Organ	Gallbladder	Small intestine	Stomach	Large intestine	Bladder
Sense Organ	Eyes	Tongue	Mouth	Nose	Ears
Taste	Sour	Bitter	Sweet	Pungent	Salty
Odor	Sour sweat	Scorched	Fragrant	Raw fish	Putrid
Verbal expression	Shouting	Laughing	Singing	Weeping	Sighing
Emotion	Anger	Joy	Pensiveness	Sorrow	Fear

origin of the body's motive forces and vital impulses. The liver corresponds to early morning and spring, as well as sour tastes and a mood of anger. It is connected with the eyes as sense organ, fingernails and toenails as external counterpart, the color green, tears as fluid, and a sour sweat/urine odor.

The heart organ field and the small intestine passage organ are connected with fire (actualized energy). The heart produces spiritual energy (shen), which contributes clarity of vision and structure to the person, and it is associated with noon-time, summer, bitter taste, a mood of joy, the color scarlet, sweaty fluid, and a burning or pungent odor.

The spleen organ field and the stomach passage organ are linked to the agent earth. The spleen is responsible for digestion and thus is a storage for surplus energy. It is the source of critical insight and is associated with the afternoon, late summer, sweet taste, a mood of pensiveness, yellow, lips and mouth, and a sweet odor.

The lung field and the large intestine passage organ are linked to the agent metal (potential settling). The lung function field is the organizing source for life's rhythms and speech and is associated with early evening, fall, acrid taste, a mood of sorrow, white, skin, the nose, fluid of nasal mucus, and a raw meat or fish odor.

The kidney organ field and the bladder passage organ are related to the agent water (actual settling). The kidney field is the storehouse of the person's natural powers and gifts and the source of endurance, hearing, and sexual potency; it is associated with winter, the time before midnight, salty taste, a mood of fear, the ears as sense organ, and a rotten odor (Reid, 1994).

The theory of arterial pathways or meridians throughout the body that link together various impulse points (*xue*) that are close to the body's surface is important both for diagnosis of sickness and for treatment. Meridians are conduits for the transmission of the various kinds of physiologic energy throughout the body. They were mapped out through centuries of experience, as physicians located the impulse points through empirical investigation and constructed the theory of pathways of energy that link these points together. These pathways are associated with the different organ fields and link each organ field with its complementary passage organs as well as other organs in a complex network (Kaptchuk, 2000; Lao, 1999). The impulse points, frequently found in cavities or recesses near the surface of the body, are significant points in each of the pathways where changes in the flow of energy can be induced. Chinese medicine has classified extensively the characteristic symptoms that arise when the normal flow of energy in each of these pathways has been disrupted.

For example, the stomach meridian, which connects with the spleen, starts near the nostrils, descends along the chest and the belly, turns outward in the groin region, and runs down the front of the leg, ending in the second toe. Pathologic symptoms associated with the disruption of energy in this meridian include shivering and groaning; as illness develops, the body may swell, accompanied by boils, high fever, and dropsy. This meridian has 45 impulse points that can serve as loci for acupuncture treatment. The pathway associated with the liver begins in the big toe, runs up the inside of the leg, around the genitals to the lower center of the abdomen, and veers to the left or right to an ending impulse point on either side of the body, with 14 impulse points altogether. Symptoms connected with energy disruption in this pathway include abdominal swelling, dry throat, and diarrhea.

The diagnosis of illness in Chinese medicine is holistic and time consuming. Every aspect of the individual's body, life, and environment is significant, for many of these factors are associated with the operation of the five agents and, thus, with the functioning of the organ fields. Traditionally, there are four types of examination: inspection, listening and smelling, questioning, and palpation. The practitioner inspects various parts of the body, including the eyes, the skin color, the various features of the tongue, even the person's demeanor and spirit. Particular attention is paid to sounds (such as voice and breathing) and odors of breath, body, and excreta because these can be clear indicators of an imbalance of energy. The physician questions the patient about the specific complaint, including the precise time of inception, and also about his or her whole physical, social, emotional, and spiritual context. A major diagnostic method is palpation, including pulse examination, palpation of the impulse points, and general palpation of the whole body. Pulse diagnosis is especially extensive in Chinese medicine. For example, there are three important pulse points on each wrist, and each pulse is characterized in terms of its quality, by such descriptions as superficial, deep, slow, rapid, depleted, overflowing, slippery, melting, or stringlike (Ergil, 1996). Each type of pulse tells something about the organ fields and their balance of energy.

On the basis of this holistic examination, the practitioner arrives at a diagnosis of the pattern of disharmony that exists. Diagnostic signs and signals traditionally are differentiated according to eight principles (Kaptchuk, 2000; Reid, 1994; Wiseman, 1995):

- Yin disorders, with fatigue, swollen tongue, labored breathing
- Yang disorders, with ruddy complexion, dry lips, dark tongue, thirst
- Interior illnesses, with high fever, abdominal pain, diarrhea
- Exterior illnesses, with shivering, headaches, stopped-up nose
- Coldness disorders, with pale skin, blue lips, light tongue, needing rest
- Heat disorders, with reddish skin, restlessness, dry lips, leathery tongue
- Lack of qi energy, with soft voice, loss of appetite, cold hands and feet, short breath
- Overaccumulation of qi energy, with belching, nausea, fever, bronchial congestion

Chinese medicine includes among pathologic agents factors such as wind, cold, summer heat, dampness, dryness, fiery heat, as well as desire, anger, worry, reflection, sorrow, fear, terror, improper diet, physical overexertion, and sexual excess.

A wide variety of remedies and treatments tailored to the specific diagnosis are used in Chinese medicine. Primary treatments are internal therapy, consisting of drug and herbal remedies, and external therapy, namely, acupuncture and moxibustion (described below). A variety of supplementary treatments can also be used, such as a prescribed diet, massage, steam baths, qigong exercises, and modification of the patient's habits. The herbal or drug remedies traditionally are classified in four natures (cold, cool, hot, warm) and five tastes (pungent, sweet, sour, bitter, and salty), and they also are differentiated according to function, such as heat-clearing, dampness-eliminating, interior-warming, blood-rectifying, spirit-quieting, and expectorants.

Chinese medicine has a number of traditional treatment strategies that differ according to the purpose of the treatment. These strategies are to induce sweating, clear away heat, induce vomiting, bring about purgation, harmonize antagonistic functions, warm the patient, cool the patient, increase the flow of energy, and dissipate the overaccumulated energy (Wiseman, 1995). Drug and herbal remedies, as well as acupuncture, are common for all of these treatment strategies. **Acupuncture** done at the impulse points along the appropriate meridian is especially useful for increasing the flow of energy or dissipating blocked energy, thus restoring balance. **Moxibustion** is used as a complement to acupuncture; it consists of burning a ball or cone of dried mugwort on one or more of the impulse points to provide heat stimulation. Related to moxibustion is cupping treatment: the stimulation of an acupuncture point by applying a heated cup that creates a vacuum. This process leaves marks on the skin, which have been misinterpreted by some Western health care practitioners as signs of abuse.

The supplementary treatments, such as prescribed diet, Chinese massage, and qigong exercises, are useful when illness is not acute, or for long-term balancing of the energy flow for health and disease prevention. Dietary practices are connected closely with the theory of yin/yang and the five agents, and families can prepare the proper balance of foods to meet changing needs, such as change of season, after childbirth, or for nourishment of the elderly. Chinese massage (*tui na*) uses hand manipulation, such as kneading, rolling, and pushing on the impulse points and other parts of the body. It can be used to balance yin and yang and to adjust qi energy flowing through the meridians. Qigong, "energy work," is an ancient Chinese meditative method combined with bodily movement to achieve a balance of qi in the body's meridian system. Slow, graceful movements, as well as mental visualization, direct the flow of qi through the desired areas to promote health and healing (Lee & Lei, 1999; McGee, Sancier, & Chow, 1996; Miura, 1989). The popular martial art, taiji-quan, derived from qigong.

An example of diagnosis and treatment for a patient who reports insomnia may be helpful. Insomnia has many causes, but suppose the patient also shows signs of restlessness, palpitations, throat dryness, backache, night sweats, a red tongue with little coating, and a thread-like pulse. This syndrome can be identified as disharmony between the heart and the kidney because restlessness, palpitations, throat dryness, and red tongue are symptoms of hyperactivity of the heart, whereas backache, night sweats, and a thready pulse show kidney yin deficiency. Normally, heart fire (yang) should warm kidney water (yin), and kidney water should nourish heart fire, but because of pathogenic factors of stress and obsessive sexual activity, disharmony has occurred. The treatment could include an herbal formula to clear fire from the heart, and another herbal remedy to nourish the kidney yin. Acupuncture could be applied to the impulse points of the heart and kidney meridians to reduce the heart fire and enhance the kidney water, and the patient could be advised to prepare certain dietary foods that nourish the heart and enhance kidney essence. In addition, the patient may be counseled to make lifestyle changes to reduce stress and avoid obsessive sexual activity. The patient may also be encouraged to practice qigong to calm the spirit of the heart and preserve the essence of the kidney (Lao, 1999).

Some modified forms of Chinese medicine have been developed in modern times. A specialized modern form is auriculotherapy, insertion of needles in points on the external ear that correspond to internal organs and meridians. Practitioners in Korea have mapped the networks of meridians onto the hands, resulting in a whole system of hand and finger acupuncture. Additional technologies such as electrostimulation and laser acupuncture have been introduced. In Western medicine, acupuncture has been widely adapted for specific purposes such as producing an analgesic or anesthetic effect or for treating drug addiction (Beal, 2000). Many Western physicians endorse the "evidence based" use of acupuncture, that is, acupuncture technique that has proven scientific results, rather than acupuncture based on the traditional Chinese theories of yin–yang, five agents, qi, and meridians (Ulett & Han,

1998). However, for East Asians, as well as some Westerners, the traditional Chinese medical theories make sense as a holistic approach to health and well-being.

HEALTH AND SPIRITUAL CONCERNS FOR EAST ASIANS

A primary concern for East Asians is their role within the family and their community relationships, which form a concrete social structure based in their spiritual traditions. Thus, sickness and health are not just an individual's concern but need to involve the family, the ancestors, and the community. East Asians feel the need to express thankfulness and gratitude and to repay others' kindness, especially to family, parents, and ancestors (Shirahama & Inoue, 2001). Family members often feel that nursing care is a family obligation, and professional nurses need to be sensitive to such feelings (Wong & Pang, 2000). Given the respect for ancestors and parents that is so important in these Confucian cultures, the idea of nursing home placement for ailing parents usually is rejected. In addition, Confucian ideals dictate that one's body be kept whole and intact as it was given from the ancestors, so organ transplantations and disfiguring surgeries are problematic. Nurses can support patients from East Asian traditions by assuring the presence of family members. Opportunities to participate in providing physical care should be offered to family members. Visitation may need to be liberal to respect patients' needs to remain connected with family and community members.

Among Japanese people, there are Shinto and Buddhist ideas that raise conflicts with some aspects of modern health care. To many Japanese, organ transplantations conflict with both Shinto and Buddhist views against removing organs before a person's life ends (McConnell, 1999; Umehara, 1994). Abortion, although widely practiced in East Asia, often causes spiritual distress so that many women feel spiritual agony and perform religious rituals to pacify the soul of the aborted fetus (Harrison, 1999; Tedesco, 1999). Shinto sensitivities among the Japanese make them particularly concerned about pollution and the need for purification. Nurses can encourage patients to express feelings to resolve conflicting emotions. Nurses can use inquiries about advance directives as an opportunity to assess patient views regarding transplantation. When patients are uncomfortable with discussing concerns with nurses, nurse should help patients identify others in whom they can confide.

Among elderly, tradition-minded East Asians, acceptance of the traditional world view of yin/yang and the five agents is often implicit. They may be suspicious of Western diagnoses and treatments that take no account of these natural forces and the treatments offered in Chinese traditional medicine (Torsch & Ma, 2000). Some of the elements of traditional medicine can be practiced without a physician, so East Asians may want to engage in activities such as dietary balancing of yin and yang foods and qigong exercises. Nurses must be aware of potential interactions between prescribed medications and herbal remedies and educate patients about their use.

Assisting patients to maintain a balance between yin and yang is of primary importance for spiritually sensitive nursing care. For example, yang activity needs to be balanced by yin rest, so after childbirth women may feel they need several days of bedrest (Chen, 2001). Because of the short stays associated with childbearing in the United States, it would be important for nurses' discharge planning to ensure that new mothers have adequate support so that they may rest at home.

PERSONAL REFLECTIONS

- How do you see yourself relating to a person who lives by one of the East Asian religions?
- Are you comfortable accepting the importance of their beliefs and practices and encouraging them to strengthen them?
- Do you feel you understand each of these religious traditions enough to be able to provide appropriate spiritual care?
- Which features of the East Asian religions do you find to make the most sense?
- Are you uncomfortable with any of the teachings and practices of the East Asian religions?
- Do you believe that your own spiritual health and awareness are important factors in enabling you to provide spiritual care for people of East Asian religions?
- Are you comfortable with the need to learn, communicate, think critically, and be willing to change your own perspectives in caring for people of East Asian religions and cultures?
- Do you feel that the holistic notions of health and healing present in the East Asian cultures could be helpful in Western medicine?
- Are you comfortable in supporting patients who want treatments in traditional Chinese medicine while maintaining their Western medical regimen?
- Do you find personal spiritual or health benefits from Eastern practices such as acupuncture or qigong?
- Would you encourage non-Asians to explore East Asian religions, spiritual disciplines, and medicinal practices?

CASE STUDY 12.1

Ken Lao is a first generation Canadian from East Asia. He is 90 years old and has received a diagnosis of terminal metastatic brain cancer. Mr. Lao has decided that he wishes no treatment to be provided, except for traditional Chinese therapies. He refuses any Western medical treatment, which has been labeled as futile in his case, and wishes to die a peaceful death at home. Mr. Lao and his family follow traditional East Asian religious practices.

Critical Thinking
- What are the primary concerns that Mr. Lao likely has as he faces the end of life?
- What are some specific interventions that would be appropriate to care for Mr. Lao and his family?
- Would it be appropriate for the nurse to discuss organ donation with the patient or family? List reasons why or why not.

(Case Study continues on page 186)

CASE STUDY 12.1 (continued)

- How might the nurse explain Mr. Lao's condition to the family in light of yin/yang beliefs?
- To what extent would the nurse expect the family to be involved in his care?
- Which types of Chinese therapies might Mr. Lao request?
- What do Confucian ideals dictate about the state of the body at and after death?

Key Points

- Eastern religions and cultures emphasize a holistic understanding of health, including body, mind, spirit, family, and nature.
- Traditional Chinese people have strong reverence for family and ancestors, and they understand the world as operating through the cyclic movements of yin/yang and the five agents; therefore, health and wholeness come both through harmony in family and social order (a key Confucian emphasis) and in balance with the natural forces and cosmic gods (a key Daoist emphasis).
- Japanese people feel a strong attachment to the sacred forces and ancestors (kami) of their people through whom life and wholeness come, and they understand the passing of life through Buddhist teachings and practices.
- Although most Korean people are Buddhist, their world views are influenced by Chinese traditions such as Confucianism and Daoism.
- The percentage of Christians in South Korea is higher than those of other countries of East Asia.
- Traditional Chinese medicine understands yin/yang and the five agents to be operating not only in the world but also in the human body, connected with bodily organs and pathways of energy (qi), with treatments of herbs and acupuncture used to restore natural harmony and health.
- Providing holistic care to people influenced by the East Asian traditions requires understanding their religious and medical traditions as well as responding to their particular spiritual concerns.

References

Beal, M. W. (2000). Acupuncture and Oriental body work: Traditional and modern biomedical concepts in holistic care—conceptual frameworks and biomedical developments. *Holistic Nursing Practice, 15*(1), 78–87.

Chen, Y. (2001). Chinese values, health and nursing. *Journal of Advanced Nursing, 36*(2), 270–273.

Ching, J. (1993). *Chinese religions.* Maryknoll: Orbis Books.

Ergil, K. (1996). China's traditional medicine. In M. S. Micozzi (Ed.), *Fundamentals of complementary and alternative medicine* (pp. 185–223). New York: Churchill Livingstone.

Harrison, E. G. (1999). 'I can only move my feet towards mizuko': Memorial services for dead children in Japan. In D. Keown (Ed.), *Buddhism and abortion* (pp. 93–120). Honolulu: University of Hawaii Press.

Kaptchuk, T. J. (2000). *The web that has no weaver: Understanding Chinese medicine* (2nd ed.). Chicago: Contemporary Books.

Kendall, L. (1987). *Shamans, housewives, and other restless spirits: Women in Korean ritual life.* Honolulu: University of Hawaii Press.

Lao, L. (1999). Traditional Chinese medicine. In W. B. Jonas & J. S. Levin (Eds.), *Essentials of complementary and alternative medicine* (pp. 216–232). Philadelphia: Lippincott Williams & Wilkins.

Lee, C., & Lei, T. (1999). Qigong. In W. B. Jonas & J. S. Levin (Eds.), *Essentials of complementary and alternative medicine* (pp. 392–411). Philadelphia: Lippincott Williams & Wilkins.

Lock, M. M. (1980). *East Asian medicine in urban Japan.* Berkeley: University of California Press.

McConnell, J. R. (1999). The ambiguity about death in Japan: An ethical implication for organ procurement. *Journal of Medical Ethics, 25*(4), 322–325.

McGee, C. T., Sancier, K., & Chow, E. P. Y. (1996). Qigong. In M. S. Micozzi (Ed.), *Fundamentals of complementary and alternative medicine* (pp. 225–230). New York: Churchill Livingstone.

Miura, K. (1989). The revival of Qi: Qigong in contemporary China. In L. Kohn (Ed.), *Taoist meditation and longevity techniques* (pp. 331–362). Ann Arbor, MI: Center for Chinese Studies, the University of Michigan.

Ohnuki-Tierney, E. (1984). *Illness and culture in contemporary Japan: An anthropological view.* Cambridge: Cambridge University Press.

Reid, D. (1994). *The complete book of Chinese health and healing.* Boston: Shambhala.

Sakade, Y. (1989). Longevity techniques in Japan: Ancient sources and contemporary studies. In L. Kohn (Ed.), *Taoist meditation and longevity techniques* (pp. 1–40). Ann Arbor, MI: Center for Chinese Studies, the University of Michigan.

Shin, K. R. (2001). Developing perspectives on Korean nursing theory: The influences of Taoism. *Nursing Science Quarterly, 14*(4), 346–353.

Shirahama, K., & Inoue, E. (2001). Spirituality in nursing from a Japanese perspective. *Holistic Nursing Practice, 15*(3), 63–72.

Tedesco, F. (1999). Abortion in Korea. In D. Keown (Ed.), *Buddhism and abortion* (pp. 121–155). Honolulu: University of Hawaii Press.

Torsch, V. L., & Ma, G. (2000). Cross-cultural comparison of health perceptions, concerns, and coping strategies among Asian and Pacific Islander American elders. *Qualitative Health Research, 10*(4), 471–490.

Ulett, G. A., & Han, J. (1998). Traditional and evidence-based acupuncture: History, mechanisms, and present status. *Southern Medical Journal, 91*(12), 1115–1121.

Umehara, T. (1994). Descartes, brain death and organ transplants: A Japanese view. *New Perspectives Quarterly, 11*(1), 25–29.

Wiseman, N. (trans.). (1995). *Fundamentals of Chinese medicine: Zhone Yi Xue Hji Chu.* Brookline, MA: Paradigm Publications.

Wong, T. K. S., & Pang, S. M. C. (2000). Holism and caring: Nursing in the Chinese health care culture. *Holistic Nursing Practice, 15*(1), 12–21.

Recommended Readings

Brannigan, M. C. (2000). *Striking a balance: A primer in traditional Asian values.* New York: Seven Bridges Press.

Clarke, J. J. (2000). *The Tao of the west: Western transformation of Taoist thought.* London: Routledge.

Eck, D. L. (2002). *A new religious America: How a Christian country has become the world's most religiously diverse nation.* New York: Harper.

Hinnells, J. R., & Porter, R. (Eds.). (1999). *Religion, health and suffering.* London: Kegan Paul International.

Mitchell, D. W. (2002). *Buddhism: Introducing the Buddhist experience.* New York: Oxford University Press.

Resources

American Association of Oriental Medicine
433 Front Street, Catasauqua, PA 18032
Phone: (610) 266-1433; (888) 500-7999
http://www.aaom.org/

Buddhanet
Buddha Dharma Education Association Incorporated, P.O. Box K1020, Haymarket, Sydney
NSW 2000 Australia
http://www.buddhanet.net/
Buddhist information and education network.

National Center for Complementary and Alternative Medicine (NCCAM)
National Institutes of Health
Department of Health and Human Services, Bethesda, MD 20892
http://nccam.nih.gov/
Official site for the National Center of Complementary and Alternative Medicine; connects consumers with the most current and reliable information on CAM.

The Pluralism Project
Harvard University, 201 Vanserg Hall, 25 Francis Avenue, Cambridge, MA 02138
Phone: (617) 496-2481
Fax: (617) 496-2428
http://www.pluralism.org/index.php
The Pluralism Project was developed by Diana L. Eck at Harvard University to study and document the growing religious diversity of the United States, with a special view to its new immigrant religious communities.

Wabash Center Guide to Internet Resources for Teaching and Learning in Theology and Religion: World Religions
Wabash Center, 301 W. Wabash Avenue, Crawfordsville, IN 47933
Phone: (765) 361-6047; (800) 655-7117
Fax: (765) 361-6051
Religion in China, http://www.wabashcenter.wabash.edu/Internet/china.htm
The Wabash Center for Teaching and Learning in Theology and Religion seeks to strengthen and enhance education in North American theological schools, colleges and universities.

13

The Role of the Nurse in the Spiritual Journey

Kristen L. Mauk

At the end of this chapter, the reader will be able to:
- Describe the relationships among person, nurse, health, and environment.
- Identify role components of the professional nurse.
- Identify role components of the professional advanced practice nurse.
- Discuss four essential processes that nurses use to promote the health of their patients.
- Discuss how nurses work within role components and through various processes to promote the spiritual health of individuals, families, and communities.
- Use the Valparaiso University College of Nursing model to analyze several given case studies.
- Describe the nurse–patient covenant.
- List several settings in which nurses may provide spiritual care.

environment
health
nurse
person
professional nursing

> . . . to redefine spiritual care, we do not need a watered-down version of past religious practices but a broader grasp of man's present search for meaning and a practical way of integrating spiritual care into everyday nursing.
>
> *Dickinson, 1975, p. 1789*

Nurses have the unique privilege of being health care providers likely to be present at the most significant, and frequently the most challenging, points in the life journeys of their patients. When one considers the nursing role, one realizes that nurses provide care during birth, in early childhood and school, through sickness and disease, and at death. Across the lifespan, nurses work with patients in various encounters: wellness checkups, community education seminars, hospitalizations, emergency procedures, home care treatments, illnesses of loved ones, care of aging parents, and deaths of friends and family members. Sharing in the life journey certainly has strong spiritual significance and implications. Other people may participate in these processes, but not in the same intimate way that nurses do, and rarely is the same close family member or friend present for each of these momentous life experiences. Although the nurse may not have the same "name" at each occasion, he or she remains the same presence of calm, patience, knowledge, and caring.

The importance of the intimate, professional, and educated care that nurses provide across the lifespan of patients cannot be overestimated. Nurses are present during many of the hallmarks of patients' lives. As individuals, families, and communities travel through life's difficult spiritual impasses, nurses join them to provide comfort, help, guidance, and support. The sharing of such critical life experiences underscores the crucial role that the nursing profession plays in the lives of many people.

The person cannot be separated from his or her spiritual self. Truly, the spirit is the core of the person. Thus, spiritual care is a part of nursing care that is integral (and perhaps even central) to all other aspects. The nurse vitally contributes to spiritual care of the person and, via the nursing process, provides competent care by working within various role components, often across multiple settings. Unit III discusses each step of the nursing process as it relates to spiritual care. However, to assist nurses to develop a skill set related to the spiritual care of patients, this chapter discusses spiritual care as though it were a separate dimension of practice.

Although it is assumed that readers of this text have a general grasp of the nursing process and the role of the nurse, the way in which nursing practice is conceptualized may vary among individuals, curricula, institutions, or facilities. Theoretical models can help explain the part that professional nurses play in care, guiding, focusing, and directing practice. This chapter presents a brief overview of a model developed by faculty at Valparaiso University (VU) College of Nursing (Valparaiso, IN) to illustrate the many role components and processes that professional nurses use, and how this model may help guide spiritual care across the lifespan. It gives enough information to illustrate the usefulness of such a framework for practice, but it is beyond the scope of this chapter to engage in deeper theoretical discussions.

In addition, nurses care for people in various settings. Whether they encounter people in the hospital, the community, the home, long-term health care facilities, or in a congregation, nurses use a unique skill set to provide quality spiritual care. Realizing that the spiritual needs of individuals and families may vary as widely as the settings in which they are found is the beginning of spiritual sensitivity.

OVERVIEW OF THE MODEL

✚ The mission of the Valparaiso University College of Nursing is to prepare critically inquiring, competent, and professional nurses who embrace truth and learning and who respect Christian values while promoting health for persons in dynamic health care environments. Such environments may be spiritually diverse, although the particular model discussed in this chapter is based on Judeo-Christian values.

Given its mission, the VU College of Nursing's Model of Professional Nursing (Figure 13-1) may be useful to understanding the roles of the nurse in spiritual care. The model incorporates the four metaparadigm concepts considered basic to any nursing framework: nurse, person, health, and environment. These four concepts are interconnected in a dynamic, ever-changing milieu influenced by a host of factors, such as socioeconomics, politics, and culture. A discussion of each concept precedes an examination of spiritual applications related to the model. Box 13.1 includes definitions of each term.

Four concentric, overlapping circles on the left side of the model represent the professional nurse. Each circle signifies a role component. The common portion of the role components forms the core of nursing, which consists of the ethical principles and values that guide nurses. These principles are based on the arts, sciences, and humanities. The core demonstrates that nurses have a scientific and ethical basis for practice.

Surrounding these role components are four essential processes that nurses use daily: critical thinking, communication, change, and lifelong learning. Each process is discussed in more detail later in this chapter.

Health is the entity that brings the nurse and client together for interaction. Thus, health is in the middle of the model to represent that connection, which is influenced by the nurse and the person, as well as the environment.

The person appears as three concentric circles and open systems. The person may be an individual, family, or community. Central to the person is a core of values and beliefs. Note that, because nurses also are persons, they come to their profession with core values and beliefs that influence their practice and sense of self.

Surrounding the entire interaction of person and nursing through health is the environment. Numerous factors influence the environment, as reflected in the model.

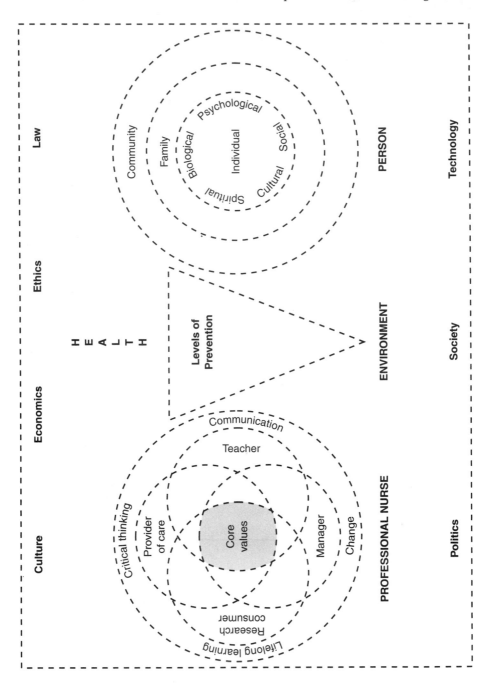

FIGURE 13.1. Valparaiso University College of Nursing's model for professional nursing.

BOX 13.1 Definitions of Major Model Concepts
Professional nursing is the process by which nurses prepared at the baccalaureate level interact with persons in the dynamic context of the environment to achieve health. **Health** is both a dynamic process and a state. As a process, health is movement toward a sense of well-being. As a state, health can be measured by personal and professional standards. The professional nurse interacts with the person using primary, secondary, and tertiary prevention strategies to improve health. The professional **nurse** uses ethical principles and values to integrate knowledge from the arts and sciences to provide competent care. He or she assumes the role components of provider of care, teacher, manager, and research consumer, using the processes of communication, critical thinking, change, and lifelong learning. **Environment** is the dynamic context in which the nurse interacts with the person. Factors influencing the environment include culture, economics, ethics, law, politics, society, and technology. **Persons** are individuals, families, or communities. Individuals are holistic beings with biologic, psychological, social, cultural, and spiritual dimensions. Families are self-defined groups of individuals who share biologic, psychological, social, cultural, or spiritual dimensions. Communities are groups of individuals or families who share common characteristics and work toward a common goal.

(From the College of Nursing at Valparaiso University, Valparaiso, Indiana, 2003. Used with permission of the faculty of the College.)

Examples include intangible elements such as culture, ethics, law, politics, society, and technology.

This entire milieu of systems is constantly changing and interacting. It forms one picture of professional nursing that illustrates how to provide spiritually competent care.

Role Components of the Professional Nurse

As identified in the VU model and discussed in detail in this chapter, the four role components of professional nursing include provider of care, teacher, manager, and research consumer. Case Studies 13.1 to 13.3 provide an opportunity for readers to use critical thinking skills to answer questions related to nurse–patient interactions rooted in the four role components at the primary, secondary, and tertiary levels of prevention. For example, Case Study 13-1 relates to primary prevention, or addressing a problem before it starts. The reader may focus on application of the role components of the professional nurse. Case Study 13-2 provides a scenario in which an APN must make some critical assessments in an acute care (secondary prevention) emergency. The reader should be able to identify application of the role components

CASE STUDY 13.1 Primary Prevention Strategies

Judy is a staff nurse on an oncology unit assigned to teach an inservice on spiritual assessment to her co-workers as part of her clinical ladder requirements. Her nurse manager suggests that Judy focus on teaching the staff how to prevent Spiritual Distress because this area has been neglected on their unit. Judy is having some difficulty devising a way to fit this into a 30-minute inservice and still make the discussion informative and interesting.

Critical Thinking
(Use the model to answer some of these questions.)

1. How should Judy begin to plan her inservice? Is this assignment realistic for a staff nurse?
2. What information would be important for Judy to include? What role components will Judy use for this task? What specific processes will she need to use?
3. What are some ways that Judy will instruct the staff to prevent Spiritual Distress? What other advice would you give to Judy in this situation?

CASE STUDY 13.2 Secondary Prevention Strategies

A woman of Indian descent brings her young son to the emergency department (ED) for treatment of a persistent stomach ache. The ED physician calls in the pediatric surgeon for a consultation. The surgeon suspects a life-threatening intestinal disorder that requires immediate corrective surgery, but he cannot make a definitive diagnosis until after a barium enema examination is done. The mother becomes hysterical and vehemently states that she will not allow her son to have "that test" done. The physician bluntly tells her, "If your son has what I think he does and we do not get that test and operate, he will be dead in 6 hours." The mother refuses to sign the consent form. The physician is irate, suspecting cultural or spiritual taboos as the reason for refusal of treatment.

The APN manager working in the ED is asked to speak with the mother. "Why do you not wish your son to have this test?" she asks the hysterical mother. The mother replies that her best friend's baby had recently come into the same hospital for a "tummy ache," and that they had done a barium enema on him, and he had died. The APN uses this opportunity to educate the mother about the test and its purpose, as well as the surgery that would need to be performed to save the child's life if the test confirms the physician's diagnosis. The APN gives the mother time to ask questions and answers each. The mother then agrees to the performance of the test and also to the subsequent surgery to save her son.

(Case Study continues on page 195)

CASE STUDY 13.2 Secondary Prevention Strategies (continued)

Critical Thinking

1. What is the major problem in this situation? What is the primary concern?
2. How could the physician have handled things differently?
3. What did the APN do that was most therapeutic? What role component did the APN most use? How did she implement the role components?
4. How does this situation relate to spirituality or spiritual assessment?
5. Were cultural or spiritual beliefs a factor in this situation? Why or why not?
6. What types of distress are present in this scenario? Are any additional interventions indicated?

---

of the APN. In Case Study 13.3, family members must deal with an elderly woman's decision to ignore medical treatment for terminal cancer (an example of tertiary prevention, or treatment of a condition that requires rehabilitation). The patient's decision not to seek care reflects the influence of environmental factors. Using the model as a guide, the reader can respond logically to the accompanying critical thinking questions.

Provider of Care

As a provider of care, the nurse may perform hands-on, direct physical care of the patient. Providing spiritual care is just as necessary but usually less direct than giving a bath or administering medication. The nurse will need to plan spiritual care just as he or she plans physical care. He or she can use the nursing process, as described in the rest of this unit, for this purpose. A brief example of each phase follows.

Assessment. The nurse will need to assess the person's spiritual status. Various tools are available for this purpose, but certain questions are common. Chapter 14 discusses a few applicable models and tools. Assessment generally involves interviewing and observing. Interview questions should be open ended and culturally and spiritually sensitive. Observations should include objective and subjective notes. The nurse should collect as much data as possible.

Nursing Diagnosis. From the assessment data, the nurse formulates a nursing diagnosis. For example, perhaps the assessment data reveal that the person is angry with God or shows signs of Spiritual Distress (Carpenito - Moyet, 2004), or perhaps the patient expresses a lack of concern regarding his or her spirituality (Spiritual Ambivalence).

Planning. Goal setting and planning follow the formulation of nursing diagnoses. One goal for the person experiencing Spiritual Distress would be to verbalize concerns and fears. A goal for the person with Spiritual Ambivalence might be to explore his or her place on the spiritual journey.

Implementation. Next, the nurse will implement appropriate interventions. Examples might include applying the therapeutic use of self, using the processes of com-

CASE STUDY 13.3 Tertiary Prevention Strategies

Ethel, an 86-year-old woman, is a widow with two children and five grand-children. Many months ago, Ethel noticed a lump in her breast but chose to ignore it, despite increased enlargement, hardness, tenderness, and eventually large amounts of purulent discharge from the breast mass. Because she highly values her independence and ability to make her own decisions, Ethel did not report these symptoms to her physician. Suspecting that her condition was serious, she purposefully hid her discomfort from family members by wearing baggy clothing to disguise physical changes in her breast, and withdrew socially to avoid questions.

When the pain became too great to manage on her own, Ethel revealed her condition to her inquiring adult grandson, who advised her to seek immediate medical care. Ethel is admitted to the acute care hospital after resisting treatment for a persistent growth in her right breast. She receives a diagnosis of advanced metastatic and inoperable breast cancer. She refuses any medical treatment and opts for hospice care at home for the remainder of her life. She is determined not to go through a long hospitalization or costly treatment for any illness. She feels she is "ready to go to be with God."

Critical Thinking
(Use the model presented in this chapter to frame the answer to the following questions.)

1. What would the nurse's assessment of Ethel in the health care setting include? Would any additional assessments be necessary as she moves to the home setting?
2. Which of the role components of the nurse will be most important in providing end-of-life care for Ethel? Would the importance of the role components be any different if Ethel had chosen to try chemotherapy or radiation treatments?
3. What is the role of the family in Ethel's care?
4. How might the nurse assess Ethel's spiritual needs at this point in her life? How would the nurse ascertain Ethel's definition of health?
5. Which of the four critical processes in the model will the nurse use in planning care for Ethel? In implementing care? In evaluating care?
6. How is the person defined in this situation?
7. What factors may have influenced Ethel's decision not to report her symptoms when they first appeared?
8. Do any spiritual diagnoses pertain to this situation? What are some of the major end-of-life tasks that Ethel might need to accomplish?
9. How does the nurse provide spiritual support in this situation to Ethel? To her family? What spiritual struggles might the family be going through related to Ethel's choice not to seek treatment?

munication, including the spiritual leader as part of the health care team, and, especially, allowing the person to verbalize concerns.

Evaluation. As always, evaluation of the effectiveness of interventions related to the person's goals would include precise documentation in terms of desired outcomes (Box 13.2).

BOX 13.2 Meeting the Spiritual Needs of Patients

Uldnall, A. (1996). A critical analysis of nursing: Meeting the spiritual needs of patients. Journal of Advanced Nursing, 23, 138–144.

This article examines the lack of significant research in the area of nursing care related to spirituality. Many of the useful studies in the literature have occurred since 1980. Oldnall describes the difficulty with defining the term *spirituality* and how persons may not practice an organized religion but still have spiritual needs to address. The author also points out that nurses may feel ill prepared to address spiritual issues because this aspect of nursing education is often lacking. In addition, although many nursing theories mention spirituality, it is not a key aspect within most frameworks. These findings indicate a need to better prepare nurses to meet the spiritual needs of patients across the lifespan.

Nursing programs in the United States today appear to be making an effort to better incorporate spiritual content into their curricula. Funding in the fields of gerontology (through organizations such as the Hartford Foundation) and end-of-life care has increased awareness of the spiritual and cultural dimensions of practice. For example, the End-of-Life Nursing Education Consortium has put together an excellent collection of educational materials and references to improve care of the dying patient and family. These materials include specific information on cultural and religious views about dying and end-of-life care, assisting nurses to address these important issues. Certainly, as Oldnall suggests, nurses may be aware of patients' spiritual needs but feel unable to give spiritual care without adequate education. Some see spiritual care as the work of the chaplain or other religious leader, although nurses have consistently felt that one cannot separate the mind and body, suggesting that the nurse's role must by its very nature include a spiritual component. The nursing profession is addressing the fact that providing care for the soul and spirit is something that nurses have often done naturally when giving holistic care. Fortunately, in today's society, we have opportunities to learn within institutions of higher learning and from each other in the area of spirituality. Thus educated, nurses may truly give holistic care so that the entire person may experience healing: body, mind, and spirit.

Teacher

In the role component of teacher, the nurse has many opportunities to assist the person to learn new skills related to spirituality. Perhaps a person wishes to learn to pray or does not know how to study the *Bible*, *Qur'an*, or *Bhagavad-Gita* but during a crisis or illness feels the need to do so. Others may explore different religions if they have not obtained spiritual satisfaction from previous practices. The nurse is often in a position to discuss spiritual questions with patients. Nurses who have developed a level of expertise and comfort also may teach other nurses to provide spiritually competent care. For example, many parish nurses have additional education and experience in this area. Likewise, hospice nurses frequently address spiritual needs for patients at the end of life. Both types of nurses can provide insight to professionals working in other areas and should be sought as resources.

Manager

As a manager, the professional nurse may be called on to coordinate complex health care situations. Overlooking the spiritual needs of the person is common when his or her physical needs are obvious and overwhelming. Some persons may have lost touch with their spiritual selves. Some may no longer be involved in a faith community, although they wish to remain spiritually connected. Others may not practice a particular faith, yet they express a desire to enhance their spirituality. However, during illness many people wish to reconnect with spiritual support systems, and nurses are in an ideal position to facilitate the rekindling of such relationships.

The nurse as manager may be required to assist families in crisis or to make decisions about whom to involve in the health care team. Family members may have to make difficult choices about placing their relatives in long-term care or end-of-life treatment. These circumstances naturally impose spiritual dilemmas and distress. Spiritual uncertainty is common as people face difficult decisions or death. The astute manager will realize such feelings affect the entire family.

Research Consumer

As research consumers, nurses stay aware of current trends and continue to read scholarly publications related to their field of practice. In the area of spirituality, nurses should avail themselves of the many publications (e.g., *Journal of Christian Nursing*) that focus on this important dimension of health care. Nurses also can take advantage of seminars and workshops offered at local, regional, or national levels.

Role Components of the Advanced Practice Nurse

Advanced practice nurses (APNs) have at least a master's level education, with skills beyond those of the professional nurse. APNs are recognized as clinical nurse specialists, nurse practitioners, nurse midwives, or nurse anesthetists. Their role components suggest their higher level of practice and clinician, educator, leader, consultant, and researcher. Each of these components will be discussed briefly here as they relate to spiritual care in advanced practice nursing. Figure 13-2 provides a model for advanced practice nursing.

Clinician

Spiritual assessments are a critical, but often overlooked, part of detailed examination. As a clinician, the APN has cultivated advanced assessment skills to provide ho-

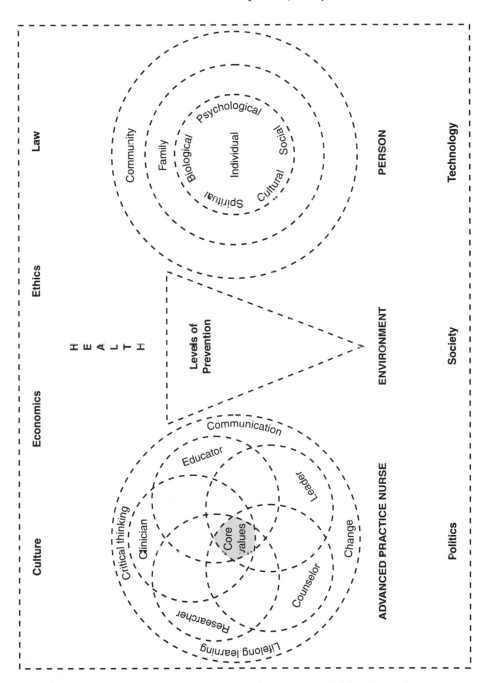

FIGURE 13.2. Valparaiso University College of Nursing's model for advanced practice nursing.

listic care. APNs often have different opportunities than do staff nurses to explore spiritual problems with patients. That is, APNs are sometimes in a unique position to address spiritual concerns. Nevertheless, the nature of their practice may limit severely the time available to do so. In some cases, they may see a link between physical ailments and spiritual crises. Astute clinicians will look for signs of Spiritual Distress and use strategies to address the underlying needs. See Case Study 13.2 for an example.

Educator

The role component of educator is interpreted as an expansion of the role of teacher. A teacher instructs, but an educator uses appropriate theories to skillfully apply the process of education. Thus, APNs are expected to have more teaching expertise than are nurses without graduate education. APNs addressing spiritual care needs may educate staff, nursing students, or both in this area. They also may be called upon to speak as members of bureaus or conferences related to the subject. As an educator, the APN is in an ideal position not only to incorporate spiritual assessment techniques into practice, but also to teach others to do the same.

Leader

As a leader, the APN takes a proactive approach in providing spiritual care and encourages others to do the same. Any APN can use the leadership role component, even if he or she is not employed in a direct management position. APNs lead other staff and peers by example. By demonstrating the importance of spiritual care and competence in their own practice, APNs promote sensitivity to those issues in others. In addition, APNs often assume leadership positions that provide them with added opportunities to effect changes in policies and procedures.

Nurses with advanced education also should be politically active and maintain membership in professional organizations. Several nationally recognized organizations have specific goals to address the spiritual needs of patients and families. One such example is Nurses Christian Fellowship, an interdenominational group within the parent organization of Intervarsity Christian Fellowship, which provides excellent resources and support for nurses focusing on spiritual care. Chapters 10 to 12 provide several Web sites related to the Eastern religions, which also might assist nurses in exploring current issues and connecting with appropriate organizations.

Consultant

The role component of consultant is important in the spiritual lives of patients and families. APNs possess the advanced education to act as professional resources for those having spiritual struggles during illness or disease. In addition, patients commonly seek from such nurse experts advice on many health-related topics. APNs should be familiar with the spiritual resources within their communities to more effectively provide information when asked. The role components of consultant and educator may overlap, as seen in the VU model (see Figure 13-2). Community leaders may seek the advice of APNs when planning programs for various groups or ask APNs to speak in faith-based settings based on their expertise. The APN who is knowledgeable about spiritual health and well-being is a valuable resource for faith-based communities.

Researcher

The role component of researcher at the APN level of practice generally is considered to encompass not only being a savvy consumer, but also actively engaging in research. With a master's level of preparation, nurses may serve as members of research teams, provide clinical expertise in research studies, and suggest research ideas and questions. Nurses with doctorates are prepared to design, conduct, analyze, and evaluate research. Thus, nurses who hold advanced degrees conduct most nursing research. APNs not only should be aware of data related to spiritual topics, but also should formulate hypotheses and researchable questions based on experience and practice.

Processes Used in Professional Nursing

According to the VU model, four major processes help guide professional nursing practice: critical thinking, communication, change, and lifelong learning.

Critical Thinking

Critical thinking is the ability to assess, reason, and arrive at a logical conclusion. The ability to think critically has become an essential expectation for nursing graduates. It is a skill that nurses can improve and hone through study and practice (Case Studies 13.1 to 13.3 include Critical Thinking questions).

Critical thinking is the foundation for appropriate and planned decision making in nursing. Within the spiritual realm, the ability to reason this way helps nurses to delve into the real problems patients are facing. Ethical decision making, a skill all nurses must develop, also involves critical thinking. Chapter 17 provides a detailed discussion of ethics related to spiritual care in nursing.

Communication

Communication is probably the most discussed process in nursing. Professional nurses must be good communicators to promote health in all dimensions. Scandrett-Hibdon (2000) states, "A counseling approach that makes the client's self-discovery the key focus is the therapeutic communication process that builds a positive, supportive relationship so the client can explore his or her personal experience and behavior" (p. 234). In the area of spirituality, creating a trusting relationship and being a good listener are essential nursing tasks. Allowing persons to express their feelings of hopelessness, frustration, or anger at God and actively listening help open the doors of communication and facilitate implementation of the role components of nursing.

Communicating acceptance and conveying a nonjudgmental attitude are ways to break the barriers to promoting spiritual health and well-being. In addition to traditional forms of communication, there is the dimension of communication with one's supreme spiritual being—communicating on a higher spiritual plane. These intensely personal experiences create an even greater challenge in communicating about spiritual needs.

For many individuals, a time of physical illness also may be a time for potential spiritual growth. However, nurses must be aware that spiritual isolation may develop from these same circumstances. Nurses can use strategies to help persons integrate faith and health activities to enhance spiritual wellness (Solari-Twadell, 1999). These strategies are discussed in Chapter 15.

Change

Facilitating change is a challenging process for nurses but one that they practice regularly. Nurses ask patients to change their behavior, their lifestyles, and their habits. Doing so may require people to give up things that are special to them on many levels. Through change processes, nurses help patients embrace healthier lifestyles. Such change may require examination of a person's core beliefs and values. Although difficult, this process often is necessary to promote health. There may be instances when the nurse is called upon to set aside his or her own beliefs to support the patient's autonomy. In cases in which religious practices are negatively affecting the physical health of one or more people, the nurse may use change processes to help people examine the consequences of their decisions and the available options.

Lifelong Learning

Lifelong learning implies that nurses never stop accumulating knowledge. This process affects all the role components. To remain informed of current research, practice, educational programs, and techniques, nurses must continue to expand their knowledge base. For example, an APN would not be prepared to act as a consultant without expertise in the area under question. Many nurses hold certification in their specialty field. Maintenance of those credentials requires continued education through several modalities, including publishing articles, accumulating continuing education credits, and pursuing an advanced degree.

Because many nurses report feeling underprepared to meet the spiritual needs of patients, lifelong learning would include pursuing knowledge on this subject. Doing so could take the form of attending a conference on spiritual care, reading a book or article on the subject, obtaining a certificate in parish nursing, or even discussing areas of weakness with an experienced role model. APNs who hold academic positions can promote lifelong learning in their students by including content on spiritual care in course work and encouraging students to continue to pursue expertise in that area.

THE NURSE–PATIENT COVENANT

The nurse–patient relationship is inherently one of trust. The term *covenant* derives from a Hebrew word meaning "binding agreement." In the first testament of the Bible, God's covenant with Israel was this type of pact. According to O'Brien (1999), the nurse–patient relationship suggests a type of covenant that may be viewed as sacred. Many experts on spirituality in nursing believe that the nurse is called to a ministry of service. Indeed, many nurses report that this vocation is a God-given calling (Barnum, 1996; O'Brien).

According to O'Brien (1999), the following theological and pastoral concepts related to covenants are applicable to the nurse–patient relationship:

- *Bonds of loyalty and responsibility.* Nurses and patients enter an unspoken arrangement of trust. The nurse is expected to be loyal to the patient and to take responsibility for his or her care.
- *Mutual obligations.* Similarly, the patient is expected to be honest in reporting symptoms and feelings to the nurse. Doing so is part of the expected mutual obligations of respect, loyalty, and honesty.

- *No conditions put on faithfulness.* The nurse is expected never to abandon the patient, regardless of personal feelings or difficulties. That is, the patient always should be able to count on the nurse to treat him or her respectfully and to act in his or her best interests, advocating on the patient's behalf. This is unconditional.
- *No expectation of a return for good services.* In addition, nurses do not expect to be rewarded for doing their work. It is their duty, responsibility, and professional obligation to provide nursing care without expecting additional reward.

Of course, not all nurses enter the profession feeling that nursing is a calling. Some choose nursing for nonspiritual reasons, such as money or the desire to work with people. Regardless of whether one agrees with the concept that the nurse–patient relationship is a sacred covenant, traditions such as saying the Florence Nightingale Pledge at nursing convocations have long served as a means to demonstrate the seriousness with which nurses enter into the intimate task of caring for others.

SETTINGS ALONG THE SPIRITUAL JOURNEY

If one views the person as being on a spiritual journey, then there may be many stops along the way, and the person may traverse some rough terrain. The settings in which persons with spiritual needs may be found are many. Familiarity with the various places where nurses may provide spiritual care is helpful. This section and Box 13.3 discuss some such settings. The short answer is nurses may provide spiritual care whenever and wherever persons are.

It is interesting to note that, although nurses in some settings may not always have the facilities or equipment available to provide the desired physical care for pa-

---

BOX 13.3   Settings in Which Nurses May Provide Spiritual Care

Acute care hospital	Occupational health clinics in
Adult day care	large factories
Assisted living	Outpatient services
Emergency air transport	Patient's home
Faith-based communities	Physician or nurse practitioner's
(e.g., church, synagogue,	office
parish)	Rehabilitation units
Group homes	Residential
Home health care	Retirement communities
Homeless shelters	School-based or community clinics
Hospice	Senior living apartments
Military bases	Skilled nursing facilities
Mission field	Subacute care facilities
Nursing homes	Wellness camps

tients, they can still provide quality spiritual care. The setting in which a person is found or placed often profoundly affects his or her sense of spiritual well-being. Nurses may identify various needs related to different settings for health care. A few are discussed here.

Acute Care Settings

When patients enter the health care system, it is often through acute care hospitals. Often, an emergency brings a person into the hospital. In this setting, nurses should expect patients to experience fear of the unknown, perhaps related to the uncertainty of their situation as they wait for a medical diagnosis. In such cases, nurses will foster hope for a positive prognosis, allow the person to express fears and frustrations, and help to bolster the support systems available.

Long-term Care Settings

When an acute crisis ends, or the problem is long term or chronic, the nurse may see patients in rehabilitation, subacute care, or extended care facilities. Facing a chronic illness or disease requires the development of a different set of coping skills—ones that many patients or families will not yet have developed. They commonly have feelings of anger, bargaining, and other forms of grief when facing a loss. Depression is common among those with long-term health problems. Anxiety, frustration, and hopelessness often loom with progressive and degenerative health concerns. Patients may express feelings of chronic sorrow with each exacerbation or setback.

Nurses will need a long-term plan for such chronic problems. A quick spiritual fix is no more appropriate than is a quick physical solution in such cases. Nurses should work with patients and their families and discuss goals to meet these complex and complicated needs. Persons who are traversing a difficult and uphill road in their physical lives also may be struggling spiritually. Nurses are in a unique position to ease the journey by addressing care holistically.

Rehabilitation

Patients in rehabilitation settings may be particularly open to discussing spiritual needs. Hope is often the "thing" that patients say keeps them going and helps them through difficult times (Easton, Rawl, Zemen, Kwiatkowski, & Burczyk, 1995; Gaskins & Forte, 1995). The nature of rehabilitation promotes the concept of hope because the goal is to maximize the patient's function to promote the highest level of holistic independence possible. Most patients in rehabilitation will return home upon discharge, so even though a long-term problem may exist, the general tone of such units is encouraging and cheerful. Nurses can use this knowledge to integrate spiritual concerns into the plan of care. Patients in rehabilitation are often ready to learn, and the environment is conducive to maximizing potential in every facet of the person's life (Derstine & Drayton-Hargrove, 2001; Easton, 1999).

Nursing Homes

Most people living in nursing homes are elderly and have unique spiritual needs related to both age and their surroundings. Older adults generally realize that mortality is a concept to deal with, particularly as they begin to lose friends within their social circle to age-related problems and begin to grieve those losses. With advanced age comes the tendency toward a process called *life review.* That is, as people approach the end of life, they reflect upon what their life has meant, how it has counted, and what they have contributed. *Reminiscence therapy,* or facilitating the recollection of positive memories, has been shown effective among older adults for this reason, even among those with degenerative brain disorders such as Alzheimer's disease (Eliopoulos, 2000). Reminiscence helps people reflect on what they have contributed to their family and society. Nurses may assist persons with this reflection process by relating reminiscence to the person's spiritual journey.

A significant number of people living in long-term care facilities are young and usually dealing with severe physical problems, such as cerebral palsy, brain injury, spinal cord injury, or multiple sclerosis. Addressing the needs of younger adults who have little hope of returning to a normal home and family environment because of complex physical health care demands is indeed a challenge.

Whether young or old, those with illness or long-term physical limitations face many challenges. They may have to fight feelings of powerlessness and depression. Nurses often help these patients struggle to make sense of their situations and to find meaning through crisis or suffering. Fostering hope, providing accurate information, and strengthening a person's support systems are interventions that all nurses can use; Chapter 15 provides a detailed discussion of numerous strategies the nurse can use in various settings. Communication about upbringing, church attendance, significant religious events (e.g., baptism, first communion, bar mitzvah, pilgrimages to holy cities, practice of self-denial and transcendence) also can help the person gain perspective on the spiritual self. Each of these rites or rituals depends on the person's religious beliefs. Unit II provides greater detail about the beliefs of many Eastern and Western religions and their practices.

Nurses also may use models such as those set forth by Orem (1995) or Miller (2000) to bolster a person's power resources. Certainly, APNs with knowledge of theory utilization in practice would be prepared to design a plan that would promote the spiritual wellness of those who perceive themselves as living in a hopeless situation. In the following chapters, specific suggestions will be discussed for assisting persons and their families through difficult times.

Hospice

Hospice is a unique setting in which nurses generally are compelled to provide spiritual care because patients at the end of life usually seek resolution and a peaceful death. One of the most defining aspects of hospice care is that patients are known to have terminal conditions. Thus, nurses who choose to work in hospice develop an expertise in caring for those struggling with the last months, weeks, days, and hours of this life. Inherently a time of great spiritual reflection and introspection, the end of life in hospice may take place in the acute care hospital, long-term care setting, or home. Hospice nurses work within an interdisciplinary team to assist dying patients and their family to achieve a peaceful death, as well as to provide bereavement support to the family after the person's death. For nurses who wish to include a strong spiritual component in their practice, hospice provides many opportunities.

PERSONAL REFLECTIONS

- How do you see yourself implementing the various role components of the nurse?
- Are you comfortable within each of the areas (provider of care, teacher, research consumer, and manager) with regard to spiritual care?
- Are you comfortable with the processes of communication, critical thinking, change, and lifelong learning? Which of these processes do you feel most proficient in? What is one strategy you can do to improve in the area in which you need improvement?
- How do you see yourself implementing the various role components of the APN within your own practice?
- Are you comfortable with acting as a clinician, educator, researcher, consultant, and leader in the realm of spiritual care? In what areas are you strongest? In what areas do you need the most improvement? What one thing can you do to strengthen your area(s) needing improvement?

Key Points

- Nurses provide holistic care to individuals, families, and communities, and such care includes the spiritual dimension.
- Both the professional nurse and the advanced practice nurse need to develop skills in providing spiritual care.
- By using the role components of nursing practice via therapeutic processes, the nurse can promote health for the person.
- The professional nurse assumes the role components of provider of care, teacher, manager, and research consumer, using the processes of communication, critical thinking, change, and lifelong learning to promote spiritual health as well as physical health.
- The advanced practice nurse assumes the role components of clinician, leader, educator, consultant, and researcher.
- Nurses may practice in a variety of settings, but the role components and processes remain relatively constant.

References

Barnum, B. S. (1996). *Spirituality in nursing: From traditional to new age*. New York: Springer.

Carpenito-Moyet, L. J. (2004). *Nursing diagnosis: Application to clinical practice* (10th ed.). Philadelphia: Lippincott Williams & Wilkins

Derstine, J., & Drayton-Hargrove, S. (2001). *Comprehensive rehabilitation nursing*. Philadelphia: WB Saunders.

Dickinson, C. (1975). The search for spiritual meaning. *American Journal of Nursing, 75*(10), 1989–1793.

Easton, K. L. (1999). *Gerontological rehabilitation nursing*. Philadelphia: WB Saunders.

Easton, K., Rawl, S., Zemen, D., Kwiatkowski, S., & Burczyk, B. (1995). The effects of nursing follow-up on the coping strategies used by rehabilitation patients after discharge. *Rehabilitation Nursing Research, 4*(4), 119–127.

Eliopoulos, C. (2000). *Gerontological nursing* (5th ed.). Philadelphia: Lippincott Williams & Wilkins.

Gaskins, S., & Forte, L. (1995). The meaning of hope: Implications for nursing practice and research. *Journal of Gerontological Nursing, 21*(3), 17–24.

Miller, J. F. (2000). *Coping with chronic illness: Overcoming powerlessness*. Philadelphia: FA Davis.

O'Brien, M. E. (1999). *Spirituality in nursing: Standing on holy ground*. Sudbury, MA: Jones and Bartlett.

Orem, D. (1995). *Nursing: Concepts of practice*. St. Louis: Mosby.

Scandrett-Hibdon, S. (2000). Therapeutic communication: The art of helping. In B. M. Dossey, L. Keegan, & C. E. Guzzetta (Eds.), *Holistic nursing: A handbook for practice* (pp. 233–246). Gaithersburg, MD: Aspen.

Solari-Twadell, P. Λ. (1999). In P. Λ. Solari-Twadell & M. A. McDermott (Eds.), *Parish nursing: Promoting whole person health within faith communities*. Thousand Oaks, CA: Sage.

Recommended Readings

Albom, M. (1999). *Tuesdays with Morrie*. New York: Doubleday.

Dossey, L. (1996). *Prayer is good medicine*. New York: Harper Collins.

Ferrell, B. R. (1996). *Suffering*. Sudbury, MA: Jones and Bartlett.

Young-Mason, J. (1997). *The patient's voice: Experiences of illness*. Philadelphia: FA Davis.

Resources

American Holistic Nurses Association
P.O. Box 2130, Flagstaff, AZ 86003-2130
Phone: (800) 278-AHNA
http://www.ahna.org

American Nurses Association
600 Maryland Avenue, SW, Suite 100 West, Washington, DC 20024
Phone: (800) 274-4ANA
http://www.ana.org

Applied Vision
P.O. Box 1344, San Carlos, CA 94070-7344
Phone: (650) 591-9307
http://www.appliedvision.com
The Caring Helper: *Videotape set and workbook to learn skills in working with people who have life-threatening illness, those who are dying, or the bereaved.*

The Catholic Communication Campaign
3321 Fourth Street NE, Washington DC 20017
Phone: (800) 235-8722
Final Blessings: *program that examines the spiritual dimensions of the dying person.*

Medical Audiovisual Communication Inc.
Niagara Falls, NY 1998
E-mail: DWC@MABC.com
A Practical Guide to Communication Skills in Clinical Practice: *CD-ROMs with pocket-size guide.*

14

Assessment and Diagnosis in Spiritual Care

Kevin Massey, George Fitchett, and Patricia A. Roberts

LEARNING OBJECTIVES

At the end of this chapter, the reader will be able to:
- Discuss the importance of assessment in spiritual care.
- Distinguish the levels of inquiry into spiritual health.
- Identify different concrete models of assessment.
- Recognize how various nursing diagnoses apply when providing spiritual care nursing.
- Apply models of spiritual screening, spiritual history taking, and spiritual assessment using the concrete example in this chapter's case study.

spiritual assessment   spiritual risk
Spiritual Distress   spiritual screening
spiritual history taking   spiritual well-being

Effective and quality health care is based on a sound practice of treating illness and disease with appropriate interventions. These interventions are determined through a rational process of assessment, observation, testing, and discovery. Nurses and physicians relieve a patient's symptoms while investigating the cause of illness. Upon discovery of the cause, they use medications or procedures that have been known to effect cure.

For many years, disciplines such as psychology and psychiatry were exceptions to this model, relying on more interpersonal means of discovery, such as the patient/therapist interview. Although personal interchanges and therapeutic relationships are still hallmarks of these disciplines, they also have developed complementary objective tools to assess, measure, and quantify conditions such as depression and anxiety.

Spiritual care is perhaps the last aspect of health care that has explored methods of measurement and assessment. The use of objective criteria and formal tools for spiritual assessment remains a matter of controversy within the field of professional spiritual care. Although nurses have contributed to the body of knowledge through research, there are no universally accepted standards for spiritual assessment.

The discipline of nursing has displayed continued interest in the pursuit of spiritual assessment. Nurses have been involved in developing important models of spiritual assessment. Nursing publications address spiritual care issues continuously, and a full understanding of the topics of spiritual care and spiritual assessment is essential for effective nursing practice. Through adequate assessment, nurses can formulate nursing diagnoses appropriate for patients.

This chapter presents the important issues regarding the measurement and assessment of spiritual conditions. It examines spiritual screening, spiritual history taking, and the fuller topic of spiritual assessment, allowing the reader to come to an understanding of how these activities contribute to patient care. The formulation of applicable nursing diagnoses for patients based on spiritual assessment is discussed.

IMPORTANCE OF ASSESSMENT IN SPIRITUAL CARE

Spiritual assessment has a central place in guiding and evaluating spiritual care. Overall assessment is necessary for caregivers to plan and implement holistic care. Assessment of the spiritual component is an equally important means of measurement and assessment. Assessment shows the skill of a profession in its own field. It demonstrates what members of the profession can see and what they can do to be contributing members of interdisciplinary teams. Assessment provides accountability to the interdisciplinary team of what nurses are doing in the midst of a total patient care plan. Finally, it provides a foundation for research that enables the field to evaluate its fundamental theories and practices.

Background of Assessment

A few years ago, several hospital chaplains were asked to describe their approaches to spiritual assessment (Emblen, unpublished study). The responses revealed great diversity in understanding and approach. For a few, the question was puzzling. Some did not know what assessment meant. Others were not aware of making assessments in their work because they simply followed institutional protocols and offered spiritual care to all patients and families. In contrast, one chaplain used a set of forms to guide patients through a self-assessment of faith using a model from Paul Pruyser, a physician whose book *The Minister as Diagnostician* (1976) formed one of the first models of spiritual assessment. Pruyser not only used an explicit method for spiritual assessment, but he also developed a set of guidelines for when he would use this tool and when he would not.

The chaplains in the survey were asked to describe how and when they made spiritual assessments. The approaches to spiritual assessment they described included a friendly greeting ("How are you today?"), a nondirective approach suggested by Carl Rogers (1957); and a direct approach ("I let them know who I am and what I represent, and I inquire how they think I can help."). There was a similar diversity when the chaplains were asked at what point they made a spiritual assessment. Some said, "Not at the first visit"; others said, "Constantly." One chaplain replied that he made an initial assessment "rapidly" to see whether to continue the visit.

The chaplains also were asked to describe the most common spiritual needs they encountered. Their responses included dynamic needs, some of which were explicitly religious (sinfulness, grace, revelation, reconciliation) and some of which were more psychosocial (alienation, loneliness, depression, hostility). They mentioned sacramental and ritual needs, such as anointing or communion. They also described the need for a relationship with the pastor.

Styles of Assessment

As demonstrated in the preceding discussion, spiritual caregivers incorporate various styles of spiritual assessment into their work. For the most part, models are informal and subjective. Subjective assessments may be useful to the person who uses them, especially if he or she is experienced. Nevertheless, other members of the care team cannot share such assessments. Thus, caregivers seem to work mysteriously, without the other team members being aware of their methods. Some caregivers may describe their assessment as being driven, or at least guided, by inspiration. Here again, such an assessment may be useful and credible to the person who claims to receive the inspiration, but no one else will be in a position to test or evaluate its accuracy.

Other caregivers use methods and styles of assessment that incorporate objective criteria, which they can document, measure, and share with the health care team to help others understand the importance of spiritual care interventions for their patients. Although this chapter highlights several models of these objective spiritual assessments, assessments performed by caregivers may be a mix of subjective approaches, inspiration, and objective analysis.

ASSESSMENT IN SPIRITUAL CARE: LEVELS OF INQUIRY INTO SPIRITUAL HEALTH

It is useful here to define clearly some different levels of assessment and their respective goals. Some refer to spiritual screening, spiritual history taking, and spiritual assessment interchangeably. In fact, each is a distinct activity with different goals that can build on one another. All are important interventions in providing spiritual care as a complement to health care.

To better understand the levels of spiritual investigation, one can form analogies between spiritual assessment and the provision of other types of nursing care. **Spiritual screening** is a basic examination to determine whether any conditions warrant further investigation. It is akin to such nursing activities as taking pulse or blood pressure. **Spiritual history taking** is similar to any other kind of history taking, such as family medical history, sexual history, or investigation into a patient's personal habits (e.g., diet). **Spiritual assessment** is a full and, in fact, invasive investigation to identify a suspected disease or condition. It is akin to some of the more advanced investigations or diagnostic tests, such as computed tomography (CT), magnetic resonance imaging (MRI), or angiogram.

These different levels of investigation are largely differentiated in terms of time and depth of inquiry. Spiritual screening is a brief intervention, ideally consisting of a few questions aimed at determining basic spiritual care needs and exploring how to satisfy them. It usually occurs upon admission, either through oral interview or a brief written survey.

Spiritual history taking is similar to spiritual screening but also distinct from it. This brief activity seeks to identify specific ways in which a patient's religious life, both past and present, affects his or her medical care. A nurse, chaplain, or physician could take a spiritual history. The findings are salient information to include in a patient's medical record.

Spiritual assessment is a full objective investigation of a patient's spiritual life and history. It is performed when specific aspects of a patient's spiritual life are presenting themselves as important to treating the patient's condition most effectively, especially in cases of suspected spiritual risk. Spiritual risk is defined more fully later in this chapter; also discussed is the urgency in identifying and treating spiritual risk.

Spiritual Screening

Basic spiritual screening seeks only to identify and categorize basic religious or spiritual needs. It can help identify whether a patient would benefit from more detailed exploration of spiritual issues. An admissions worker, chaplain, spiritual care volunteer, or nurse, depending on the setting, could conduct spiritual screening. A series of simple questions can form a spiritual screening activity. Box 14.1 provides an example.

Danger of Spiritual Risk

The single most important thing that providers can accomplish through spiritual screening is to identify spiritual risk. **Spiritual risk** is defined as being at risk for poor health outcomes as a result of underdeveloped, conflicted, overwhelmed, or negative spirituality. Focusing on a person's spiritual resources and spiritual needs provides another way to think about spiritual risk. Spiritual risk is having many spiritual needs, yet few spiritual resources with which to address them.

BOX 14.1 Spiritual Screening

- Do you wish to express a religious or spiritual identity or preference at this time?
- Do you belong to a formal religious group?
- Would you like your religious or spiritual community notified of your admission to hospital?
- Would any specific religious or spiritual needs or resources (e.g., religious reading material, candles, sacraments, prayer, prayer rugs) be helpful to you during your hospital stay?
- Do you have any concerns about which you would like to speak with a chaplain?

Evidence for Spiritual Risk

An example of the concept of screening for spiritual risk is found in Oxman, Freeman, and Manheimer's study (1995) of 232 older adults undergoing heart surgery. As indicated in Table 14.1, patients with greater impairment in activities of daily living (ADLs) and a history of previous cardiac surgery were at greater risk for not surviving 6 months after their last surgery. These risk factors probably come as no surprise. But many might be surprised by the next two risk factors. Patients with greater so

TABLE 14.1 Predictors of Mortality in Older Adults Undergoing Elective Heart Surgery

Variable	All Cases (n=232)	Patients who Died (n=21)
Age		
70+ y	110	15 (14%)
55-69 y	122	6 (5%)
Impairment in ADL		
Severe	28	8 (29%)
Not severe	204	13 (6%)
Previous cardiac surgery		
Yes	18	7 (39%)
No	214	14 (7%)
Participation in social groups		
No	135	17 (13%)
Yes	97	4 (4%)
Strength and comfort from religion		
None	74	12 (16%)
Little or great deal	158	9 (6%)

Percents reported are row percent.

cial isolation and those who reported they received no strength and comfort from religion also were at increased risk for not surviving 6 months after their surgery.

Some researchers correctly point to this study as demonstrating the positive benefits of finding strength and comfort in one's faith. The study also demonstrates the dangers of spiritual risk for the patients who reported they received no strength and comfort from religion. Further analysis of the data indicates that these patients have a threefold increase in risk for postoperative mortality compared with those who reported receiving a little or great deal of strength and comfort from religion. Viewed from this perspective, the study identified an important measure of spiritual risk for poor postoperative survival for older adult clients having heart surgery.

Benefits of Screening for Spiritual Risk

Spiritual screening can be an important means of identifying patients with spiritual risk because limitations are inherent in the three usual major ways that chaplains make decisions about which patients to visit: patient and family request, staff referrals, and regular new patient rounds. Patients with spiritual risk are less likely to request spiritual care for themselves. Staff may tend to refer only "religious" patients to see chaplains. New patient rounds are time consuming and not a reliable method of identifying patients with spiritual risk.

Interventions for Spiritual Risk

By implementing programs in which interdisciplinary teams use spiritual screening tools to identify and refer patients with potential spiritual risk, nurses and chaplains can reduce the time currently spent in case finding and increase the time available for spiritual care with patients with spiritual risk. Chaplains will have the time for intensive work with patients at spiritual risk if they can spend less time case finding. Using guided conversation, experiences of reconciliation, personal life storytelling, ritual experiences, and pastoral presence, chaplains can provide spiritual care that can address and reverse spiritual risk.

Spiritual risk is a complicated and serious condition that sometimes cannot be effectively reversed. Some cases of spiritual risk are so intractable that they are ultimately terminal. For example, one man experienced a chemical addiction that began after he accidentally killed his brother in a hunting accident. For the man, the inability to experience forgiveness contributed directly to his chemical addiction. Years of drug rehabilitation never assisted this patient, who spoke continuously of his sense of self-blame and guilt. Years of intensive spiritual care also failed to assist him to experience relief from his guilt. Advanced medical care could not heal this patient's damaged kidneys and liver. When this patient died, his situation could only be described as a terminal case of spiritual risk.

Fortunately, many cases of spiritual risk can be addressed and relieved. The use of screening for the timely identification of patients with spiritual risk contributes to the success of spiritual care.

Spiritual History Taking

Health care professionals have learned to leave their comfort zones in history taking, understanding that a full history of every aspect of a patient's life is crucial to a comprehensive care plan. For example, taking a sexual history often is uncomfortable at first for many clinicians, but clinicians routinely and appropriately incorporate sexual history into a full history. Likewise, spiritual history is appearing on the radar of healers who wish to understand their patients' needs as fully as possible.

Several models of spiritual history taking have appeared in recent years, most of which medical professionals, not spiritual care professionals, have developed. The specific goal of history taking is to capture salient information as a complement to other observable symptoms to form a comprehensive care plan. Such a care plan attends to any of the patient's spiritual needs and allows providers to understand how spiritual concerns can complement or complicate a patient's condition.

This chapter reviews three models of spiritual history taking: SPIRIT, FICA, and HOPE. Models such as these can be useful in organizing thoughts while seeking to gather important central information about a patient's spiritual life and how it may be involved in health. Through a spiritual history, a nurse or other health care provider may identify themes and issues that may point to a state of spiritual risk for which a patient may benefit from further spiritual assessment and spiritual care interventions to address the risk.

A nurse may develop other personal ways to organize a spiritual history taking effort. Any means of gathering the salient information is valid. As nurses become more accustomed to taking spiritual history, no doubt, other methods and means of recording information will arise.

SPIRIT Model

Dr. Todd Maugans (1996) presents a method of spiritual history taking based on the acronym SPIRIT (Box 14.2). He developed this model for physicians to use when considering spiritual issues with patients. Maugans offers some sample questions for each of the areas with which the model is concerned. Providers may need to tailor the questions outlined here as appropriate to the patient's cognitive development and cultural background.

S—Spiritual belief system
- What is your formal religious affiliation?
- Name or describe your spiritual belief system.

P—Personal spirituality
- Describe the beliefs and practices of your religion or personal spiritual system.
- Describe the beliefs or practices you do not accept. Do you accept or believe ... (specific tenet or practice)?
- What does your spirituality/religion mean to you?
- What is the importance of your spirituality/religion in daily life?

B O X 1 4 . 2   SPIRIT Model of Spiritual History Taking

S = Spiritual belief system
P = Personal spirituality
I = Integration and involvement in a spiritual community
R = Ritualized practices and restrictions
I = Implications for medical care
T = Terminal events planning (advance directives)

I—Integration with a spiritual community
- Do you belong to any spiritual or religious group or community? What is your position or role?
- What importance does this group have to you? Is it a source of support? In what ways?
- Does or could this group provide help in dealing with health issues?

R—Ritualized practices and restrictions
- Are there specific practices that you carry out as part of your religion/spirituality (e.g., prayer, meditation)?
- Are there certain lifestyle activities or practices that your religion/spirituality encourages or forbids? Do you comply? What significance do these practices and restrictions have to you?
- Are there specific elements of medical care that you forbid on the basis of religious/spiritual grounds?

I—Implications for medical care
- What aspects of your religion/spirituality would you like me to keep in mind as I care for you?
- Would you like to discuss religious or spiritual implications of health care?
- What knowledge or understanding would strengthen our relationship as physician and patient?
- Are there any barriers to our relationship based on religious or spiritual issues?

T—Terminal events planning
- As we plan for your care near the end of life, how does your faith affect your decisions?
- Are there particular aspects of care that you wish to forgo or have withheld because of your faith?

FICA Model

Puchalski and Romer (2000) developed a model based on the acronym FICA (Box 14.3) that assists in capturing vital information about a patient's spiritual and religious background. The FICA model is memorable and user friendly, while flexible enough for use with a diverse population. Some specific questions the nurse can use to discuss issues for each of the components are as follows:

- F: What is your faith or belief? Do you consider yourself spiritual or religious? What things do you believe in that give meaning to your life?

B O X 1 4 . 3   FICA Model of Spiritual History Taking

F = Faith or beliefs
I = Importance and Influence
C = Community
A = Address

- *I*: Is faith important in your life? What influences does it have on how you take care of yourself? How have your beliefs influenced your behavior during this illness? What role do your beliefs play in regaining your health?
- *C*: Are you part of a spiritual or religious community? Is this of support to you and how? Is there a person or group of people you really love or who are really important to you?
- *A*: How would you like me, your health care provider, to address these issues in your health care?

Figure 14-1 gives an example of a completed FICA assessment in a chart note.

HOPE Model

Drs. Gowri Anandarajah and Ellen Hight (Anandarajah & Hight, 2001) offer another model based on the acronym HOPE (Box 14.4). They present the following sample questions to accompany the model:

H = Sources of hope, meaning, comfort, strength, peace, love, and connection

We have been discussing your support systems. I was wondering, what is there in your life that gives you internal support? What are your sources of hope, strength, comfort, and peace? What do you hold on to during difficult times?

Spiritual History

F = *Southern Baptist*

I = *Pt's faith very important to her. She practices prayer regularly.*

C = *Pt belongs to a congregation who will visit her regularly in hospital.*

A = *Pt wishes to see a chaplain during stay. She states that regular prayer and spiritual conversation will help her cope. She invites persons caring for her to remember her in their prayers.*

I will refer pt to be seen by Spiritual Care staff to complement care.

Mary Stevens, RN

FIGURE 14-1 Sample spiritual history taken during admission according to the FICA model.

What sustains you and keeps you going? For some people, religious or spiritual beliefs act as a source of comfort and strength in dealing with life's ups and downs; is this true for you?

If answer is "Yes," go on to O and P questions.

If answer is "No," consider asking: Was it ever? If the answer is "Yes," ask: What changed?

O = Organized religion

Do you consider yourself part of an organized religion? How important is this to you? What aspects of your religion are helpful and not so helpful to you? Are you part of a religious or spiritual community? Does it help you? How?

P = Personal spirituality and practice

Do you have personal spiritual beliefs that are independent of organized religion? What are they? Do you believe in God? What kind of relationship do you have with God? What aspects of your spirituality or spiritual practices do you find most helpful personally (e.g., prayer, meditation, reading scripture, attending religious services, listening to music, hiking, communing with nature)?

E = Effects on medical care and end-of-life issues

Has being sick (or your current situation) affected your ability to do the things that usually help you spiritually? (Or affected your relationship with God?) Is there anything that I, as a nurse, can do to help you access the resources that usually help you? Are you worried about any conflicts between your beliefs and your medical situation, care, decisions? Would it be helpful for you to speak to a clinical chaplain/community spiritual leader? Are there any specific practices or restrictions I should know about in providing your medical care (e.g., dietary restrictions, use of blood products)?

If the patient is dying: How do your beliefs affect the kind of medical care you would like me to provide during the next few days/weeks/months?

Spiritual Assessment

Although spiritual screening and spiritual history taking offer important ways to assess patients, a spiritual assessment is indicated when more depth is desired. The goal of assessment, alluded to earlier, is to form a complete picture of a patient's spiritual condition. With such information, providers can give intentional and comprehensive treatment for a patient's spiritual condition, especially spiritual risk. No single model of assessment has been embraced as a standard. This chapter discusses the

---

BOX 14.4   HOPE Model of Spiritual History Taking

H = Sources of hope, meaning, comfort, strength, peace, love, and connection
O = Organized religion
P = Personal spirituality and practice
E = Effects on medical care and end of life issues

strengths and weaknesses of two spiritual assessment models: Pruyser's Model and the 7 × 7 Model.

Pruyser's "Model"

Paul Pruyser's 1976 book *The Minister as Diagnostician* is one of the most influential works on spiritual assessment. Ironically, Pruyser was not a pastor but a psychologist who had a strong interest in spiritual care and counseling. He frequently was a consultant to spiritual care and counseling training programs, professional organizations, and theological schools. Many in spiritual care knew him as a friend and colleague and respected him as a scholar and writer.

Quotes are around the word "Model" because Pruyser did not actually set out to create a specific model of spiritual assessment. His aim in writing *The Minister as Diagnostician* was not to teach pastors how to do spiritual assessment but to encourage them to be more deliberate about including spiritual assessment as part of their work. Although Pruyser did not intend for his book to become a manual for spiritual assessment, the seven themes he identifies in his fifth chapter have become the foundation of more specific models of spiritual assessment.

Pruyser frames his work as an effort to change pastors' self-deprecating description of themselves as jacks-of-all-trades and masters of none. In Pruyser's view, each professional discipline has a distinct perspective on the human condition. No one profession can claim to have the only real or true perspective. Rather, each profession has a partial view. The greater the number of different perspectives brought to a person's problems, the more likely it is to generate an adequate understanding of that person.

After the Second World War, Pruyser observed that pastors had no distinct diagnostic framework to contribute to the multidisciplinary dialogue occurring in health care. Rather, they seemed strongly attracted to the language of psychological diagnosis. When he talked with pastors, Pruyser reported they said "their basic theological disciplines were of little help to them in ordering their observations and planning their ameliorative moves" (1976, p. 21). This distressed Pruyser, who thought pastors ought to claim a distinct diagnostic perspective. To assist this process, he briefly reviewed the ways pastoral diagnosis was performed in earlier periods in the church. However, when he concluded this review, he criticized the authoritarian and legalistic approach to pastoral diagnosis it revealed. Turning to the modern period, Pruyser reviewed the influence of Carl Rogers' (1957) client-centered type of therapy on pastors. He saw Rogers' work as having contributed to pastors' lack of interest in pastoral diagnosis.

Pruyser believed that when people turned to pastors, they wanted to review their problems from a theological perspective. Yet, Pruyser acknowledged, pastors "have a hard time finding appropriate theological categories for approaching their patients and responding to their needs" (1976, p. 55). To help, Pruyser offered some "Guidelines for Pastoral Diagnosis" in Chapter 5 of his book. The guidelines are in the form of seven theological themes. Pruyser suggested that as pastors listen to their parishioners, they also listen for the ways the story the person shares relates to the themes. Box 14.5 lists Pruyser's seven themes and key elaborating questions for each theme.

Following his description of these themes, Pruyser (1976) described the relationship between the parties in the pastoral diagnostic process as a *diagnostic partnership*. For Pruyser, pastoral diagnosis did not mean labeling people. It meant assisting them in their process of spiritual self-assessment. Regarding the pastoral diagnostic process, Pruyser wrote, "The person is entitled to define for himself [sic], with the help of the expert he seeks out, the nature of his condition, his situation, his self, in the perspective which he finds most relevant" (p. 83). Throughout the rest of the

---

BOX 14.5   Pruyser's Guidelines for Pastoral Diagnosis

1. AWARENESS OF THE HOLY
- What, if anything, is sacred, revered
- Any experiences of awe or bliss; when; in what situations; any sense of mystery, of anything transcendent
- Any sense of creatureliness, humility, awareness of own limitations, any idolatry, reverence displaced to improper symbols

2. PROVIDENCE
- What is God's intention toward me?
- What has God promised me?
- Belief in cosmic benevolence related to capacity for trust
- Extent of hoping versus wishing

3. FAITH
- Affirming versus negating stance in life
- Able to commit self, to engage
- Open to world or constricted

4. GRACE OR GRATEFULNESS
- Kindness, generosity, the beauty of giving and receiving
- No felt need for grace or gratefulness
- Forced gratitude under any circumstances
- Desire for versus resistance to blessing

5. REPENTANCE
- The process of change from crookedness to rectitude
- A sense of agency in one's own problems or one's response to them versus being a victim versus being too sorry for debatable sins
- Feelings of contrition, remorse, regret
- Willingness to do penance

6. COMMUNION
- Feelings of kinship with the whole chain of being
- Feeling embedded or estranged, united or separated in the world, in relations with one's faith, one's church

7. SENSE OF VOCATION
- Willingness to be a cheerful participant in creation
- Signs of zest, vigor, liveliness, dedication
- Alignment with divine benevolence or malevolence
- Humorous and inventive involvement in life versus grim and dogmatic

book, Pruyser discussed the role of religious language in pastoral diagnosis and ways a pastor and psychiatrist can work together to provide care (rather than one professional always referring the case to the other). In his final chapter, Pruyser included five case vignettes to illustrate the process of pastoral diagnosis.

Pruyser's work provided the basic impetus for assessment as well as a framework for later models of spiritual assessment. His challenge to clergy to claim their distinct role has never been fully embraced. The voice of theological observation remains outside the partnership role it could fill in the medical setting.

In summary, Pruyser's pioneering work on pastoral diagnosis gave pastors and health care providers a set of theological categories for spiritual assessment, which have been widely adapted for various ministry contexts. The model's conception of spirituality is sophisticated and complex. Generally, it makes possible a distinctly spiritual, yet dynamically informed, spiritual assessment. Pruyser's work is a model for balancing the autonomy of the person with a dynamic assessment approach.

7 × 7 Model for Spiritual Assessment

The spiritual assessment model that has enjoyed the widest circulation and influenced many other approaches is the 7 × 7 Model for Spiritual Assessment. This section presents this model in detail, along with how to analyze a specific case using the model, to contribute to an understanding of patient spiritual health and the contribution of spiritual assessment to the spiritual care of patients.

Work on the 7 × 7 model began in the fall of 1985. Julia Quiring Emblen, then a professor of nursing at Rush University in Chicago, wanted to give surgical nurses a tool they could use to assess their patients' spiritual needs. She talked with hospital chaplains, first with Russell Burck, later with George Fitchett, knowing they could have some helpful resources.

Professor Emblen, Carol Farran (another member of the nursing faculty), and Chaplains Burck and Fitchett discussed the strengths and weaknesses of the various approaches to spiritual assessment with which they were familiar. None of them was quite sure what they would recommend. The four met regularly for more than 2½ years. During that period, they developed a set of guidelines for evaluating models of spiritual assessment.

Their work led to the development of their own approach to spiritual assessment, the 7 × 7 model (Farran, Fitchett, Emblen, & Burck, 1989). Under Julia Quiring Emblen's leadership, they also carried out a research project on the ways different professionals, primarily nurse educators, identify spiritual needs. Their regular meetings and collaborations ended in 1988. The results of their work during that time have been presented at several professional meetings and reported in many publications. Ironically, although they accomplished much, they never developed the simple spiritual assessment tool that Professor Emblen originally requested. What they did produce was a rich and useful spiritual assessment tool for comprehensive in-depth exploration into patients' spiritual health and its effects on their health care.

The 7 × 7 model has two major subdivisions, each of which has seven dimensions (Fitchett, 1993; Fitchett & Burck, 1990). Some of the dimensions in the model are more familiar and easier to understand than others. Box 14.6 summarizes the organization of the model.

Holistic Dimensions. The spiritual life in general and spiritual needs and resources at any particular moment are influenced strongly by what is happening in the rest of one's life. The power of these dimensions to influence spiritual well-being is one reason for attending to them through spiritual assessment.

But there is another reason as well. Spirits are not separate from bodies, emotions, and thoughts. Each individual is one whole person. Ways of thinking about oneself often limit a person to consider only one dimension at a time, but that does not mean those dimensions are separate or discrete. Wholeness, the way in which a person expresses the spiritual aspects of who he or she is in all life aspects, requires that spiritual assessment be whole person assessment. Thus, when caregivers begin spiritual assessment they first review the information they have about all aspects of the person's life.

Medical Dimension. The first holistic dimension that caregivers consider is the physical or medical dimension. The concern is whether what is happening in the person's life at this level is affecting his or her spiritual well-being or functioning. This is usually readily apparent. Major changes in health, such as a stroke and subsequent paralysis or a below-the-knee leg amputation related to diabetes, frequently have noticeable effects on a person's spiritual life.

Sometimes, concerns at this level emerge not from what has happened but what might happen. An example would be determining whether episodes of memory loss are early signs of Alzheimer's disease. Physical or medical assessment is also important in caring for people with disabilities.

A person whose mood or behavior has changed without obvious cause should be encouraged to have a thorough medical assessment. Different things, including disease, diet, and reactions to medication, can cause such changes. Spiritual care will take different directions, depending on whether someone is dealing with a temporary and easily reversible biologic change or with a severe, permanent, or even progressive loss of physical health.

In this dimension of holistic assessment the caregiver's role is usually adjunctive. In most cases, he or she may do little more than make a referral for medical attention if that has not already happened. Sometimes, the role includes helping people make choices about treatment options for themselves or a loved one. Sometimes, the role includes advocacy within the health care system on behalf of people who are being treated unjustly.

Psychological Dimension. Next, the caregiver considers three closely related dimensions of psychosocial functioning: psychological, family systems, and psychosocial.

BOX 14.6   7 × 7 Model for Spiritual Assessment

HOLISTIC DIMENSIONS
Medical dimension
Psychological dimension
Psychosocial dimension
Family systems dimension
Ethnic and cultural dimension
Societal issues dimension
Spiritual dimension

THE SPIRITUAL DIMENSION
Beliefs and meaning
Vocation and consequences
Experience and emotion
Courage and growth
Ritual and practice
Community
Authority and guidance

Although the model reviews each separately, providers can group them together during the assessment.

In considering the psychological dimension, caregivers would like to know if patients are currently receiving treatment for any psychological problems and, if so, what that treatment is. They want to know something about their patient's personality and general approach to life. They also are interested in knowing if patients have had any major psychiatric illnesses, and, if so, what it was, how it was treated, and how it was resolved.

Obviously, any problems people have in this area often greatly influence their spiritual lives and needs. Those providing spiritual care must be aware of such problems to work in tandem with any mental health professionals patients are seeing, or to make referrals for careful psychological assessments in cases of suspected problems in mental health.

Family Systems Dimension. A family systems perspective is familiar to many pastoral workers, some of whom may have received advanced training in it. This perspective helps caregivers focus on the way that a patient's family relationships (either current immediate family or patterns traceable through several generations) may shape his or her current problems.

Psychosocial Dimension. The psychosocial dimension is next. Colleagues in social work examine this perspective routinely. Here caregivers are interested in learning about the patient's past and present. Where was this person born and raised? Who was in his or her family? What were childhood, adolescence, and adulthood like for this person? Were there any major crises in those years? Within this context, providers also want to know how much schooling a person completed and his or her employment history.

This perspective also focuses on where people are in the present. What is their current living situation? Where do they live? Is their housing adequate? With whom do they live? What are those relationships like? Are they responsible for others? Caregivers are interested in what patients do with their time, if they are working, what kind of work they do, and whether they find it fulfilling. Caregivers also inquire about other things patients do with their time and whether they have any important leisure interests. They also assess whether financial resources are adequate to meet needs.

Ethnic and Cultural Dimension. The next aspect considers the person from the perspective of race, ethnicity, and culture. Racial and ethnic backgrounds strongly influence behavior. The assessment process needs to include this perspective to appreciate people within this context and to avoid inappropriately imposing values from one's own culture.

Societal Issues Dimension. The sixth dimension of holistic assessment in the 7 × 7 Model is called the societal issues perspective, which usually is the least familiar to caregivers and often the most difficult to explain. It is a way of learning whether dysfunctional and oppressive social and cultural systems are causing or compounding the person's distress.

The most powerful diagnostic tools of traditional helping professions explain the causes of people's problems in terms of the individual person, his or her body, or his or her behavior. Although these approaches are helpful, they don't consider the possibility that the "sickness" of a social institution or cultural pattern is causing or contributing to a person's misery. If health care providers neglect the societal issues perspective, they risk looking for individual causes for social and cultural problems, blaming the victims, or both. The societal issues perspective allows providers to learn the fullest possible picture of the person and his or her situation and to avoid creating a diagnostic perspective that forces caregivers into individual-level explanations for social and cultural problems.

People at a power disadvantage in society, including women, racial minorities, those with low incomes, and those with disabilities, are at increased risk for social or cultural oppression. In working with such patients, caregivers will do well to include a careful societal issues assessment.

The Spiritual Dimension. To describe the explicitly spiritual dimension of human life, the seventh dimension of the model, several aspects are assessed.

Beliefs and Meaning. The first aspect focuses on beliefs and meaning, or the ways the person finds meaning and purpose in his or her life. Some people can express directly the sources of meaning and purpose. Some use religious language to describe that meaning, whereas others do not. Some people would say, for instance, that knowing they are children of God gives life meaning. Others would attribute their sense of purpose to their enjoyment of life.

Sometimes people cannot say in a few short sentences what gives their lives meaning and purpose, but they can tell a story or two about themselves. In those stories they convey what gives their lives meaning. Paying attention to objects with symbolic significance to a patient can be helpful to learning about their important beliefs. For some, those objects are related to religious traditions, pictures, or statues. For others, symbolic objects are nonreligious, such as a family heirloom or summer home.

How a person handles the symbolic nature of religious objects and language is another point that caregivers consider in this aspect of spiritual assessment. However, attending to what people say about what gives their lives meaning is not always the best way to learn how they handle religious meaning. People also convey important information through how they behave, what they do with energy and vitality, and what they avoid.

If a caregiver wants to know what gives meaning and purpose to people, he or she can listen to what they say, but he or she also can watch how they live their lives and then make inferences. Sometimes a caregiver will find that what people say about the meaning in their lives is consistent with their behavior. Other times, inconsistencies will be obvious. A caregiver may observe sources of meaning of which patients themselves are unaware. They might even disagree if someone pointed out what they had seen. This is what it means to take a dynamic perspective on the spiritual dimension. Caregivers take seriously both what people say and what is observed, which may or may not be consistent with what people have told the caregivers.

In learning about another person's beliefs and meaning, it is also important to attend to any significant changes that have occurred in those beliefs. Further, it is important to know about any current situations that threaten to disrupt important sources of meaning.

For many people, past and present contact with religious traditions shapes the ways they find meaning in life. In this dimension, caregivers want to know if the person has participated in any religious traditions in the past or is participating in any at present. Caregivers assess how that participation has shaped that person's beliefs and the way he or she finds meaning in life.

Vocation and Consequences. The next aspect of spiritual assessment in the 7 × 7 Model focuses on a person's vocation and consequences. These are the duties and obligations that a person feels called to fulfill. This aspect is closely linked to the previous one, beliefs and meaning. Sometimes one's sense of the duties and obligations in life stems consciously and directly from the beliefs that give meaning to life. That is, sense of duty is a consequence of beliefs. At other times the connection may be more unconscious or indirect.

In this aspect of the spiritual assessment, caregivers also reflect on the patient's sense of right living: the shoulds and oughts that shape behavior and the judgments about others. Many religious traditions have specific prescriptions and prohibitions on behavior. The assessment here focuses on the role these play in the life of the person the caregivers are assessing.

Assessment includes gaining a sense of whether people feel they are fairly able to fulfill the duties and obligations that are important to them, or whether they are frustrated or guilty about being unable to fulfill them. In spiritual care situations of change or crisis, it is important to be sensitive to changes in the person's perception of being able to fulfill duties and obligations. In other situations, when a person's motivation seems blocked or he or she seems unable to fulfill important goals, it is possible that the person feels a duty to suffer or make a sacrifice. Potential growth in meeting expectations could be seen as conflicting with the need to find meaning through suffering and sacrifice; thus, an impasse could result.

Experience and Emotion. The third aspect explores experience and emotion. This portion of the assessment attends to the person's reports of any direct encounters with the divine or the demonic. Survey research indicates that about 30% of people in the United States claim to have had a core spiritual experience (Kass, Friedman, Leserman, Zuttermeister, & Benson, 1991). In this category, caregivers would include near-death experiences. People who have had such experiences are often hesitant to reveal them to others. However, the authors know from those who have described them that these experiences often have profound and lasting effects. Direct contacts with demonic or evil powers seem to be less common, but they are no doubt at least as equally powerful in their impact on a person's life.

The 7 × 7 Model also focuses on the overall emotional tone of the person's spiritual life, which may be influenced strongly by any direct religious experiences a person has had. It summarizes the emotional tone that accompanies the person's living out of his or her sense of the meaning of life and the consequent duties and obligations. This mood has consistency over time, despite the emotions that may come and go in response to passing events. It is easy to confuse this aspect of the spiritual dimension with the holistic dimension of psychological assessment described earlier, but they are distinct.

Courage and Growth. The next aspect focuses on the person's courage and growth. The use of the term *courage* in this context has been influenced by Paul Tillich's (1952) classic book *The Courage to Be*. In this context, courage is not a matter of being brave or tough in threatening situations. Rather, it is the ability to enter into spiritual doubt, to tolerate times when we reject as false or inadequate some or all of what we have believed previously, not knowing if a new sense of belief will emerge to replace it (Tillich, 1952). It is the courage to enter the dark night of the soul. It is also the courage to experience a conversion, turnaround, or breakthrough.

Another approach is to observe what a person does when new experiences challenge existing beliefs. Must people disavow the new experiences not to have their beliefs threatened? Must they strain their perception of new realities, or existing beliefs, for them to fit? Or can they let go of existing beliefs, even when it is unclear what new beliefs might emerge to provide security? Can the person entertain the possibility of new beliefs? Does his or her history reveal a capacity for spiritual growth or development? If so, has that growth been slow and gradual, or more sudden? Have there been experiences of spiritual rebirth or conversion? Or has there been an arrest in the growth of faith, or a long, sustained plateau?

In the development of the 7 × 7 Model, faith development was not incorporated as a norm. Rather than creating multiple assessment models based on stages of spiritual development and age, a more descriptive approach was preferred, seeing whether there is evidence of change and growth in a person's spiritual life, and if so, attempting to describe it.

Rituals and Practices. The next aspect of spiritual assessment in the 7 × 7 Model focuses on rituals and practices. Here attention is directed to any rituals or practices by people that give expression to a sense of meaning and purpose in life or that are part of their fulfillment of their sense of their duties and obligations.

In the assessment of rituals and practices, it is important to note any important changes. It is also important to determine if any significant changes are about to happen that would interfere with a person's ability to perform the rituals and practices.

Life in Community. The next aspect of spiritual assessment focuses on a person's life in community. Is the person part of one or more formal or informal communities of shared belief and meaning in life, shared ritual and practice? In this portion, it is important to determine to what extent the communities a person is part of might be resources for support in times of need. Are they large and vital communities, or are they threatened and depleted? Are they flexible, resourceful, and adaptive, or defensive and rigid?

Other interests in the area of a person's community also are worth considering. What role, for instance, do people typically play in their communities of shared meaning and purpose? Are they open, guarded, or conflicted? Can they give and receive affection and support in any of their communities? Based on his reading of family systems theory, Burton (1988) names four roles a person may typically take in a family or a family-like group: mover, opposer, follower, and bystander. This can be a useful structure for this portion of the assessment.

Authority and Guidance. The final aspect of spiritual assessment in the 7 × 7 Model focuses on authority and guidance. Three aspects are important to this portion. First, caregivers want to know if the person will give them enough authority to enable them to help him or her, if needed. Second, them want to know if the person looks upon himself or herself as having some authority to help meet the questions and challenges of life. Third, caregivers want to know what other significant sources of authority in this person's life they must consider. The question of authority is linked to several aspects of the spiritual life already described. It focuses on where people find the authority for their beliefs, meaning in life, sense of vocation and duties, and rituals and practices. The question of authority takes center stage when people face conflict between duties or beliefs, or when they face doubts or confusion. Where a person turns for comfort and guidance at such times says a good deal about where spiritual authority resides for him or her.

One common place people look for authority and guidance are special texts, including traditional religious or holy books. They also may seek it in other people, some of whom may be ordained or otherwise consecrated individuals, and others of whom are trusted mentors, family members, or friends. Some may be worthy, and others unworthy, of the authority and trust given to them. People also may see themselves as having the inner resources and authority with which to meet challenges. People who look to several different authorities may find divergent opinions at a particular point, an important consideration when assessing this dimension.

CASE STUDY: IN THE GARDEN WITH ANDREA

One of the best ways to learn how to do spiritual assessment is to review an actual case study application. The authors have chosen the case of a patient whom they call Andrea, from a case in which Reverend Patricia Roberts worked to illustrate how a chaplain, nurse, or other spiritual care provider can use the 7 × 7 Model of spiritual assessment to inform and guide his or her spiritual care. Case Study 14.1 is Rev. Roberts' report of her second visit with Andrea.

(Text continues on page 236)

CASE STUDY 14.1 In the Garden with Andrea

It was a busy, stressful Saturday on-call. I had just finished discussing advance directives with a patient on the oncology unit where I work when one of the nurses, Mamie, said, "I need your help with something. We're going outside for awhile. Do you have a few minutes to spare?" "Sure," I responded, as I followed Mamie into a patient's room.

The patient was Andrea, a 56-year-old woman with breast cancer that had metastasized to her bones. She had been hospitalized this time for more than 6 weeks and was experiencing one complication after another from her treatment. Her prognosis was not good and she knew it. Her husband was so fearful that he would not allow her to talk to him about her dying. Andrea's depression seemed to grow with each passing day. Nothing could comfort or distract her for very long.

I had one previous visit with Andrea. During that visit, she looked down and would not discuss her feelings with me. She looked like she wanted to give up. She said she wanted nothing to do with religion. She vehemently refused prayer and through her tears asked to be left alone. Her husband, holding her hand, asked for some privacy. I left with a great sense of hopelessness and loss. On this Saturday Andrea was too weak to sit up in a wheelchair, so

(Case Study continues on page 228)

CASE STUDY 14.1 In the Garden with Andrea (continued)

Mamie had gone to great lengths to borrow a moving bed from the transplant unit and to make all the other necessary preparations for this trip.

Mamie: "I asked Patty to help take you out for awhile. She just happens to be the only one available right now, so she was 'volunteered' for the job, OK?"

Andrea: "Oh, you don't want to bother with this, do you?" (She seemed none too thrilled with Mamie's choice of helper.)

Patty: "Oh, it's no bother, Andrea. I have lots of time today. I'm on-call, and nothing is happening right now. So I'll just go along for the ride."

Andrea was ready. Mamie and I wheeled the bed down the hallway toward the elevators.

Andrea: (incredulously) "Where are we going? I thought you just meant that you were taking me out of the room. Where are we going?"

Mamie: "Oh, we're just taking a little trip outside, that's all."

As the rest of the plan sunk in, the change in Andrea's face was remarkable. Suddenly, she had a look in her eyes of anticipation, amazement, and hope that had not been there before. The trip through the lobby and down the elevators to the main doors was fun. We joked about getting the bed to move as we wanted. We all began to smile, a lot. At last we were outside. It was a gorgeous spring day. The sun was shining, not a cloud in the blue sky. The wind was brisk, but warm and inviting. We maneuvered the bed so that Andrea could see some tulips planted on the hospital grounds and an adjacent field with lots of green grass. In a small way, I was able to appreciate the feeling of being out in the fresh air because by that time I had been on call and inside the hospital for many hours. I could just imagine how this would feel to someone who had been inside for 6 weeks.

I didn't have to imagine very hard though, because it was written all over Andrea's face. She raised her face to the sun, eyes closed, as the spring breeze caressed her face. The smile on her lips told the story more than her words or mine ever could. We just stood by and took it all in, all three of us. Mamie and I made some casual remarks about the weather, the flowers, the grass, but we really didn't need to say a word. After a few minutes, Mamie sat down on a picnic bench behind us.

Andrea: "This is so wonderful, so, so wonderful." (Tears formed in the corners of her eyes. They didn't seem like only sad tears, more a mixture of sad and happy.) "I have been so depressed. I am just so confused about all of this, you know? Patty, I did everything right. I exercised. I ate right. I watched my cholesterol. I got mammograms regularly. I did everything they say you're supposed to do, and what happens? I get cancer anyway." (Pause.) "I guess it has caused me to lose faith."

Patty: "It would be hard not to lose faith. It just doesn't seem fair does it?"

CASE STUDY 14.1 In the Garden with Andrea (continued)

Andrea: "NO! It isn't fair. Not at all. I did everything right. Everything I was supposed to do for my health. I walked. I exercised a lot. I did everything I was supposed to do. And I worry so much about my husband. We don't have any kids. Who will take care of him? I'm going to leave him alone. How will he be after I die? I know I'm dying. He doesn't like to talk about it, but I know I am. What do I have to look forward to? More treatment? More days in the hospital? For what? I'm just not sure. I'm not sure of anything. Except that I'm angry. I'm SO VERY ANGRY at God for doing this. So very angry."

Patty: "I understand what you mean. Why? Why should you have to suffer like this?"

Andrea: "That's right! Why? Why me? I just can't figure it out. And I get so depressed that I just want to give up on life altogether, you know? And I'm so very angry at God. So angry. I refuse to speak to Him. You know what I mean?"

Patty: "Yes. I do know. I happen to be angry at God right now myself."

Andrea: "You are?"

Patty: "Yes. My 23-year-old son was just in a serious auto accident and nearly died. I asked the same questions you did. Why? Why my son? What had he done to deserve this? He's a good kid, doing all the right things, and now this. He might have died. And I was furious, absolutely furious, at God for allowing it to happen. I wanted to know why. I guess we don't get to have those answers though."

Andrea: "Oh, so you DO know! And you got angry about it, too? Wow. Someone like you?"

Patty: "Well, I do feel the anger too."

Andrea: "So you know what it's like to be so very angry inside that you cannot even speak to God? You can't even pray, right? I just refuse to speak to God. I'm so very angry that I refuse even to speak. I'm not trying anymore. He's not listening anyway."

Patty: "I went through a period when I wouldn't speak to God either. Lately though I have seemed to want to go ahead and BE angry. I mean, God is God, right? God made me. I guess I think He ought to be able to handle the fact that I'm angry. In some ways, I think He ought to hear about it. I guess I think God knows about my anger anyway. So I just let 'im have it! It feels kind of good, too, to let it all hang out, so to speak. But that's what has been right for me. It might not necessarily be so with you."

Andrea: (Reflected for a long while in some silence as I waited for her to speak.) "It feels so good to be able to say this to someone, to say the

(Case Study continues on page 230)

CASE STUDY 14.1 In the Garden with Andrea (continued)

words, you know? I really appreciate your understanding. It helps me to know that someone else feels like this. I guess I thought I shouldn't have these feelings at all, like I wasn't being faithful, and that just made me feel worse. It really helps me to know you do understand. Just to say this to someone feels so good. I've been holding it all inside for so long. So very long."

Patty: "I think I would be angry if I were in your place."

Andrea: "Yes. It's hard to survive this illness and all its effects. For awhile I was able to keep up my spirits, but I am really struggling now. I guess I realize that the battle is being lost, and I need to find out how to die. How I need to die, that's what's on my mind."

Patty: "How do you think you need to die?"

Andrea: "I think I have to stop treatment and go home. I don't want any more treatment. I want to die with some dignity. What is this life I have right now, anyway? What kind of life is it when the biggest thing I can look forward to is some more treatment and more pain? I don't want to keep on going like this."

Patty: "Do you think you can say this to your husband sometime? I know he's very scared about losing you."

Andrea: "Yes, he is. And I have not wanted to tell him that I want to give up. He is so insistent that I try, that I not give up."

Patty: "It must be hard to keep up the pretense."

Andrea: "Yes." (She sighed.) "It's very hard. It takes all the energy I've got to keep him from seeing how depressed I really am. And crying? Forget about it. I do my crying when he's not there."

Patty: "That sounds very lonely."

Andrea: "Yes it is." (Tears formed in her eyes once more but only for a moment.) "But right now, I'm here. I'm out in the sunshine. This feels so very good to me! Where's Mamie, where'd she go?"

Patty: "She's sitting right behind us on the picnic bench, just enjoying the sun. From where I stand I can see Mamie." (I smiled at her, and she gave me a knowing smile right back. For a few more precious moments, we were all silent, just taking in the sights, smells, and sounds of creation. It was an unforgettable moment of beauty, peace, and transcendence.)

Andrea: "I guess it must be getting time to go back. I just can't tell you how much this has meant to me, you know! I didn't even know that she was planning on taking me all the way outside." (She smiled widely.) "What a tremendous gift! I can't believe she did this!"

CASE STUDY 14.1 In the Garden with Andrea (continued)

Patty: "Yes, I agree. This has been a wonderful gift. Mamie is a very special person, isn't she? You know, Andrea, I guess if I really look hard, I can find grace here. I mean, to me, if I wanted to be able to find God somewhere, I could find God in Mamie and the incredible gift she has given you in this moment. I mean, that's gotta be grace, that she would go to such great lengths to do this one very loving, very kind act of caring. I feel very fortunate to have been here to be part of it, very fortunate."

Andrea: "Yeah. You're right. This is the best I've felt for a long, long while. Such a little thing, to enjoy the fresh air for just a few minutes. And yet, it has been so very, very good for me. I can't thank her enough. Mamie, where are you?"

At this, Mamie came up to receive a hug from Andrea. As I watched them, I was the one with tears in my eyes.

Reflection
Before beginning work on a spiritual assessment of Andrea or any other patient, it helps to take a minute to reflect on one's emotional response. Personal feelings about patients can color assessments. It is best to be aware of such feelings so that nurses can consider their effects.

What feelings were evoked for you as you read the conversation between Andrea and Patty? I, Patty the minister, felt shut out and helpless in my first visit with Andrea. The day of the surprise trip outside, as I caught hold of what Mamie had in mind, I remember being slightly anxious about Andrea's acceptance of my inclusion in the plan. Soon I was swept up in the adventure of it all. Once outside, I could feel the palpable presence of a sacred moment in the making. As I watched and listened, I felt so sad for Andrea, not just because of her illness, but because of the circumstances surrounding her at that moment. She was trapped inside a hospital with too much treatment, suffering, and pain and not enough fresh air, acceptance, and sunshine. I remember being truly humbled by participating in this grace-filled moment. I also admired, and still do, Mamie's kindness, compassion, and action.

Spiritual Assessment
As seen in Box 14-6, the 7×7 Model for Spiritual Assessment has two major sections. The first section is the holistic assessment. Caregivers begin with a review of the medical dimension, which is the central feature in Andrea's case. She has metastasized breast cancer, and her recent treatment has been fraught with complications. She is beginning to recognize that her prognosis is not good. "I know I'm dying," she says early in the visit and later confirms this. "I guess I realize that the battle is being lost." As with many patients, the progression of her illness, the change in the proportion of good days and bad days, leads Andrea to recognize this difficult truth. "What kind of life is it when the biggest thing I can look forward to is some more treatment and more pain?" The case gives us the impression that her conversation in the

(Case Study continues on page 232)

CASE STUDY 14.1 In the Garden with Andrea (continued)

garden with Patty is one of the first times Andrea has verbalized this reality, that she is just beginning to shift from understanding herself as someone battling her disease to someone who needs to "find out how to die."

The second dimension is psychological. In Andrea's case, this dimension is also very important. Patty observes that during her 6 weeks of treatment and complications, Andrea's depression seemed to grow each passing day. The depth of her depression moved Mamie to go to great lengths to get her a breath of fresh air and a few moments of sunshine. In her conversation in the garden, Andrea also shares intense angry feelings, confusion, and some grief. Her recognition that "the battle is being lost" has evoked many intense emotions in Andrea.

Next is family systems. Andrea is married; she and her husband have no children. We do not know if other important family members are in the picture. Andrea states that her husband is so fearful that he will not allow her talk to him about her dying. She indicates the toll this is taking on her, "It takes all the energy I've got to keep him from seeing how depressed I really am." It is clear that the communication problems in this key relationship are adding to Andrea's distress.

The psychosocial dimension is next. In this case, we have little additional information to help us understand who Andrea is besides a patient with advanced cancer. Further psychosocial information may help us better understand Andrea's needs and the resources she may have to help her cope at this difficult time.

Religion and spirituality are often profoundly intertwined with race, ethnicity, and cultural background, so it is important to include these dimensions. Andrea is Caucasian, but no other ethnic or cultural aspects of her case have emerged thus far.

The social issues dimension may be less familiar than the five dimensions we have just reviewed. It is where we examine the effects of social policies and institutions on Andrea and her situation. Most approaches to diagnosis or assessment focus on the individual, or perhaps the individual in the family system. We include this dimension to remind us that we live in a social context and that features of that context sometimes make things easier or harder for the people, like Andrea, with whom we are working. In this case, as we know it thus far, there do not appear to be any major social issues complicating matters for Andrea.

The seventh and last dimension of the holistic assessment is the spiritual dimension, which is also the second major division of the 7 × 7 Model. We now examine the seven specific spiritual dimensions.

The first is beliefs and meaning. What are Andrea's key religious or spiritual beliefs? What gives her life meaning and purpose? We don't yet know Andrea's religious background, but based on what she shares with Patty, it appears that she holds beliefs in an omnipotent, just God. This teaching is common in many different Christian traditions. At this time, we do not know

CASE STUDY 14.1 In the Garden with Andrea (continued)

what other religious or spiritual beliefs may be important to Andrea. Part of the religious/spiritual crisis that often results from serious illness is a crisis in a person's sense of meaning and purpose. At this point it is hard to say what gives Andrea's life meaning and purpose. In recent weeks she has sacrificed much of her own emotional comfort to care for her husband. As she thinks about her death she is anxious about "Who will take care of him?" Her relationship with her husband may be a significant source of meaning and purpose for Andrea. As we get to know her better, we may get a fuller picture of her key beliefs, what gives her life meaning and purpose, and the effects of her worsening health on this dimension of life.

The second spiritual dimension we consider is vocation and obligations. This is the place in our model where we explore the moral dimension of a person's life. What duties and obligations does Andrea hold for herself and others? Is her changing health causing changes in her sense of duties and obligations? This appears to be a key dimension in our understanding of Andrea's spiritual needs and resources, with six moral themes evident in her conversation with Patty.

The first moral theme Andrea expresses is confusion about what she should do. She finds herself not "sure of anything," "really struggling now" to keep up her spirits. She is asking herself if it is her duty to battle, to fight her illness and keep her spirits up, or may she begin to "find out how to die"? Andrea is not alone in asking this question. Many patients who contend with life-threatening illnesses come to a point at which they recognize the diminishing returns of additional treatment and wonder if it is permissible to shift their focus from an effort to cure their illness to getting ready to die with dignity.

For many patients, this moral decision is not theirs to make alone. It must be addressed in the context of felt duties to others, especially family members and caregivers.

The second theme in the moral dimension of Andrea's story is that she confronts this decision in the context of her care for her husband. She knows that thinking about her possible death is difficult for him: "I have not wanted to tell him that I want to give up. He is so insistent that I try, that I not give up." Andrea feels an obligation to her husband, and perhaps her caregivers, to continue treatment and not give up prematurely. At the same time, she feels the time may have come to focus on getting ready to die with dignity.

The tension between these choices may be accompanied by a feeling of guilt, of letting her husband and/or health care team down if she opts for a palliative approach. Andrea also struggles to protect her husband from her distress. "And crying? Forget about it. I do my crying when he's not there." How can Andrea continue the duty she feels to care for and protect her husband in light of her declining health? For Andrea and for many others, just as there is a good way to live, there is a good way to die.

(Case Study continues on page 234)

CASE STUDY 14.1 In the Garden with Andrea (continued)

The third theme in the moral dimension of Andrea's story is her interest in learning how to die. When Patty asks her, "How do you think you need to die," it becomes evident that Andrea has some clear, specific images of what her dying should be like. It should be marked by dignity that will be facilitated by no additional futile, painful treatment and the peace and security of her home.

The fourth theme that emerges in our assessment of Andrea's moral dimension is more explicitly religious. She is enraged that God is being unfair to her. She believes that God should reward a good life with health and longevity. However, God has not rewarded her good life, her exceedingly good life, with good health. God is treating her unfairly, unjustly.

Andrea says, "I'm so very angry at God. So angry. I refuse to speak to Him." The intensity of her anger toward God and her turning away from God suggests that Andrea feels God has betrayed her, broken a promise or covenant Andrea felt existed between them. Andrea's anger with God raises the fifth theme in the moral dimension of her story. "I guess I thought I shouldn't have these feelings at all, like I wasn't being faithful, and that just made me feel worse." It is very common for religiously affiliated and active people to feel that faithfulness precludes anger with God. Andrea's internalization of this belief suggests a depth of earlier religious training that appears to stand in contrast to her current rejection of religion.

Andrea's belief that God should reward her because of her good behavior points to the sixth and final theme in the moral dimension of her story— grace. Unlike the preceding moral themes we have described, Andrea is not raising questions about grace, the term in the Christian tradition that refers to the unearned love of God. We don't hear about experiences of grace in Andrea's life in the small portion of her story that she shares with Patty. Rather, she appears to operate out of the belief that you should get what you earn, what you work for. Patty points out that Mamie's efforts to arrange the visit to the garden might be a moment of grace. Andrea seems to have experienced it as such: "What a tremendous gift!" It would help to know how rare such moments have been in Andrea's life.

The third spiritual dimension we consider is experience and emotion. This is where we consider whether the person reports any direct spiritual experiences and if so, what impact they have had upon them. In this conversation Andrea doesn't report any direct spiritual experiences. Perhaps this contributes to her belief that you only get what you have earned. People often need to develop trust in a caregiver before they are comfortable sharing any spiritual experiences they have had. We might learn more about this as we get to know Andrea better.

The fourth spiritual dimension in the 7 × 7 Model is courage and growth. This is the place in the model where caregivers look at whether there has been, or appears likely to be, any change in the way the person makes mean-

CASE STUDY 14.1 In the Garden with Andrea (continued)

ing and finds purpose in life. For example, has Andrea had an experience of radical doubt, an experience of the dark night of the soul, in which there was a profound change in her faith? Andrea's anger with God, her feeling that God is not being fair and not listening to her are frequently important elements in experiences of deep spiritual crises and transformations, elements of what has been described as "searching faith" (Westerhoff, 1976). However, by deciding not to talk to God ("I'm not trying anymore. He's not listening anyway."), Andrea has suspended the process of entering into and resolving her spiritual crisis.

The fifth spiritual dimension that caregivers assess is rituals and practices. What rituals and practices shape and express Andrea's key beliefs and her sense of meaning and purpose in life? From the little that we know about her, it does not appear that Andrea currently has any public or private religious rituals or practices that are important to her. In fact, Patty reports that during her first visit Andrea "vehemently refused prayer." Andrea's current rejection of prayer may be related to her experience that God is not listening to her. It is hoped we will be able to clarify this as we get to know Andrea better. Although Andrea may have little use for religious rituals, she may have personal practices that help her feel peaceful or centered. The pilgrimage to the hospital garden appears to have offered Andrea a refreshing moment of sunshine and catharsis. As we get to know Andrea better, it will be important to learn more about any other rituals or practices that are important to her.

The sixth spiritual dimension in our model is community. Who are the people with whom Andrea shares her beliefs and her sense of meaning and purpose in life? With whom does she share her sense of duties and obligations? With whom does she share any rituals or practices that help her feel peaceful or centered? It appears that Andrea is not part of any formal religious community.

Her story, as we know it thus far, does not include any family or friends other than her husband. This key relationship also appears to be a stressful one, in which Andrea feels she must sacrifice her own needs in order to care for him. Although she initially rejected Patty, learning of their shared anger with God has been important to Andrea. "I really appreciate your understanding. It helps me to know that someone else feels like this."

The final spiritual dimension we consider in our model is authority and guidance. In times of crisis and doubt, to whom does Andrea turn for support and direction? We don't know Andrea well enough to answer this question confidently. Some things in her story, such as protecting her husband, suggest she may be a strong, self-reliant woman. Her response to Patty on their first visit suggests that she doesn't welcome the authority clergy traditionally represent. Yet, the case also suggests she may be open to Patty's authority when it is grounded in their shared personal experiences of distress and anger with God.

(Case Study continues on page 236)

CASE STUDY 14.1 In the Garden with Andrea (continued)

Conclusion

As can be seen here, the process of developing a spiritual assessment using the 7 × 7 Model is lengthy and complex; however, caregivers can summarize a spiritual assessment based on the description. A summary could be used in a chart note to share this spiritual assessment with other members of the care team. An example follows:

Andrea is starting to face the reality of her death and wonders if it would be permissible for her to give up struggling and prepare to die with dignity. She is, for the most part, quite alone in this important and stressful process. Her husband is uncomfortable with her talking about dying, and she feels she must protect him. Further, she feels God has been unfair in allowing her to become ill, despite her exceptionally good health practices. She is enraged with God and refuses to speak to Him. Although she was initially rejecting toward the chaplain as a representative of religion, today's visit to the hospital garden became the occasion of a cathartic conversation and perhaps the start of a trusting relationship in which we can work together on these important issues.

DIAGNOSIS IN SPIRITUAL CARE

Nurses have a longstanding record of interest in their patients' spiritual needs. As mentioned, nursing has been a leader in the development of models for spiritual assessment. This interest is evidenced in the substantial number of publications related to spiritual assessment published during the last nearly 30 years. One of the most developed models for nursing spiritual assessment stems from the work of the North American Nursing Diagnosis Association (NANDA). Since its first conference in 1975, NANDA has developed a list of almost 100 conditions that nurses are qualified to diagnose and treat (Carpenito-Moyet, 2004). The conditions include biologic problems (decreased cardiac output, constipation), psychological conditions (chronic low self-esteem, dysfunctional grieving), and interpersonal problems (social isolation, interrupted family processes).

NANDA defines a nursing diagnosis as:

A clinical judgment about an individual, family, or community that is derived through a deliberate, systematic process of data collection and analysis. It provides the basis for prescriptions for definitive therapy for which the nurse is accountable. It is expressed concisely and includes the etiology of the condition when known. *(Kim, McFarland, & McLane, 1989, p. xi).*

Each diagnosis has three parts: a label and definition; a statement of etiology (cause) or related factors; and a list of defining characteristics, specific observable signs, and symptoms associated with the diagnosis (Kim et al., 1989).

Nursing diagnoses are linked to the nursing process. The steps are similar to those outlined for the clinical ministry process. Nurses use them to move from assessment to treatment.

BOX 14.7 Nursing Diagnosis of Spiritual Distress

Definition: The state in which the individual or group experiences a disturbance in the belief or value system that provides strength, hope, and meaning to life.

MAJOR DEFINING CHARACTERISTICS
- Experiences a disturbance in belief system

MINOR DEFINING CHARACTERISTICS
- Questions meaning of life, death, and suffering
- Questions credibility of belief system
- Demonstrates discouragement or despair
- Chooses not to practice usual religious rituals
- Has ambivalent feelings (doubts) about beliefs
- Expresses that he has no reason for living
- Feels a sense of spiritual emptiness
- Shows emotional detachment from self and others
- Expresses concern—anger, resentment, fear—over meaning of life, suffering, and death
- Requests spiritual assistance for a disturbance in belief system

RELATED FACTORS

Pathophysiologic
Loss of body part or function
Terminal illness
Debilitating disease
Pain
Trauma
Stillbirth, miscarriage

Treatment Related
Abortion
Isolation
Surgery
Medications
Blood transfusion
Dietary restrictions

Situational
Death/illness of significant other
Divorce, separation from loved one
Embarrassment of or barriers to practicing spiritual rituals
Beliefs opposed by family, peers, or health care providers

(Adapted with permission from Carpenito-Moyet, L. J. [2004]. *Nursing diagnosis: Application to clinical practice* [10th ed.]. Philadelphia: Lippincott Williams & Wilkins.)

At the third national NANDA conference (1978), the association approved Spiritual Concerns, Spiritual Distress, and Spiritual Despair as nursing diagnoses. At the fourth national conference (1980), NANDA combined these into one category: Spiritual Distress (Ellerhorst-Ryan, 1985, p. 93). Like any nursing diagnosis, Spiritual Distress (distress of the human spirit) has three components: a definition, related factors, and defining characteristics (Box 14.7).

The definition of Spiritual Distress and its defining characteristics are the extent of the formal NANDA diagnosis. Secondary materials related to this and other nursing diagnoses have been published. For example, *Pocket Guide to Nursing Diagnoses* includes a two-page prototype care plan for a homeless client with alcoholism and a nursing diagnosis of Spiritual Distress. It includes patient goals, expected outcomes, and associated nursing interventions (Kim et al., 1989).

Doenges and Moorhouse (1988) have written a *Nurse's Pocket Guide* that, in addition to the NANDA diagnoses, describes desired patient outcomes or evaluation criteria and specific nursing interventions. The specific outcomes and interventions listed are those commonly found in adult patients in acute or long-term care settings and are provided to help nurses formulate patient care plans. Desired patient outcomes for the diagnosis Spiritual Distress include "discusses beliefs/values about spiritual issues" and "verbalizes increased sense of self-esteem and hope for future." Examples of nursing interventions include "determine patient's religious/spiritual orientation," "establish environment that allows free expression of feelings and concerns," and "help patient find a reason for living" (Doenges & Moorhouse, pp. 351–353).

Carpenito-Moyet (2004) has written a guide to the application of nursing diagnoses in clinical practice that spiritual caregivers may find interesting and helpful. She suggests five simple but thorough questions that nurses could add to a nursing psychosocial assessment to facilitate spiritual assessment (Box 14.8). Her discussion of Spiritual Distress includes a seven-page table of beliefs and practices related to health and illness for most major religions, along with pediatric and geriatric considerations (Carpenito-Moyet). The wonderfully useful table includes non-Christian groups. There is also a helpful list of principles and rationales for how and why nurses should be involved in spiritual care. Like Doenges and Moorhouse (1988), Carpenito-Moyet also provides specific goals and interventions for two forms of Spiritual Distress: Spiritual Distress Related to the Inability to Practice Spiritual Rituals and Spiritual Distress Related to Conflict with Prescribed Therapy.

In the case study with Andrea, much evidence from the assessment would lead nurses to include a diagnosis of Spiritual Distress in the care plan. Andrea expressed anger at God, feeling that God had been unfair, thus disturbing her previous belief system.

NANDA recognizes that nurses are important caregivers who can identify people at risk for Spiritual Distress. The diagnosis Risk for Spiritual Distress is defined as "the state in which the individual or group is at risk of experiencing a disturbance

---

B O X   1 4 . 8   Assessment Questions for Diagnosis of Spiritual Distress

- What is your source of spiritual strength or meaning? What is your source of peace, comfort, faith, well-being, hope, or worth?
- How do you practice your spiritual beliefs?
- Are there any practices that are important for your spiritual well-being?
- Do you have a spiritual leader?
- Has being ill or hurt affected your spiritual beliefs?

(From Carpenito-Moyet, L. J. [2004]. *Nursing diagnosis: Application to clinical practice* [10th ed]. Philadelphia: Lippincott Williams & Wilkins. Used with permission.)

BOX 14.9 Defining Characteristics of Nursing Diagnosis of Readiness for Enhanced Spiritual Well-being

Inner strength that nurtures
Inner peace
Sacred source
Sense of awareness
Trust relationships
Unifying force
Intangible motivation and commitment directed toward ultimate values of love, meaning, hope, beauty, and truth
Trust relationships with or in the transcendent that provide bases for meaning and hope in life's experiences and love in one's relationships
Has meaning and purpose to existence

(From Carpenito-Moyet, L. J. [2004]. *Nursing diagnosis: Application to clinical practice* [10th ed.]. Philadelphia: Lippincott Williams & Wilkins. Used with permission.)

in their belief or value system that provides strength, hope, and meaning to life" (Carpenito-Moyet, 2004). The risk factors are the same as those indicated for Spiritual Distress.

Another applicable NANDA diagnosis when providing spiritual care is Readiness for Enhanced Spiritual Well-being, which is defined as "an individual who experiences affirmation of life in relationship with a higher power (as defined by the person), self, community, and environment that nurtures and celebrates wholeness" (Carpenito-Moyet, 2004). The defining characteristics can be seen in Box 14.9. With its emphasis on well-being and growth, related factors are not warranted.

Data collected during spiritual assessment might support other NANDA diagnoses. Nurses, appreciating the complex holistic nature of human beings, would recognize the spiritual component of the diagnoses listed in Box 14.10.

Nurses have applied their research skills to their work on spiritual diagnosis. An example is Weatherall's (1985) validation study of NANDA's defining characteristics for spiritual distress. Weatherall reviewed 34 articles on spiritual issues written by

---

BOX 14.10 NANDA Diagnoses Associated with Spirituality

Anxiety	Risk for loneliness
Ineffective coping	Powerlessness
Disturbed energy field	Disturbed self-esteem
Interrupted family processes	Social isolation
Fear	Chronic sorrow
Grieving	Risk for suicide
Hopelessness	Risk for violence

nurses between 1959 and 1984. She also gathered case reports and care plans for 13 patients with Spiritual Distress, as diagnosed by their nurses. She counted the "cues" in each article and case report and compared them to the 22 NANDA defining characteristics. She found strong support in both the literature and patient cases for only three of the NANDA characteristics: questions meaning of suffering, verbalizes concern about relationship with deity, and verbalizes inner conflict about beliefs. She also found support for two characteristics not in the NANDA list, hopelessness and relationships with other people. Weatherall concludes, "It is difficult to say that the characteristics are strongly supported and valid" (p. 12).

Although NANDA's list of diagnoses was developed for use by nurses, nothing in its formal description prevents other spiritual care providers from making fruitful use of it. In fact the NANDA Model's link to the nursing process, with its clear description of the steps of clinical reasoning and therapeutic action, makes it useful for multidisciplinary caregivers to enhance their clarity of thinking about spiritual assessment, care plans, and interventions.

The list of defining characteristics appears to be a major strength of NANDA's model. The specificity directs the caregiver's attention to explicit expressions of Spiritual Distress. The model is less helpful in directing attention to signs of spiritual ill health that may not be causing distress to the patient, such as substance abuse. Like any list, this one is not exhaustive.

A central strength of the NANDA list is its practicality. The model enables a caregiver to attend quickly to areas of spiritual pain and to begin to plan ways to address them. Its list of the possible areas of spiritual distress includes areas of concern that caregivers frequently encounter in clinical practice. Inclusion of related factors and etiology also adds to the list's practicality. It quickly focuses attention on possible causes of spiritual distress that specific interventions could address.

The model appears quite user friendly. The specificity of the defining characteristics implies that little training is required to conduct the data-gathering phase of the assessment. This model makes it easy to communicate to other professionals and to the patient and family the data providing the basis for an assessment of spiritual distress. One of the model's virtues is the behaviorally specific and practice focus nature of the defining characteristics.

Other models with similar levels of concreteness and simplicity rely on a structured or semistructured interview for data gathering. Although Carpenito-Moyet (2004) provides a ministructured interview to guide data gathering, the formal model does not include or suggest a structured interview. Rather, assessment could proceed in a more informal conversational mode, as in traditional spiritual care. The nurse could later organize observations during the interview and report findings in light of the model's defining characteristics. However, the defining characteristics also lend themselves to use as a checklist, which would make an effective baseline measure of Spiritual Distress against which the nurse could measure progress or lack of it. Such a tool would be useful in quality assurance programs and in research about spiritual care.

In summary, the NANDA model for spiritual assessment, although developed for nurses, could be useful for other spiritual caregivers. Using the term Spiritual Distress, the model also focuses on religious distress caused by separation from accustomed spiritual practices, conflict between beliefs and recommended therapy, and doubts created by intense suffering. The model is multidimensional, considering beliefs, practices, and key relationships. The defining characteristics are very specific and can be useful in both clinical practice and research.

CONCLUSION

This chapter presents various examples and models for spiritual screening, spiritual history taking, and spiritual assessment. No model or approach has become a standard for spiritual care, which points to the relative novelty and underdevelopment of these resources. This frontier-like feel is exciting because it encourages and invites caregivers from many disciplines to innovate, experiment, and participate in developing and perfecting these approaches and resources when providing spiritual care. Nurses should be at the forefront by acting as patient advocates through incorporation of spiritual assessment into nursing practice.

The future of spiritual assessment must certainly include research. Any clinical intervention or method of measurement ought to be subject to scrutiny to determine its effectiveness when compared with other means of care. The development, refinement, and widespread use of spiritual assessment and nursing diagnoses certainly will improve the spiritual care provided to those seeking health care. This important resource to nursing and medical care will complement and improve whole-person wellness well into the new century.

PERSONAL REFLECTIONS

- What are my feelings regarding the role of the nurse in spiritual assessment?
- How would familiarity with spiritual assessment improve my nursing care? Which of the models presented would I choose to care for patients I encounter? Could this model appeal to me because it fits with my own perceptions about spirituality?
- What would I do if I determined my patient was at spiritual risk? How would I advocate for this patient?
- What steps can I take to become more comfortable performing a spiritual history?
- How can I distinguish my own spiritual experiences from those of my patients?
- What nursing diagnoses related to spiritual distress and spiritual well-being have I encountered in my practice?

Key Points
- Spiritual assessment is important for providing appropriate spiritual care.
- There are different levels of inquiry into spiritual health, i.e. spiritual screening, spiritual history taking, and spiritual assessment.
- Spiritual risk is an important concern for patients' health care.
- NANDA diagnoses include Spiritual Distress and Potential for Enhanced Spiritual Well-being.

References

Anandarajah, G., & Hight, E. (2001). Spirituality and medical practice: Using the HOPE questions as a practical tool for spiritual assessment. *American Family Physician, 63*, 81–89.

Burton, L. (1988). *Pastoral paradigms.* Washington, DC: The Alban Institute.

Carpenito-Moyet, L. J. (2004). *Nursing diagnosis: Application to clinical practice* (10th ed.). Philadelphia: Lippincott Williams & Wilkins.

Doenges, M. E., & Moorhouse, M. F. (1988). *Nurse's pocket guide: Nursing diagnoses with interventions* (2nd ed.). Philadelphia: FA Davis.

Ellerhorst-Ryan, J. (1985). Selecting an instrument to measure spiritual distress. *Oncology Nursing Forum, 12*(2), 93.

Farran, C., Fitchett, G., Emblen, J. Q, & Burck, J. R. (1989). Development of a model for spiritual assessment and intervention. *Journal of Religion and Health, 28*(3), 185–194.

Fitchett, G. (1993). *Assessing spiritual needs: A guide for caregivers.* Minneapolis: Augsberg.

Fitchett, G., & Burck, J. R. (1990). A multi-dimensional, functional model for spiritual assessment. *The Care Giver Journal, 7*(1), 43–62.

Kass, J. D., Friedman, R., Leserman, J., Zuttermeister, P., & Benson, H. (1991). Health outcomes and a new index of spiritual experience. *Journal for the Scientific Study of Religion, 30*(2), 203–211.

Kim, M. J., McFarland, K., & McLane, A. (1989). *Pocket guide to nursing diagnosis* (3rd ed.). St. Louis: Mosby.

Maugans, T. A. (1996). The SPIRITual History. *Archives of Family Medicine, 5*(1), 11–16.

Oxman, T. E., Freeman, D. H. Jr., & Manheimer, E. D. (1995). Lack of social participation or religious strength and comfort as risk factors for death after cardiac surgery in the elderly. *Psychosomatic Medicine, 57*, 5–15.

Pruyser, P. (1976). *The minister as diagnostician.* Louisville, KY: Westminster John Knox Press.

Puchalski, C., & Romer, A. L. (2000). Taking a spiritual history allows clinicians to understand patients more fully. *Journal of Palliative Medicine, 3*(1), 129–137.

Rogers, C. R. (1957). The necessary and sufficient conditions of therapeutic personality change. *Journal of Consulting Psychology, 2*(21), 96.

Tillich, P. (1952). *The courage to be.* New Haven, CT: Yale University Press.

Weatherall, J. D. (1985). *Validation of the nursing diagnosis spiritual distress.* Unpublished master's thesis, University of Illinois, Chicago.

Westerhoff, J. (1976). *Will our children have faith?* New York: Seabury Press.

Recommended Readings

Carson, V. B. (Ed.). (1989). *Spiritual dimensions of nursing practice.* Philadelphia: WB Saunders.

Emblen, J. Q., Fitchett, G., Farran, C., & Burck, J. R. (1992). Identifying parameters of spiritual need. *The Care Giver Journal, 8*(2), 44–50.

Fish, S., & Shelly, J. A. (1978). *Spiritual care: The nurse's role.* Downers Grove, IL: InterVarsity Press.

Granstrom, S. L. (1985). Spiritual nursing care for oncology patients. *Topics in Clinical Nursing, 7*(1), 39–45.

Pargament, K., et al. (1988). Religion and the problem-solving process: Three styles of coping. *Journal for the Scientific Study of Religion, 27*(1), 90–104.

Richardson, S. (2000). Making a spiritual assessment. *Nursing Spectrum, 14*(2IL), 18–21.

15

*P*lanning, Implementing, and Evaluating Spiritual Care

Kristen L. Mauk, Cynthia A. Russell, and Nola A. Schmidt

LEARNING OBJECTIVES

At the end of this chapter, the reader will be able to:

- Identify patient outcomes for people experiencing spiritual distress.
- Plan care for patients in spiritual distress.
- Develop nursing interventions for supporting spiritual well-being.
- Identify interventions from the Nursing Interventions Classification (NIC) that would be most appropriate in providing spiritual care.
- Describe several alternatives to traditional therapies that may help enhance spiritual wellness.
- Explain the relationships among documentation of spiritual care and assuring quality care, addressing economic issues, and maintaining a legal document.
- List strategies to improve charting about spiritual care.
- Discuss the importance of documentation for parish nursing.
- Evaluate interventions for promoting spiritual wellness and easing spiritual distress.

acupuncture
animal-assisted therapy (AAT)
art therapy
complementary and alternative
    medicine (CAM)
document
drama therapy
evaluate
evaluation
HIPAA
hope instillation
humor therapy
implement
JCAHO

massage
meditation
music therapy
Nursing Interventions Classification (NIC)
Nursing Outcomes Classification (NOC)
pet therapy
plan
prayer
spiritual distress
tai chi
therapeutic arts
therapeutic touch
yoga

As discussed in Unit II, patients of various faiths and denominations may share common basic beliefs. However, religious practices within belief systems vary so widely that nothing can replace a thorough spiritual assessment as part of the nursing care plan. Chapter 14 provides suggestions for assessment and nursing diagnosis. The next step in meeting the spiritual needs of patients and their families is to set goals, which is called *outcome identification*.

PATIENT OUTCOME IDENTIFICATION AND PLANNING

After assessing patients and identifying the spiritually related nursing diagnoses, nurses identify specific patient outcomes to direct the planning phase of the nursing process. Nurses must individualize the outcomes for the patient to target nursing diagnoses related to the spiritual care needed to improve the patient's health status. The nurse, in conjunction with the patient, develops one or more patient-appropriate outcomes for each nursing diagnosis. These should be specific to each diagnosis and provide a measurable statement of the outcome desired within a designated time frame. Well-defined patient outcomes help guide the plan of care and facilitate its evaluation.

Standardized classification systems, such as the **Nursing Outcomes Classification (NOC)**, can be useful for the nurse working with spiritually distressed patients (Johnson, Maas, & Moorhead, 2000). This resource for outcomes specially directed toward spiritual well-being, hopelessness, risk for spiritual distress, and spiritual distress is an exceptional reference for nurses because it lists outcomes associated with the NANDA diagnoses applicable to spiritual care. Including patients in planning outcomes is critical to the success of the entire process. The challenge for nurses is to appreciate the person as an individual and respect each person's faith-based beliefs and practices. Many traditional nursing interventions promote spiritual well-being, but this chapter focuses on several strategies beyond what is typically learned in basic nursing education. As suggested in previous chapters, the spiritual aspect of the person is intangible and often best assisted by interventions that communicate to the soul and spirit. Spiritual distress is often best relieved by soothing the spirit with more universal languages, such as music. Several interventions are discussed in the following section.

STRATEGIES FOR IMPLEMENTATION

The third edition of the *Nursing Interventions Classification* (NIC), created by the University of Iowa and the National Institute of Nursing Research, provides suggestions for interventions related to nursing diagnoses, including a few spiritual ones. The NIC is described as "the first comprehensive classification of treatments that nurses perform" (McCloskey & Bulechek, 1996, p. 41). NIC defines a nursing intervention as "any treatment, based upon clinical judgment and knowledge, that a nurse performs to enhance patient/patient outcomes" (McCloskey & Bulechek, p. xvii).

NIC provides a standardized language of nurse-initiated and physician-initiated nursing interventions that include direct and indirect care. NIC interventions are composed of three parts: the label, a definition, and a set of activities that a nurse does to carry out the intervention. A short list of background readings is also provided (http://www.library.ucsf.edu). Interventions are included for physiologic, psychosocial, and spiritual needs. The spiritual aspects are integrated into and across domains and classes. Interventions cross all levels of prevention. The system of classification is under continual development, with interventions in new settings (indirect care or care of communities) being added.

Although it provides nurses with a common language, the NIC is not the only terminology that nurses use. Few NIC terms have been adopted for use in research or clinical articles in the realm of spiritual care. Nevertheless, a common language for nursing builds a database that serves as a foundation for the discipline and moves forward the science of nursing. Box 15.1 lists 43 interventions from the NIC list that nurses may use frequently for providing spiritual care. A list of activities associated with each of these interventions is available in *Nursing Interventions Classification* (McCloskey & Bulechek, 2000). For example, the intervention of music therapy includes such activities as "determine the patient's interest in music," and "make music tapes/compact disc and equipment available to patient" (McCloskey & Bulechek, 1996, p. 391).

The remainder of this chapter provides general and commonly used terms to refer to various strategies that nurses use to provide spiritual care. Although this chapter does not exclusively use NIC terms, the reader can link the discussion to NIC by referring to Box 15.1.

The term **complementary and alternative medicine** (CAM) has gained wide use in recent years. CAM therapies include those not approved by the Food and Drug Administration (FDA); not routinely taught in medical schools; used in different doses or for conditions different from those for which the therapy has received FDA approval; and not covered by most insurance policies (Greene, Berger, Reeves, & Moffat, 1999). Many of the therapeutic interventions nurses use, especially those who consciously attend to patients' spiritual needs, may be considered CAM therapies.

BOX 15.1   Selected NIC Interventions Commonly Used in Providing Spiritual Care

Active listening	Hope instillation
Activity therapy	Learning facilitation
Anger control assistance	Meditation milieu therapy
Animal-assisted therapy	Music therapy
Anticipatory guidance	Play therapy
Anxiety reduction	Presence recreation therapy
Art therapy	Reminiscence therapy
Calming technique	Self-awareness enhancement
Caregiver support	Self-esteem enhancement
Communication enhancement	Simple guided imagery
Coping enhancement	Simple massage
Counseling	Simple relaxation therapy
Crisis intervention	Spiritual support
Decision-making support	Support group
Emotional support	Support system enhancement
Environmental management: comfort	Teaching: group
Environmental management: safety	Teaching: individual
Exercise promotion	Therapeutic touch
Family integrity promotion	Therapy group touch
Family involvement	Truth telling
Family support	Values clarification
Grief work facilitation	

Nurses often use the techniques described in this chapter to complement, supplement, or even provide the basis for care the patient needs.

About 40% of Americans have used some form of CAM because they believed it to be beneficial and were generally satisfied with it (Greene et al., 1999; Kreitzer & Snyder, 2002). Patients who used CAM shared such characteristics as being better educated and having more symptoms than did patients who did not use CAM (Sullivan, 2000).

In a review of the literature, researchers found the most frequently used activities beyond traditional medicine for patients with acquired immunodeficiency syndrome (AIDS) were: aerobic exercise, prayer, massage, acupuncture, meditation, support groups, visualization and imagery, breathing exercises, spiritual activities, and other exercise (Greene et al., 1999). Older adults with cancer were found to use exercise, herbal therapy, and spiritual healing most often. The 33% (n = 699) of patients in one study who reported using complementary therapies were most likely to be female patients with breast cancer and patients with higher levels of education (Wyatt, Friedman, Given, Given, & Beckrow, 1999). Because CAM has been found to "reduce stress, anxiety, and lifestyle patterns known to contribute to cardiovascular disease" (Kreitzer & Snyder, 2002, p. 73), many patients with cardiac problems have used CAM. The CAM strategies most supported by physicians because of significant research evidence include mind–body techniques, herbal therapy, nutrition and vitamin therapy, acupuncture, massage, and spiritual interventions (Sullivan, 2000). This chapter discusses a few of the more common forms of spiritual interventions, many of which may be considered by the general public and some health professionals to fall under CAM. However, since the beginning of professional nursing, many nurses have used these strategies as a traditional part of the daily care of their patients.

Prayer

Prayer is simply defined as talking to God. Wangerin states, "Simply, prayer is communication. We talk with God, not just to him. First, we speak, while, second, God listens. Third, God speaks, while, fourth, we listen" (1996, p. 29). Dossey argues, "A complete definition of prayer can never be given...if prayer has its roots in the unconscious" (1996, p. 6). Mother Teresa believed "Real prayer is union with God" (1998, p. 8). She said, "Prayer is the very life of oneness, of being one with Christ. Therefore, prayer is as necessary as the air, as the blood in our body, as anything, to keep us alive to the grace of God" (p. 9).

Prayer can be done privately or with others in corporate worship or small groups. In some faiths, prayer at certain times of the day is mandatory. Others believe that prayer is an attitude that one can carry throughout the day. 1 Thessalonians 5:17 instructs, "Pray without ceasing." Certain religions or denominations prohibit followers from praying with those of different beliefs. Despite other differences, people of all faiths have historically believed in the power of prayer and used it to intercede for the sick. According to Williamson, "Prayer and meditation reconnect us with our Source" (1998, p. 20).

✚ Followers of Christ from Biblical times believed in the ultimate power of God to answer the prayers of His children. Many Christians today take comfort in the hope of healing that is promised in James 5:13–18 (notice the numerous references to the power of prayer):

> Is any among you afflicted? Let him pray. Is any merry? Let him sing psalms. Is any sick among you? Let him call for the elders of the church; and let them pray over him, anointing him with oil in the name of the Lord; And the prayer of faith shall save the sick, and the Lord shall raise him up; and if he have committed sins, they shall be forgiven him. Confess your faults one to another and pray one for another, that ye may be healed. The effectual, fervent prayer of a righteous man availeth much. Elijah was a man subject to like passions as we are, and he prayed earnestly that it might not rain; and it rained not on the earth by the space of three years and six months. And he prayed again, and the heaven gave rain, and the earth brought forth her fruit.

The connection of prayer to health has been studied in many settings. However, because prayer is difficult to define or measure, "scientific" evidence is lacking. Yet to those who have experienced healing from disease or personal tragedy, prayer may be an unexplainable source of power. Dossey states, "It is simply a fact that patients sometimes improve dramatically following prayer" (1996, p. 9).

The effects of prayer on patient outcomes are a relatively new area of research. The rigor of the methodology for such studies can be difficult to justify and evaluate. Nevertheless, some researchers have reported findings that prayer may decrease lengths of stay in the critical care unit and mortality of patients with cardiac disorders (Kreitzer & Snyder, 2002). Patients who found strength and comfort in religion were less likely to die after heart surgery than were those who did not (Kreitzer & Snyder). In one study, patients with AIDS cited prayer as the spiritual ritual they used most frequently (Greene et al., 1999). Another study showed that patients undergoing rehabilitation used prayer as a positive coping mechanism after discharge to the home setting, reporting it to be highly effective (Easton, Rawl, Zemen, Kwiatkowski, & Burczyk, 1995). Patients with cancer also have used prayer. In addition to using prayer as a strategy for coping with cancer in general, there is evidence that people with cancer use prayer to cope with distressing symptoms and procedures. Older patients with cancer agreed that prayer made them feel better, less anxious, less depressed, and comforted (Wyatt et al., 1999). Research measuring the relationships between prayer experience and such psychological factors would clarify and extend our understanding. Prayer was reported as a strategy frequently used by patients in many other situations, such as recovering from stroke, undergoing surgery, or heart problems (Dossey, 1996; Easton, 1999; Easton & Andrews, 1999).

Nursing strategies for facilitating prayer must be designed with sensitivity to the uniqueness of each patient. Once prayer has been identified as important to the patient, ask "What helps you pray?" As discussed in Unit II, patients of various faiths may have items that they commonly use during prayer, such as a rosary, prayer beads, or a book of prayers. These items should be kept near the bedside, within the patient's reach at all times. The nurse occasionally may need to limit visitors so that a patient may have time to pray.

Keeping a prayer journal is another strategy for helping patients who value prayer as a spiritual support. This type of journal is similar to a diary in which the person records prayer requests, thoughts about time with God, or both. The prayer journal often becomes a personal reflective notebook, with the person returning to the journal to see which prayers have been answered and how. Because the person can see results from the prayers offered for others or himself/herself, the journal becomes a source of encouragement and fosters the belief that prayer is effective in changing life circumstances for the better. Schlintz (2001) listed the following reasons for keeping a prayer journal:

- To develop a relationship with God and others
- To discover ourselves
- To discern the will of God
- To design a consistent, meaningful devotional life
- To deepen our prayer life

Both patients and nurses can use a prayer journal.

Patients may ask nurses to pray for or with them as a form of comfort. Nurses should feel free to pray with patients if this is an appropriate and requested intervention to meet a spiritual need. In times of severe spiritual turmoil or distress, referral to a trained chaplain or other appropriate professional counselor is advisable.

Presence

Nurses often provide the greatest amount of spiritual care to patients without employing multiple strategies or interventions but by simply being with the patient. The gift of presence, being with a patient in the time of need, can provide a tremendous spiritual benefit. Many nurses have an intuitive sense that their physical presence is the best medicine at certain times. They often combine presence with other modalities, such as therapeutic touch. For example, during a painful medical procedure, the nurse may hold the patient's hand, providing calm reassurance. When a patient is being told about an unexpected serious health condition, the nurse can be present in the room to comfort and console the patient and family, answering questions as needed after the initial shock subsides. The physical presence of the caring nurse is an essential spiritual intervention that many patients need.

Hope Instillation

"Hope instillation" is an NIC term. However, a search of the literature reveals little research or clinical articles that use this term, although hope has been widely studied as a concept in nursing. The reader is referred to Chapter 1 for a discussion of the concept of hope and ways it has been researched.

NIC defines **hope instillation** as "facilitation of the development of a positive outlook in a given situation" (McCloskey & Bulechek, 1996, p. 321). Most activities that NIC suggests to foster hope in patients relate to the following areas: showing acceptance of the patient, emphasizing the positive in the situation, being honest, promoting therapeutic relationships including those with the family, encouraging self-care, providing accurate information to both patient and family, educating, and fostering a healing environment. NIC lists many activities related to each theme. The reader is encouraged to explore the complete list for further information (McCloskey & Bulechek, 2000). Each key area for intervention should be viewed within the framework of the person's spirituality and religious practices. Hope instillation fosters the belief that things may get better, that these trials may be temporary, and that some improvement may be just around the corner. It is the power of positive thinking in action.

Miller (2000) has done extensive work on the concept of hope. In a chapter entitled "Inspiring Hope," Miller states that hope is a power resource that patients can use to promote wellness. According to Miller, hope at its best arises out of suffering, personal loss, and despair; hope is multidimensional and complex. Box 15.2 lists the crit-

---

BOX 15.2 Miller's Critical Elements of Hope

- Mutuality and affiliation (trusting interpersonal relationships)
- Sense of the possible (not giving into despair)
- Avoidance of absolutizing (not having an all-or-nothing attitude with regard to what is hoped for)
- Anticipation (expecting good things in the future)
- Establishing and achieving goals (objects of hope)
- Psychological well-being and coping (elements that sustain energy needed for hope)
- Purpose and meaning in life (having something to live for)
- Freedom (feeling that there is a way out—avoiding hopelessness)
- Reality surveillance (keeping hope alive by searching for reasons to continue to hope)
- Optimism (a prerequisite)
- Mental and physical activation (energy that battles despair)

(Explanations in parentheses were adapted from Miller, J. F. [2000]. *Coping with chronic illness: Overcoming powerlessness.* Philadelphia: FA Davis.)

---

ical elements of hope according to Miller. Miller recommends categories for intervention, which can be read about in *Coping with Chronic Illness: Overcoming Powerlessness* (2000). Table 15.1 simplifies and makes practical some nursing interventions to instill hope based on the categories from Miller's analyses of her grounded theory study.

TABLE 15.1   Nursing Interventions to Instill Hope Based on Miller's Categories

Strategies to Maintain Hope	Practical Application
Cognitive strategies	Assess the patient's mental coping strategies; promote the idea that the patient can make it through this difficulty; encourage use of scriptures for meditation; encourage use of positive coping strategies that worked in the past; promote positive thinking.
Determinism	Remind the patient that there is always hope; emphasize patient strengths; promote a positive attitude that does not give up.
Philosophy of life and world view	Remind the patient that growth occurs from struggles; assess patient's daily way of dealing with difficulties, then emphasize the positive aspects of this.
Spiritual strategies	Prayer; facilitate use of religious articles and attendance at worship services if possible; involve the spiritual leader and provide other spiritual support.
Relationship with caregivers	Foster warm, sincere relationships that encourage the person to continue to positively cope; promote the use of positive coping strategies; let caregivers know you are on their side and cheering for them.
Family bonds	Promote family involvement in care; strengthen family ties and help with resolution of strained relationships; point out reasons based on the family (such as children needing the parent) for the person to continue to live.
Sense of being in control	Provide information and education to enhance knowledge of the disease/illness process and what to expect; provide opportunities for decision making even in the smallest of areas; return as much control as possible to the patient.
Goal accomplishment	Help the patient set reasonable goals and assist with writing short-term and long-term ways to meet them.
Other	Humor, relaxation, music therapy, and other CAM activities may also be used to instill hope.

(Adapted with permission from Miller, J. F. [2000]. *Coping with chronic illness: Overcoming powerlessness*. Philadelphia: FA Davis.)

The essence of nursing is an attitude of hope. Most nurses would not be in the field if they did not have a sense of hope that their actions could improve patient outcomes. Nurses must not forget that they are messengers of hope for patients who may be in despair. Those in spiritual distress may have lost hope, so an important part of any nurse's job when providing spiritual care is to instill hope.

Acupuncture

Ⓢ **Acupuncture** is a part of Chinese medicine that has been used for approximately 5000 years. Through needles that pinpoint specific parts of the body, acupuncture seeks to restore the balance and flow of chi (the life force or energy). Chi (also written qi or ch'i) is important because it helps maintain the balance of the yin and the yang (opposing forces) in the body. Yin and yang often are symbolized by black/white, dark/light, evil/good, and cold/hot. An imbalance of chi results in illness.

Only an experienced and trained acupuncturist should perform this type of CAM. The general procedure begins with an extensive medical history, followed by a physical examination that includes thorough evaluation of the person's pulses and meridian lines. The acupuncturist inserts needles at specific points. Sometimes, he or she uses additional therapies, such as moxibustion (burning an herb on or near the skin) to enhance the treatment. A full treatment usually lasts 15 to 60 minutes as the patient rests with the needles in place (Dean, Mullins, & Yuen, 2000). After the treatment session, herbal remedies, massage, or a special diet may be recommended.

Acupuncture has been shown to affect the release of endorphins, which directly influence brain chemistry. It has been used to manage pain and nausea, asthma, infertility, and chronic fatigue (Sullivan, 2000). The American Academy of Medical Acupuncture reports the therapy can treat many other conditions, such as injuries related to sports, nerve pain, cancer, allergies, high blood pressure, digestive diseases, depression, and other psychological disorders (Dean et al., 2000).

Ⓢ Nurses should be alert to the likelihood that patients who practice Eastern religions may use acupuncture as a major or adjunctive treatment for illness, pain, or disease. Regardless of the nurse's personal opinion about the safety or clinical effectiveness of certain practices of Chinese medicine, respect for the patient's beliefs is essential. Open communication about the patient's preferred methods of medical and nursing care is required to provide a holistic plan of care that meets the patient's needs and goals.

Herbs and Vitamin Therapy

In Europe, herbal therapy is integrated into traditional medicine, but in the 1940s and 1950s herbal therapy was almost abandoned in the United States and replaced with pharmaceutical agents (Sullivan, 2000). Recently, interest in herbal and vitamin therapies has re-emerged in the United States.

Vitamins are commonly used in the United States as a regular treatment to promote or enhance health. Health food stores sell a variety of herbs and vitamins for the treatment of various ailments. Nurses need to take a thorough history and ask specific questions about the patient's habits regarding vitamins or herbal medicines. Supplemental vitamins often are essential to promote health, particularly in frail, elderly patients or pregnant or breast-feeding women. Vitamin and mineral supplements, such as vitamins E, C, and B complex and zinc, have been shown to increase fertility in both men and women and have been linked to a host of other benefits. Many people take vitamin C to ward off colds. Vitamin B complex is thought to help improve mood and fight depression. Vitamin E aids healing, helps prevent heart disease, and may help in the treatment of certain types of diabetes and arthritis (Sullivan, 2000). Vitamins C, D, E, and A help build strong bones and promote good eyesight. In other parts of the world, vitamins may be necessary because economic or geographic problems prohibit access to enough nutrients to sustain life and prevent disease, but in the United States, much of the need for vitamin supplements is the result of poor eating habits in today's society. The use of too much vitamin supplementation can be hazardous to one's health.

The use of vitamins may help enhance a person's health, not just through promotion of physical well-being, but also by fostering a sense of control over one's own health through active participation. That is, choosing to use vitamin supplements and selecting which particular vitamins to take promote a sense of ownership of one's health. Thus, such health-promoting and disease-preventing activities also enhance spiritual wellness because they increase feelings of well-being and autonomy.

Herbs also have been shown to help in the treatment of many common disorders. In Germany, 90% of the most frequently used medications for depression are brands of St. John's wort (Sullivan, 2000). Herbal remedies often are used to combat depression by elevating mood and enhancing a sense of well-being. People may use herbs to try to meet unrecognized spiritual needs. It is important for nurses to assess the connection between the herb and what patients feel its benefits are to them personally. In this way, nurses may better address any underlying concerns and evaluate additional appropriate strategies for managing them.

Other herbs are used for their positive physical effects. Saw palmetto is thought to help benign prostatic hypertrophy. Avocado–soybean unsaponifiables herbal therapy has been identified as beneficial in the treatment of osteoarthritis, but evidence for other herbal therapies is insufficient and inconclusive (Little, Parsons, & Logan, 2002).

Many herbs found in local health food stores are not FDA approved. Thus, there is no guarantee of their potency or regulation of their purity. Unfortunately, many patients are seen in emergency departments and hospitals each year who have supplemented traditional prescription medications with an herbal remedy containing a similar drug, causing toxicity and overdose symptoms. Herbs also may interfere with certain prescribed medications. For example, St. John's wort can decrease the effectiveness of some medications, such as theophylline. Thus, it is essential for nurses to ensure that the physician or primary health care provider is informed of a patient's use of vitamins and herbs because they may alter the medically prescribed regimen. The nurse should not impose judgment regarding the use of these remedies, but all care providers should be informed of their use.

Massage

Covering each of the nearly 100 different types or techniques of **massage** is beyond the scope of this text. Several of the most common massage therapies should be familiar to readers: portable, reflexology, shiatsu, Swedish, sports-related, and massage used in combination with aromatherapy. Most nurses have been educated to use simple massage techniques in patients' daily care. A licensed massage therapist generally receives 500 hours of education, including supervised practice (Greene, 2000). Use of certain fragrances and oils with massage is believed to enhance the experience as they are absorbed and smelled.

Each type of massage has a specific focus. The portable or onsite massage is popular with busy professionals. The massage therapist generally brings a portable table on which the patient relaxes, or a chair massage of just the shoulders and neck can be done in an abbreviated session to relieve work-related tensions. Reflexology is based on the Eastern belief that reflex points in the hands and feet connect the entire body and that stimulation of a specific area on the hand corresponds to a healing effect on a certain organ of the body. Reflexology is a learned skill and can be used by some trained professionals to promote healing of various parts of the body. Shiatsu is thought to decrease pain and stimulate the flow of energy in the body by application of pressure to specific points. Swedish massage, one of the most familiar and widely practiced, uses certain strokes primarily for the purpose of general muscle relaxation, decreasing stress, and easing tension. First developed in 1812 by Professor Ling of Sweden, this massage system is based on scientific manipulations with the purpose of affecting the neuromuscular system and promoting circulation. Trainers use sports-related massages on professional athletes to prevent injuries.

The benefits of massage are generally well accepted. With regard to the spiritual self, massage may relieve pain, improve function, promote relaxation, increase energy, enhance mood, and reduce anxiety (Greene, 2000). Massage has been shown to help patients with arthritis, sleep disorders, and many other problems.

Most nurses were taught basic massage techniques in their nursing programs and can use massage to promote relaxation in patients. For the average adult patient, the simple intervention of a therapeutic back rub brings the benefits previously described. Because the human spirit is so closely connected to a patient's mental and emotional state, massage can evoke a relaxing state that enhances self-esteem and promotes a general sense of well-being. Massage is contraindicated in certain patients, such as those with deep vein thrombosis, those with especially fragile skin or contagious skin conditions, and those at risk for bleeding. Nurses use certain types of massage with caution in patients with diabetes or pregnancy, although nurse midwives have long used massage techniques to ease the pain of labor.

Therapeutic Touch

Therapeutic touch (TT) is one aspect of treatment that emerged in relationship to the perceived benefits of human touch. Studies have reported TT reduces anxiety, promotes sleep, decreases stress and pain, and increases the rate of healing. According to two comprehensive integrative reviews with meta-analyses of TT research, there seems to be a moderate, positive relationship with several variables (Peters, 1999; Winstead-Fry & Kijek, 1999). For example, TT may have a moderately positive effect on reducing anxiety in certain patient populations, and some studies support the hypothesis that TT can reduce stress and postoperative pain. It may even enhance wound healing. However, many of the studies on TT had serious methodological flaws. More rigorous research should be undertaken to determine the efficacy of TT.

Meditation

Meditation can be defined as "an activity synthesizing the mind and spirit in the present moment" (Greene et al., 1999, p. 66). More simply, it means slowing down or taking pause. Meditation may be stimulating and may create a sense of peace and well being (de Alberdi, 1998). Meditation has been around for thousands of years; it is not a new concept to most health care professionals. It often has been linked to the spiritual self, whether by focusing on the concepts or words of a faith or by centering of the self to refocus. Trieschmann, who used meditation in rehabilitative practice, states: "The addition of meditation and the discipline of spirituality will enhance one's experience of the religion of the ancestors if that is a meaningful part of the person's life" (2001, p. 32).

Meditation also has been found to have specific physiologic benefits. Herbert Benson found that "Meditation evokes a state of the autonomic nervous system that is correlated with a reduction in stress reactivity, as measured by lowering of the heart rate, blood pressure, pulse rate, respiration rate, and levels of the stress hormone plasma cortisol" (Kreitzer & Snyder, 2002). Meditation has helped patients with cardiac problems to improve their cardiovascular status. It is also one of the strategies frequently used by patients with AIDS who have longer survival times (Carson, 1993). In addition, meditation is often combined with other CAM strategies, such as yoga, tai chi, or aromatherapy.

Yoga

Yoga, derived from the Sanskrit word meaning "union," is an integrated system developed to promote spiritual enlightenment and physical well-being. With origins in India more than 4000 years ago, yoga brings together a person's mind, body, and spirit into a unified whole. Central to the practice of yoga is the use of postures, stretches, and breathing techniques. Many forms of yoga are found in the United States, but perhaps the most popular type is Hatha yoga. Hatha yoga focuses on the use of asanas, or specific postural shapes, that pair with steady breathing. People practicing yoga are encouraged to calm their minds and be open to enlightened awareness. Achievement of this goal is more likely with systematic and regular practice.

Although yoga is perhaps best recognized for its physical benefits (increased flexibility, enhanced muscular strength and tone, improved balance, and improved generalized body systems), its emotional and spiritual benefits are equally impressive. These include relaxation, improved concentration, enhanced self-worth and confidence, a sense of inner peace, the ability to stay calm under pressure, and improved mental alertness. As a noncompetitive activity, the practice of yoga promotes personal growth and self-exploration. Each of these ties positive physical benefits to the strengthening of the spiritual or inner self.

With the popularity of yoga increasing across the country, the nurse should be familiar with community resources for patient referral. The Internet can be a helpful tool for locating area practitioners and practice sites. Because of the great variation in forms of yoga and differences in abilities of the providers, the nurse must remind patients to "shop around" until they find a good fit. The key to yoga's usefulness as a spiritual tool is consistent practice. This occurs only if patients integrate the activity into their daily life. Suggest participation with a partner or friend to create an even greater bond with this practice.

Tai Chi

Ⓢ Developed in China 3000 years ago, **tai chi** is a systematic method of movement that promotes spiritual centering and mental focus, in addition to exercise and martial arts training. As a form of traditional Chinese medicine, tai chi's goal is to ensure the flow of chi or "life energy" within the body (Woodham & Peters, 1997). A balance of chi is necessary for the body to maintain health.

Advocates for the use of tai chi suggest that regular participants might experience enhanced mood and well-being, increased relaxation, and improved physical strength (Chin, 1995). The health benefits of tai chi as a nursing intervention are multidimensional. Research has supported the use of tai chi for the reduction of stress (Jin, 1992; Lan, Lai, & Chen, 1998), health improvements for patients with health failure (Fontana, Colella, Baas, & Ghazi, 2000), the reduction of pain (Ross, Bohannon, & Davis, 1999; Wu, Bandilla, & Iccone, 1999), and the reduction of fall risk and associated improvement of balance (Province, Hadley, & Hornbrook, 1995).

Often described as "meditation in motion," tai chi is an intervention amenable to people of all ages and physical abilities. Tai chi has been a treatment modality for some patients at the Rehabilitation Institute of Chicago recovering from chronic or disabling health problems. Older adults especially can benefit from engaging in the practice of tai chi. Studying with a master teacher and attending classes helps participants learn philosophy, breathing techniques, and the proper form of tai chi. Weekly sessions and daily practice result in maximum health benefits for the participant. Although six primary forms of tai chi exist, yang is the most common form practiced worldwide (Chin, 1995). Yang style is extremely gentle, using a series of postures to create a rhythmical exercise movement. This style is available in long form (108 postures) or short form (24 postures). In addition to the physical benefits of such exercise, the calming effect of achieving balance and an improved flow of energy or chi can soothe the soul and spirit.

Therapeutic Arts

Therapeutic arts are generally thought to include drama, music, art, and dance. Each field may be used to enhance a patient's sense of well-being and promote emotional and spiritual wellness. Nurses should be alert to the possibility that individuals in their care may have already established a routine of incorporating such activities into their daily life as a health-promoting strategy. Therapeutic arts also are often used to reduce stress and anxiety for caregivers and nurses.

Before the days of heightened cost-containment consciousness, hospital arts programs were "thriving because the wellness within the patients responding as listeners, viewers, poets, dancers, or creators of some sort is sparked by the art that entices them, if only briefly, to leave a diseased state and refresh their souls and spirits" (Pratt, 1992, p. 3). However, in today's society, the potential benefits of these programs are sometimes lost in the politics of health care as budgetary restrictions often call for the elimination of activities deemed "less essential." Health care professionals should be mindful that the therapeutic arts often cross the barriers of culture and language and can be used with a variety of patients or for personal health enhancement. As Miles states, "medicine and the arts have always been linked. ... Any of the art forms offer activity that is all about personal choices (including whether or not to participate—a choice not open in the medical part of patient care) and help retain a sense of self-esteem" (1992, p. 26, 28).

Drama Therapy

Drama therapy evolved from the experience of teachers, actors, and therapists who realized that sometimes nontraditional therapies that included the arts worked better with patients than did traditional approaches. In its purest sense, drama therapy can be a strategy used in professional psychotherapy. For most of the general public, drama therapy provides benefits for those who feel spiritual rejuvenation and release through acting.

The use of drama as therapy is intentional, systematic, and goal oriented. **Drama therapy** integrates drama and psychotherapy to facilitate personal change. It can be used with individuals, families, or groups. The National Association for Drama Therapy (n.d.) defines drama therapy as "the systematic and intentional use of drama/theater processes, products, and associations to achieve the therapeutic goals of symptom relief, emotional and physical integration, and personal growth." Kavanaugh (1995) states: "Drama therapy brings a sense of renewal. It helps residents to forget about their pains and troubles and become creative and productive" (p. 5).

The California Institute of Integral Studies (n.d.) offers one of the few U.S. graduate programs in drama therapy. Such programs focus on educating professionals to use drama therapy as an enhancement to traditional mental health services. Registered drama therapists ascribe to professional, ethical, and moral standards similar to those of other health care professionals. Techniques used in this type of therapy may include role playing, pantomime, puppetry, improvisation, combinations with music and/or dance therapy, creating original sound/movement/drama pieces, and group theater work.

Many different groups and individuals may benefit from drama therapy: elderly residents in nursing homes, those in mental health facilities, the disabled, or others who just want to enhance self-exploration. The theatre provides an outlet in which persons can be more than themselves, release emotions, and role play. The benefits of drama therapy may include symptom relief, personal growth, improved quality of life, increased self-awareness, enhancement of self-expression, increased self-esteem, better interpersonal and social skills, improved coping skills, decreased stress, and increased spontaneity (California Institute of Integral Studies, n.d.).

Drama therapy can facilitate patients' abilities to tell their stories, help resolve conflicts, improve relationship skills, and explore creativity. Participation in community theater can provide similar benefits for individuals who find drama therapeutic. Nurses in long-term care facilities or senior centers can facilitate modified forms of drama therapy.

Music Therapy

The American Music Therapy Association (http://www.musictherapy.org) defines **music therapy** as "the prescribed use of music by a qualified person to effect positive changes in the psychological, physical, cognitive, or social functioning of individuals with health or educational problems." Unfortunately, this definition is limiting, suggesting that only those educated as music therapists are qualified to use music therapy with patients. Nurses who work in the spiritual care area realize that many therapeutic uses of music do not require a certified music therapist. However, the most qualified person to offer music therapy meets the qualifications of the AMTA. Individuals must complete an approved college music therapy curriculum that includes an internship, after which they are eligible to take the national examination offered by the certification board for music therapists. Their education includes both music and therapy-related courses. Successful completion of these requirements leads to certification (as a music therapist-board certified [MT-BC]).

Music is often called the universal language because it crosses the boundaries of age, generation, class, and culture. Music also has a healing property: "Every culture in the world has used sound and music to heal" (Gerber, 1998, p. 69). Frohnmayer (1994) states: "Think, then, of music as a bridge over damaged paths in our brains and between our earthbound selves and our spiritual lives" (p. 27).

The goals of music therapy are not generally musical in nature: music is used not to create musicians, but to meet patients' needs, such as anxiety reduction, pain relief, reminiscence, or communication. Other goals of music therapy may include a change in mood or emotions, promotion of imagery, promotion of healing, or transitioning from life to death. Music therapy can refer to the patient's participation in the music or to the use of music performed by others to achieve patient goals.

Several instruments are commonly used in music therapy in which the patient participates. Drums provide immediate accessibility and do not take much expertise to play (Janowiak, 1993). Therapeutic goals may be met in a more timely manner because little practice or preparation is required to learn to play drums. Other percussion instruments, such a simple dulcimers or hand bells, and using the voice to sing also encourage patient participation.

The harp has long been thought to be the music of angels. King Saul's troubled spirit was soothed when David played the stringed instrument for him. Harp players are often summoned to the bedside of dying patients to provide a peaceful transition to their eternal home. Because the harp is a difficult instrument to play, someone else most likely would play it while the patient listens. However, some harpists maintain there is therapy in playing the harp, both because of the physical movement involved and because the vibrations that go through the musician's body while playing are healing in nature.

The human voice also can be soothing, with or without additional accompaniment. Toning, chanting, humming, and singing are all uses of the voice as an instrument. The act of playing or singing that engages the person in the act of making music is thought to be more therapeutic in many cases than merely listening. Box 15.3 lists benefits of music therapy.

Because music should be geared to the population being addressed, nurses should ask patients which types of music they prefer. The setting also must be considered. For example, if the patient finds loud hard rock music relaxing, headphones may need to be used to avoid disturbing others. Most likely, the music found to be most soothing to individuals is moderate, calming, and rhythmic. Much preferred music reflects the person's ethnic or cultural background. For example, African-Americans may prefer to listen to spirituals or jazz, whereas Hispanics may have a favorite Latino artist. "Music is the voice of the human spirit" (Frohnmayer, 1994, p. 26), and nurses need to foster the types of music that give expression to the patient's individual choices and personality.

Music therapy has been used in a variety of settings. For example, music has been used with premature infants with good results. Findings suggest that "music has statistically significant and clinically important benefits for premature infants in the NICU" (Standley, 2002). Music has been shown to enhance the mood of patients during cardiac rehabilitation exercise sessions (Murrock, 2002). As an alternative to restraint use, music may increase positive behaviors among hospitalized patients (Janelli, Kanski, & Wu, 2002). In patients undergoing colonoscopy, music therapy decreased anxiety, heart rate, and blood pressure (Smolen, Topp, & Singer, 2002).

B O X   1 5 . 3   Potential Benefits of Music Therapy

- Can lower heart rate, blood pressure, and respiratory rate
- Produces a calming effect
- Often an integral part of guided imagery therapy
- Can be used in combination with biofeedback
- Eases pain, sometimes resulting in use of less pain medication
- Can boost the immune system
- Conveys one's culture, values, or beliefs without words
- Is a universal language
- Assists persons to work through conflict
- Can produce a sense of camaraderie by breaking social and cultural barriers and crossing generations
- May promote imagery or transcendence
- Playing instruments or dancing to music can exercise joints
- Reconnects people with their past, aids in reminiscence or end-of-life

---

One situation in which music is being used more frequently is the end of life. It has been used as an appropriate intervention for oncology nurses in improving quality of life in dying patients. Musical selections that are carefully chosen can "help alleviate pain, anxiety, and nausea, and induce sleep" (Halstead & Roscoe, 2002). One study found that using music therapy with the homeless and indigent who were actively dying decreased anxiety and brought about a peaceful transition at death (Mramor, 2001). In this study, the music was live, sung a cappella or played on a keyboard, and sometimes sung with an instrumental accompaniment. The most effective types of music to facilitate dying with this population were lullabies, music with spiritual themes, favorite songs of the person, original songs, or popular music. Recorded music was helpful, but live music was preferred.

Whether nurses assist patients to use music in a participatory or observant way, "music demonstrates the connection between thought and emotion, physical and mental activity" (Frohnmayer, 1994, p. 26). It is an effective tool to effect change and help meet patient goals, and can bring about change individually or collectively. As Frohnmayer states, "Music is the spiritual glue that binds the human community" (p. 26).

Art Therapy

Although perhaps used less often than other therapeutic arts, art therapy has been shown to have distinct benefits with specific groups of patients. Arts and crafts groups are often a part of the social program of many senior centers. Churches, synagogues, and parishes may offer art classes such as painting or pottery to attract community members. Although some may not consider the benefits that such informal situations provide, there is little doubt that participants enjoy fellowship and camaraderie as much as the artistic expression. Art can be used in a more structured way in a variety of health care settings. Art therapy can be used in conjunction with behavior therapy for patients with cognitive and mental disorders. According to Sterritt and Pokorny (1994), "art therapy is now widely used in psychiatric hospitals, for assessment of individuals and families, and in special education programs for learning disabled and retarded in nursing homes, halfway houses, and drug programs. Yet there has been little research on the use of art therapy by health care professionals" (p. 156).

Therapists have long used art to help observe problems in children who are unable to verbalize. Certain symbols that occur when children draw have been linked to specific feelings they may be unable to express. For example, a child who draws a large, isolated, empty tree in a picture of his back yard may be feeling loneliness. When children draw pictures of their family, issues are often revealed regarding relationships and events that may be causing problems for that child.

"Art may help fight disuse, decrease isolation, and facilitate communication" in those with Alzheimer's disease and related disorders (Sterritt & Pokorny, 1994, p. 155). These researchers found that creative artistic expression by the elderly helped to decrease depression and enhance self-esteem by providing a sense of control over an experience. Art therapy can be used concurrently with reminiscence therapy and may often facilitate the expression of feelings. When done in a group setting, art therapy also can facilitate communication and social interaction (Sterritt & Pokorny).

Art therapy has also been used successfully with children who have dyslexia or other problems. Persons with communication problems often experience poor self-esteem and emotional frustration. By assisting patients with individual ways to express themselves, nurses can decrease the emotional and spiritual trauma that can be created in a world of words that isolates those with learning disabilities. For example, the Ron Davis method for helping people with dyslexia learn to read incorporates the use of clay in orienting the person to letters and shapes. Working with clay seems to help those with cognitive, orientation, or spacial/perceptual difficulties in many ways. Regarding symbol mastery for words by those with reading disabilities, Davis states that "building the forms of the letters in clay not only helps break the habit of heavy concentration, but allows the person to do something creative as a learning activity" (1997, p. 223).

Nurses can easily and informally incorporate art therapy into their program. Small interventions, such as providing supplies for patients and families to engage in artistic activities, can be used. However, for persons with specific needs who would benefit from formal art therapy, the help of a trained professional in the field is advisable.

Humor Therapy

The positive benefits of **humor therapy** have been widely accepted. Proverbs 17:22 states that "a merry heart doeth good like a medicine." Hulse states: "Humor has been defined as both an emotional and a cognitive process that is unique to an individual and appeals to the comic sense" (1994, p. 88). The physiologic benefits of laughter include improved oxygenation, stimulation of the many muscles used in laughing, increased energy levels, and release of endorphins. After hearty laughter, a period of relaxation follows. Research has shown that humor, especially laughter, is positively correlated with an increase in secretory immunoglobulin A in both adults and children (Lambert & Lambert, 1995).

Humor is known to provide relief from stress, anxiety, and pain. In 1977, Norman Cousins described how using humor and laughter cured him of disease. His therapy was to spend at least 10 minutes per day in hearty laughter, often evoked by watching humorous shows on television, such as the Marx Brothers or the Three Stooges. Cousins found that by doing so, he was able to sleep without pain for a time and eventually was free of his illness.

Johnson (2002) studied the use of humor related to spirituality and coping in breast cancer survivors. Her research showed that breast cancer survivors used humor as an effective coping strategy to deal with their diagnosis. In addition, survivors said that humor was part of their spirituality, helping them to find meaning and purpose in life. Humor was also viewed as a part of the recovery process. Johnson's study also showed that nurses' use of humor with these patients helped to build a more trusting nurse–patient relationship.

Creating humor in the health care setting is not difficult. Often, nurses naturally foster a light-hearted attitude to deal with their own emotions in a stressful situation. Within such settings as long-term care facilities, nurses can do much to bring humor to residents or patients. Specific suggestions for incorporating humor into nursing practice are listed in Box 15.4.

Nurses can use humor to help patients meet their goals, but at times humor may be inappropriate, such as when concentration needs to be focused on problem solving or grief, and laughter would detract from the work at hand. In addition, the nurse must assess the receptiveness of the individual to humor because not all persons find it therapeutic. Patients who are paranoid may misinterpret humor, and those who are depressed may feel that the nurse has not considered their feelings (Davidhizar & Bowen, 1992).

Pet Therapy and Animal-Assisted Therapy

Pets provide companionship and affection and have been used in a working capacity throughout history. Recent research has demonstrated that animals can provide many therapeutic benefits physically, socially, and psychologically to humans in various settings, including prisons, homes, hospitals, and nursing facilities (Spence & Kaiser, 2002). Benefits associated with animals include decreased blood pressure and heart rate, increased feelings of relaxation, decreased stress, and improved self-esteem and socialization (Johnson & Meadows, 2002).

The main goal of traditional **pet therapy** is socialization, usually through a formal or informal visitation program. In contrast, "**animal-assisted therapy** (AAT) is the utilization of animals as a therapeutic modality to facilitate healing and rehabilitation of patients with acute or chronic diseases" (Therapet Animal Assisted Therapy Foundation, http://therapet.com), suggesting a higher level of involvement of both person and animal. In AAT, a licensed therapist rigorously screens and uses the animal as a treatment tool to achieve specific goals.

The benefits of socialization and companionship have led some researchers to examine pets as a significant support system for some patients. Cohen (2002) suggested that for many people, pets function as family members and are considered inside the family circle. Pets often meet the need for companionship for those who might otherwise experience social isolation and loneliness. The household dog or cat also provides opportunities for nurturing and communication that might otherwise be absent. Johnson and Meadows conducted a study among healthy Latino elders and suggested that "pet visitation may be required as an important part of the plan

BOX 15.4 Tips for Incorporating Therapeutic Humor into Nursing Practice

- Have a baby photo contest for patients or staff. See who can match the baby with the grown-up.
- Have a humor board in the staff bathroom where staff can post jokes, stories, or write notes.
- Start a humor board in the hallway or dining room. Put funny comics or pictures on it and change it weekly.
- Invite a clown to visit your floor. Many cities have clowning groups whose members are specifically trained to clown for the sick or for children.
- Keep tapes of humorous movies, old and new, for visitors and patients to watch.
- Start a bookshelf in the lounge and stock it with joke books or funny stories.
- Decorate the unit or the person's room with a humorous play on a theme for the month.
- Institute a "play time" for visitors and patients/residents.
- Hold a carnival or fun-fair.
- Invite a local comedian to entertain at your facility.
- Have local dance companies bring their children's classes over for an informal recital. (Children who are just learning to dance are quite entertaining).
- Use decorations that are uplifting and light-hearted, such as balloons, mobiles, baskets, hand-painted pictures on the walls. Use "happy" colors and comforting scenes.
- Hold a therapy session and have a staring contest to see who can stare the longest without smiling.
- Have the local elementary school children come to the facility for a game of Bingo. Have fun and silly prizes donated from local merchants.
- Smile a lot during your daily routine.

of care for older Latinos" (2002, p. 618) because many considered their pets to be family members.

An animal may participate with a person in pet therapy at many levels. The most basic function would be to provide companionship and affection, allowing patients to pet and stroke the animal. A higher level of therapy would be the use of dogs that are trained to allow patients to groom them, hold them, and engage in closer care of them. Such dogs must be disciplined enough that they can pass a rigorous test to ensure that any sudden pulling of the hair or startling would not result in biting or other harmful behavior. Some occupational therapists use these trained pets to assist patients with upper extremity exercises.

A unique example of a recent trend in AAT is therapeutic horseback riding, the goal of which is to promote rehabilitation of people with physical, emotional, and learning disabilities through activities related to horses. Certain riding stables have such programs and use community volunteers to assist persons individually with riding activities. The potential benefits of horseback riding include improved muscle tone, better balance and posture, improved coordination, a sense of emotional well-being and independence, and a sense of normalcy, not to mention just plain fun! Individuals who might benefit from equine-assisted therapy include adults or children with cerebral palsy, autism, stroke, brain injury, muscular dystrophy, multiple sclerosis, or spina bifida. Therapeutic riding has also been incorporated into plans of care for at-risk teens and those who abuse drugs or alcohol.

Dolphins have been used in a relatively new, yet promising, AAT. It combines interaction with an animal with the therapeutic effects of aquatics, in which range of motion and movement against minimal resistance is employed.

One of the highest levels of AAT is having a service dog that is trained for the sole purpose of being a helper to man as a full-time job. Groups such as Canine Companions for Independence facilitate the breeding, raising, and training of service dogs to assist those with functional limitations. Dogs are bred to become service animals and are socialized to humans by living with families dedicated to this purpose. After about 16 months of social orientation with a family, the dogs are put through rigorous training to obey numerous commands and ignore environmental distractions. When training is complete, the animal is matched to a person requiring a service dog, and the pair engage in training together for a 2-week period at camp to get to know one another before the dog is taken home. The dogs most frequently assigned to those with physical disabilities are retrievers; border collies are often used by those with hearing impairments. German shepherds used to be the standard breed to assist the visually impaired, but some researchers maintain that any dog with the right disposition can be trained to assist people.

The role of pets in relationship to health promotion has been widely studied across various disciplines, but criticism has historically focused on the lack of scientific rigor with which such research has been done. Most studies support the theory that pets provide social and emotional support. Nevertheless, many researchers do not believe that animals provide an equal substitute for human interaction. Kaiser, Spence, McGavin, Struble, and Keilman (2002) studied the response of six nursing home residents to both a "happy person" visit and a visit from a dog. Although the sample size was small, the study results suggested that positive and happy interactions with a human were as effective and desirable as those with a dog. The authors state, "In fact, some evidence suggests that it is the person associated with the visiting animal, not the animal itself, that is responsible for the reported beneficial effects" (p. 672).

Regardless of how nurses view the current research, pets are an important part of the lives of many patients seen in health care settings. Nurses should always ask about the presence and significance of pets in a patient's life. The benefits associated with even the lowest level of involvement with pets can be therapeutic to individuals or families. Consider the use of fish tanks in physicians' or dentists' offices, which are intended to bring a calming influence to the waiting room. Aviaries with many different types of birds are at the center of some activity rooms in long-term care facilities. A pet dog or cat may live at the nursing home and be cared for by all the residents.

The creative therapeutic use of animals to promote health and wellness among people may be considered nontraditional in health care. However, the positive effect of pet therapy in any sense on the spiritual and emotional well-being of persons should always be considered.

EVALUATION

Evaluation sets the stage for ongoing reassessment, diagnosing, planning, and intervening. **Evaluation** involves two steps: evaluating goal achievement and reviewing the plan of care (Murray & Atkinson, 2000).

Evaluating Goal Achievement

Evaluation of goal achievement requires nurses to review the patient goal statements in the care plan and determine if the goals were met, partially met, or unmet (Murray & Atkinson, 2000). This part of the nursing process is significantly easier when patient goals include objective measures. For instance, nurses find it easy to evaluate patient goals related to physical health, such as "The patient's blood pressure will remain less than 140/90 mm Hg until discharge." But evaluating patient goals related to spiritual health is more difficult because one cannot "observe" the spirit. It is important for nurses to recognize that they might have to write goals to include subjective, rather than objective, patient data. For instance, nurses often implement spiritual care to reduce a patient's spiritual distress, so they may state a related goal as "The patient will verbalize decreased anger with God in 2 weeks." Evaluation of such a goal requires nurses to ask the patient to report feelings of anger and to inquire about any feelings of spiritual distress. Observable signs of reduced spiritual distress, such as a more positive affect or more positive encounters with others, also can provide evidence that the goal was met. If the nurse evaluates these subtle signs without the patient actually stating so (with only the nurse's subjective observation), the evaluation of the goal is incomplete. Inclusion of patient and family perceptions of the degree to which goals are met is important. Collaboration between patients and nurses during evaluation can facilitate healing by communicating to patients that they are valued and their faith beliefs and practices are respected.

Another helpful way to think about the evaluation step is to consider which patient outcomes were desired. The *Nursing Outcomes Classification* (NOC) (Johnson & Maas, 1997) delineates outcomes consistent with North American Nursing Diagnosis Association (NANDA) diagnoses. In spiritual care, the primary diagnoses are Readiness for Enhanced Spiritual Well-being and Spiritual Distress (see Chapter 14). Nurses can evaluate suggested outcomes for these diagnoses (Table 15.2) using standardized surveys that allow patients to rate various statements using a five-point Likert scale (Johnson & Maas). The NOC also includes outcomes and surveys for other NANDA diagnoses associated with spiritual care, such as Hopelessness and Ineffective Coping.

Reviewing the Plan of Care

Once they have evaluated goals, nurses move to the second step of evaluation, reviewing the plan of care. Thus, the process returns to additional assessment as nurses

TABLE 15.2	Nursing Classification Outcomes (NOC) for Spiritual Care	

Nursing Diagnosis	Suggested Outcomes	Additional Associated Outcomes
Spiritual Well-being, Potential for Enhanced	*Hope* Quality of life Spiritual well-being Well-being	*Dignified dying* Grief resolution Psychological adjustment Life change
Spiritual Distress	*Dignified dying* Hope Spiritual well-being	*Anxiety control* Grief resolution Psychological adjustment: life change Quality of life Suicide Self-restraint Well-being Will to live

(Adapted with permission from Johnson, M., & Maas M. [Eds.]. [1997]. *Nursing outcomes classification* [NOC] [pp. 366–367]. St. Louis: Mosby.)

re-examine the data in light of new observations. They update information about patients' spiritual health and make decisions about spiritual care while respecting their belief systems. If evaluation indicates that the patient has met goals and the problem no longer exists, the nursing diagnosis is no longer applicable. If the problem is not resolved, nurses may choose to add a new goal that is mutually agreeable with the patient and health care providers. When goals are partially met or unmet, nurses can re-evaluate the nursing diagnoses to ascertain what diagnoses are accurate in light of new findings or add new nursing diagnoses.

Once nurses have determined which diagnoses are still appropriate, they can adapt the plan of care by revising former goals or adding new ones. While reviewing the plan of care, nurses evaluate the success of the previously implemented spiritual care interventions. Beginning nurses should note that the effectiveness of nursing interventions is determined at this point and not in the first step of evaluation. Novices sometimes make the mistake of reviewing nursing interventions, rather than patient goals, in the first step of evaluation. Nurses can retain useful interventions and eliminate ineffective ones while adding new spiritual care interventions that assist in achieving patient goals. Once reviewed, the updated plan of care is ready for implementation and later evaluation.

DOCUMENTATION

As with all nursing care, documentation of spiritual care is critical for providing quality patient care, addressing economic issues, and maintaining a legal document. Because documentation can be overwhelming, nurses may tend to overlook the documentation of spiritual care. Broten (1991) discussed spiritual care with 15 patients, who identified 63 spiritual care interventions their nurses provided. However, when the patient-reported interventions were compared with the information in patient charts, it was determined that only 25% (n = 16) of the interventions had been documented. Although this study, with its small sample size, had limitations, the finding is consistent with other studies regarding documentation of nursing care (Brooks, 1998; Broten; Davis, Holman, & Sousa, 2000). Thus, nurses must develop an awareness of and appreciation for the importance of documentation in facilitating spiritual care.

Providing Quality Patient Care

The Joint Commission on Accreditation of Healthcare Organizations (**JCAHO**, 2001), an organization that sets standards for quality patient care, has specified the minimal requirements for a spiritual assessment: determining the patient's denomination, beliefs, and spiritual practices that are important to the patient. For health care organizations to be compliant with this standard, they must define the content and scope of spiritual assessment and the qualifications of those performing the assessment. Documentation by such persons needs to be consistent with the policies the health care organization sets forth to demonstrate how it meets these minimal requirements.

Meeting minimal JCAHO requirements is a step toward assuring quality patient care, but it does not guarantee that the spiritual care of patients will improve. Because JCAHO standards include only spiritual assessment, the process could end after assessment, with implementation not occurring. Yocum (2002) writes that properly documenting patient assessments and interventions can provide "future readers the tools they need to ensure timely continuity of care for the patient" (p. 60). Yocum suggests asking these questions when charting is completed: "If I were the next nurse responsible for this patient's care, would these notes enable me to make good nursing decisions? Could I tell if the patient's condition has changed, I met his needs, and I fulfilled my duty to him?" (p. 60). Some hints for quality charting related to spiritual care are provided in Box 15.5.

Addressing Economic Issues

Documentation of nursing practice also is critical for economic reasons. For Medicare and Medicaid reimbursement, peer review organizations (PROs) examine patient charts after the patient has been discharged (Raymond, 2001, 2002). A PRO hires nurses and physicians as reviewers who use government criteria to determine whether health care services were used appropriately. The PRO determines the type of risk (minimal, moderate, and significant) to the patient based on documentation. Minimal risk involves documentation issues that do not affect patient care. Documentation indicating that a patient was placed at risk for a complication or adverse event, without permanent injury or death, can be cited as moderate risk. When a patient has been placed at risk for disability, disfigurement, or death, the PRO cites the organization for significant risk. Medicare and Medicaid funding may be withdrawn from health care organizations that have repeated citations. Because omissions or errors in documentation can lead reviewers to assume that risk existed when it did not, health care organizations can lose money if documentation is consistently inadequate.

Patient outcomes observed by insurance companies drive the reimbursement of nursing care. To encourage insurance companies to reimburse for nursing services related to spiritual care, nurses must demonstrate through documentation that spiritual

BOX 15.5 Tips for Quality Charting of Spiritual Care

- Document patient spiritual beliefs accurately. Proper documentation of spiritual beliefs reflects respect for the patient and facilitates implementation of appropriate interventions and avoidance of disrespectful interventions. Example: Patient is a vegetarian and does not eat meat based on religious beliefs. Patient eats beans with lunch and dinner.
- Mean what you say and say what you mean. Avoid generalizations or vague notes, such as "patient is spiritually distressed." Be clear about what it is that you want others to know. Example: Patient expressed anger toward God because of illness but also described feeling guilty because "I shouldn't be angry at God." Encouraged patient to discuss feelings about this, and patient indicated would like to speak to rabbi. Contacted Rabbi Goldberg, Star of David Synagogue, who stated will visit this evening."
- Follow professional standards for nursing care. When care deviates from legal, professional, or organizational standards, provide a valid reason for the alteration. Example: The patient had indicated that she missed her pet cat and wished she could see him. Bringing pet to hospital visit could have therapeutic effect on patient's spirit. After discussion with Barbara Brown, nursing supervisor, arrangements were made to have daughter, Beth, bring pet into hospital for visit.
- Name anyone who becomes involved in the patient's care. Because providing quality spiritual care for patients is interdisciplinary, be sure to include anyone who becomes involved. This could include organizational chaplains or clergy, parish nurses or lay visitors from the patient's faith community. Example: Discussed discharge plans with Elaine Sculley, RN, parish nurse from Christian Community Church, who will be following up with patient at home.
- Use approved abbreviations. Use the abbreviations approved at your organization because using unapproved abbreviations can lead to confusion. For instance does "sc" stand for spiritual care or sickle cell? The same goes for flow sheets. If the size of the box cannot accommodate the information needed to be documented, make a narrative note.
- Write legibly. Writing so others can read your notes minimizes the risk of errors, thereby contributing to quality spiritual care.

(Adapted with permission from Yocum, R. F. [2002]. Documenting for quality patient care. *Nursing 2002, 32*([8], 58–64.)

care is effective. Furthermore, providing spiritual care takes time and effort by the nurse. If only 25% of the work nurses perform is indicated in the patient records, it is difficult for administrators and managers to make claims about needing resources to provide more staff so that spiritual care can be provided. Changes in reimbursement occur only if documentation data indicate that providing spiritual care is cost effective.

Philanthropists and foundations that provide grants are increasingly interested in supporting spiritual care and funding research about health and spirituality. Administrators, researchers, and grant writers must provide strong rationales for why their organization deserves to receive such funding (known as soft monies). Having substantial documented data can strengthen the organization's position for receiving such monies.

Maintaining a Legal Document

The patient's chart is a legal document, so documentation of patient care is essential. During 1999, more than 70 cases involving some type of documentation error led to discipline by the Texas State Board of Nurse Examiners against licenses of registered nurses (Jacobson, 2000). Accurate record keeping is essential for nurses to protect themselves from litigation (Rodden & Bell, 2002): "poor records mean a poor defense and no records mean no defense" (Tingle, 1998, p. 245). Because patient records can be entered as evidence in trials that occur years after the fact, documentation is essential for establishing the context of the situation. A nurse whose charting is unclear, incomplete, illegible, or lacking appropriate grammar and spelling can be discredited as a professional, regardless of the effectiveness of the spiritual care provided.

Although statutes vary from state to state, nurses can be prosecuted for poor documentation. Incomplete record keeping, falsifying records, mishandling of records, or failure to protect patient confidentiality are documentation issues not consistent with the standard of care set forth in nurse practice acts (Yocum, 2002). For more information about state nurse practice acts and regulations, visit the web site for the relevant state board of nursing or http://www.ncsbn.org.

Organizations also must be compliant with regulations implemented under the Health Insurance Portability and Accountability Act of 1996 (**HIPAA**). HIPAA legislation aims to: "(a) assure health insurance portability by eliminating job-lock due to pre-existing medical conditions, (b) reduce healthcare fraud and abuse, (c) enforce standards of health information, and (d) guarantee security and privacy of health information" (Stevens, n.d.). HIPAA requires that the United States Department of Health and Human Services (2002) set national standards for electronic health care transactions to improve efficiency by reducing paperwork and address the privacy of health care records. The effects of this legislation on documentation and the protection of health information are unfolding.

Documentation Issues for Parish Nurses

Parish nurses have unique concerns related to documentation because their nursing practice does not occur in a health care organization, but parish nurses are required to document in accordance with their state's legislated nurse practice act. The tendency of some parish nurses to maintain inadequate records of encounters with members of their faith community is not in keeping with standards of nursing practice. Fortunately, the International Parish Resource Center offers the publication *Parish Nurse Documentation: Applying NANDA, NIC, and NOC* (Burkhart, 2002), which includes documentation forms easily used or adapted by parish nurses in their communities of faith.

It is important for parish nurses to maintain records for economic reasons as well. In most faith communities, the parish nurse is a volunteer position. Parish nurse positions are unpaid in part because of the economic structure of faith communities, but also because the discipline of nursing has failed to document the success of parish nursing. Some parish nurses reason that because they are volunteering, their time is better spent with patients than in documenting and reporting; however, this reasoning is what keeps them in volunteer positions. If parish nurses can demonstrate to their faith communities the value of their services through documentation and reporting of outcomes, faith communities are more likely to invest finances in those services. If parish nurses report their activities to central databases, arguments for economic support in the form of grants to parish nursing can be made to state and national governments.

Parish nurses are also accountable for the professional standards set by the American Nurses Association (ANA) in collaboration with the Health Ministries Association (HMA) (HMA & ANA, 1998). Policies about parish nursing practice and the use of volunteers in the community of faith, such as the policy on infection control in the Sunday nursery, are intended to address legal issues. Parish nurses also must maintain patient privacy and confidentiality of records.

Conclusion on Documentation

Imagine how powerful it would be if nurses could report that length of stay was reduced by 1 day and that patient satisfaction increased 12% for patients receiving quality spiritual care. The discipline of nursing will be able to make such a claim only through proper documentation. Documentation may seem like a task that is not central to providing spiritual care, but it is. Nurses must be diligent in charting the process of the spiritual care they provide so that the data can be used to demonstrate the improvement in patients' health. Documentation can serve to justify the amount of nursing time spent providing spiritual care and perhaps influence the reimbursement system, thereby increasing staffing. In addition, documentation can make the case for funding research about spiritual care. Always remember: "If it wasn't documented, it wasn't done."

PERSONAL REFLECTIONS

For the professional nurse:
- What do you think about the use of the various complementary/alternative therapies discussed in this chapter?
- Which of the therapeutic interventions mentioned have you used most often? With which are you most comfortable?
- How do you think that complementary/alternative therapies fit into the overall medical and nursing plans of care for patients? How important are interventions such as prayer, meditation, or talking?
- If one of your patients tells you that he or she believes a certain nontraditional activity will help him or her recover, but you do not personally approve of it, what should you do?
- How do you feel about pet therapy being allowed in health care settings that strive for a "clean" environment to foster healing?

(continues)

PERSONAL REFLECTIONS (*continued*)

- Consider the last time you entered data in a chart. How would you feel if a photocopy of the chart were placed on an overhead for everyone in a courtroom to see?
- Do you believe that information is power? Can data from documentation really change policy?
- If you were the nurse manager of a cardiac unit in which many patients expressed the desire to use alternative therapies to help with their healing, what proactive approach could you take?
- The clinical nurse specialist on your transplant unit asks you about the possibility of participating in a study of the recovery time benefits related to animal-assisted therapy for patients undergoing liver transplant. How do you respond? What concerns come to mind?
- A group of therapists at the large rehabilitation center where you are chief executive nursing officer want to start a tai chi program for inpatients. You are asked to participate on a committee to examine the feasibility of this program. What information will you bring to this discussion? What benefits will you explain? What commitment would this take from nursing staff? From therapists? From administration? How does current research on tai chi related to personal health enlighten this discussion?
- If you were reviewing grant applications for spiritual care, what kind of information would you want to know before you awarded money to an organization? How much of a role would documentation play in your decision?
- How familiar are you with the nurse practice act for the state in which you practice?

CASE STUDY 15.1

Emily, 90 years old, was recently placed in a freestanding hospice center by her family. One month ago, Emily received a diagnosis of inoperable metastatic breast cancer. The physicians told her family (one son and one daughter, both married with several children and grandchildren) that Emily may have 2 months or less to live and that her cancer had spread to the brain and bone. She has been set up to receive hospice care in a private room, where she has few visitors.

Emily had lived at home alone with her seven cats since the death of her husband 14 years ago. She had been an active, healthy woman and had not felt it necessary to visit her physician regularly unless she "had a problem." Pain in her back had caused her to seek treatment, but once her diagnosis was made, Emily chose to "let nature run its course." Emily did not attend

(Case Study continues on page 270)

CASE STUDY 15.1 (continued)

church or engage in socializing, preferring to watch TV, cook, listen to the radio, and spend time with her cats. She describes herself as a spiritual person but not religious. The hospice nurses notes that Emily seems worried and agitated, especially in the evening. She repeatedly asks about her cats and who is caring for them. She expresses concern about who will care for them once she is gone and how she wishes to see them again.

Emily's family insists that she stay at the hospice center because they feel that she will get better care and pain management. They feel the burden of care in her own home would be too great, costly, and unrealistic. Both of Emily's children live far away and feel that they are unable to leave their own families to help Emily at home. No other family members are willing or able to care for Emily at the end of her life. Emily wishes that she could go to her own home to die so that her cats could be with her. She tells the hospice staff that her pets mean as much to her as her own children.

Critical Thinking

- What can the hospice nurses do to help Emily achieve her end-of-life goals?
- Is it realistic to think that Emily might be able to die at home as she wishes? If so, how might this be accomplished? If not, what other options might be suggested to achieve Emily's desired outcomes?
- What is the role of Emily's cats in her life?
- What types of complementary/alternative therapies might be appropriate for Emily?
- What are some other spiritual interventions that should be planned for this patient? How should the nurse document the plan of care and subsequent outcomes for this patient?

CASE STUDY 15.2

Tiger is a 9-year-old African-American boy with sickle cell anemia. He is in the fourth grade at a public school. Tiger has many friends but has told only his closest friends about his disease. He has been in the hospital twice during the past 6 months for bouts of pain associated with his illness. Tiger is an only child who lives with his divorced mother in a small urban apartment. He sees his father every other weekend and expresses having a close relationship with both parents, but he tearfully states: "My mom and dad hate each other and fight all the time." This appears to cause him great emotional stress. Tiger uses prayer as his main way to cope with the various problems caused by sickle cell anemia, especially pain. He tells the nurses that it also helps when his mother "puts her hands on his head and prays." In the past, deacons from his church anointed him with healing oil and made a circle

(Case Study continues on page 271)

CASE STUDY 15.2 (continued)

around his bed to pray, which helped Tiger feel better. During this admission, Tiger is particularly anxious and crying out in pain. He tells the nurse that he is afraid he is going to die and wants both parents at his bedside.

Critical Thinking
- In addition to the usual medical and nursing treatments for a child with his condition, what spiritual interventions would be appropriate for Tiger?
- How would you handle his request to have both of his parents present at his bedside?
- What are Tiger's main coping strategies?
- What practical suggestions could you make to help Tiger and his family through this hospitalization?
- What is the role of the church and spiritual leader in this case?
- What are the essential issues to document in this case?
- What long-term coping strategies could you help to foster for this family?
- What resources could be used in addition to those already in place?

Key Points

- NIC and NOC provide a common language for nursing interventions and outcome classifications. Nurses may use NIC and NOC to facilitate specific spiritual care planning, implementation, and evaluation. NIC and NOC are one common method for labeling and planning care but are not necessarily used universally.
- Patients of various faiths use many complementary and alternative therapies. These include prayer, therapeutic touch, acupuncture, herbs, yoga, tai chi, meditation (and other forms of stress management), the therapeutic arts (drama, music, art), humor, and animal-assisted therapy. Nurses should be aware of the benefits of these therapeutic modalities and be open to their appropriate incorporation in the nursing care plan.
- Nurses evaluate outcomes in terms of how well the goals mutually established with the patient were met. If the desired outcomes are not being met, re-evaluation of nursing interventions is indicated, and the plan of care should be modified accordingly.

References

Brooks, J. T. (1998). An analysis of nursing documentation as a reflection of actual nurse work. *MEDSURG Nursing, 7*, 189–198.

Broten, P. J. (1991). Spiritual care given by nurses and spiritual well-being of terminally ill cancer patients. *Dissertation Abstracts International, 52*(05B), 2497. (UMI No. AAG9131135)

Burkhart, L. (2002). *Parish nurse documentation: Applying NANDA, NIC, and NOC.* St. Louis: International Parish Nurse Resource Center.

The California Institute of Integral Studies. (n.d.). *Drama therapy* (pp. 1–3). Available at: http://www.ciis.edu. Accessed March 3, 2001.

Carson, V. B. (1993). Prayer, meditation, exercise, and special diets: Behaviors of the hardy person with HIV/AIDS. *Journal of the Association of Nurses in AIDS Care, 4*(3), 18–28.

Chin, R. M. (1995). *The energy within: The science behind every Oriental therapy from acupuncture to yoga.* New York: Marlowe.

Cohen, S. P. (2002). Can pets function as family members? *Western Journal of Nursing Research, 24*(6), 621–638.

Cousins, N. (1977). *The healing heart.* New York: Bantam.

Davidhizar, R., & Bowen, M. (1992). The dynamics of laughter. *Archives of Psychiatric Nursing, 6*(2), 132–137.

Davis, A. L., Holman, E. J., & Sousa, K. H. (2000). Documentation of care outcomes in an academic nursing clinic: An assessment. *Journal of the American Academy of Nurse Practitioners, 12,* 497–502.

Davis, R. D. (1997). *The gift of dyslexia.* New York: Berkley.

De Alberdi, L. (1998). Meditation for health. *Positive Health, 32,* 9–10.

Dean, C. F., Mullins, M., & Yuen, J. (2000). Acupuncture. In D. W. Novey (Ed.), *Clinician's complete reference to complementary/alternative medicine* (pp. 191–202). St. Louis: Mosby.

Dossey, L. (1996). *Prayer is good medicine.* New York: Harper Collins.

Easton, K. L. (1999). The post-stroke journey: From agonizing to owning. *Geriatric Nursing, 20*(2), 70–75.

Easton, K. L., & Andrews, J. C. (1999). Nursing the soul: A team approach. *Journal of Christian Nursing, 16*(3), 26–29.

Easton, K. L., Rawl, S. M., Zemen, D., Kwiatkowski, S., & Burczyk, B. (1995). The effects of nursing follow-up on the coping strategies used by rehabilitation patients after discharge. *Rehabilitation Nursing Research, 4*(4), 119–127.

Fontana, J. A., Colella, C., Baas, L. S., & Ghazi, F. (2000). T'ai chi as an intervention for heart failure. *Nursing Clinics of North America, 35,* 1031–1046.

Frohnmayer, J. (1994). Music and spirituality: Defining the human condition. *International Journal of Arts and Medicine, 3*(1), 26–29.

Gerber, S. (1998). The sound of healing. *Vegetarian Times,* (March), 69–73.

Greene, E. (2000). Massage therapy. In D. W. Novey (Ed.), *Clinician's complete reference to complementary and alternative medicine.* St. Louis: Mosby.

Greene, K. B., Berger, J., Reeves, C., & Moffat, A. (1999). Most frequently used alternative and complementary therapies and activities by participants in the AMCOA study. *The Journal of the Association of Nurses in AIDS Care, 10*(3), 60–73.

Halstead, M. T., & Roscoe, S. T. (2002). Restoring the spirit at end of life: Music as an intervention for oncology nurses. *Journal of Oncology Nursing, 6*(6), 332–336, 352–353.

Health Ministries Association & American Nurses Association (HMA & ANA). (1998). *Scope and standards of parish nursing practice.* Washington, DC: American Nurses Association.

Hulse, J. R. (1994). Humor: A nursing intervention for the elderly. *Geriatric Nursing, 15,* 88–90.

Jacobson, J. (2000). RN practice demands excellent documentation. *RN, 31*(3), 4–5.

Janelli, L. M., Kanski, G. W., & Wu, Y. B. (2002). Individualized music—a different approach to the restraint issue. *Rehabilitation Nursing, 27*(6), 221–226.

Janowiak, J. (1993). A drum in every hospital. *Music Inc.,* November.

Jin, P. (1992). Efficacy of T'ai chi, brisk walking, meditation, and reading in reducing mental and emotional stress. *Journal of Psychosomatic Research, 36,* 361–370.

Johnson, M., & Maas, M. (Eds.). (1997). *Nursing outcomes classification* (NOC). St. Louis: Mosby.

Johnson, M., Maas, M., & Moorhead, S. (Eds.) (2000). *Nursing outcomes classification* (NOC) (2nd ed.). St. Louis: Mosby.

Johnson, P. (2002). The use of humor and its influences on spirituality and coping in breast cancer survivors. *Oncology Nurse Forum, 29*(4), 691–695.

Johnson, R., & Meadows, R. L. (2002). Older Latinos, pets, and health. *Western Journal of Nursing Research, 24*(6), 609–620.

Joint Commission on Accreditation of Healthcare Organizations (JCAHO). (2001, July 31). *Spiritual assessment.* Available at: http://www.jcaho.org/accredited+organizations/hospitals/standards/hospital+fs/assessment++of+patients/index.htm. Accessed December 21, 2002.

Kaiser, L., Spence, L. J., McGavin, L., Struble, L., & Keilman, L. (2002). A dog and a 'happy person' visit nursing home residents. *Western Journal of Nursing Research, 24*(6), 671–683.

Kavanaugh, K. (1995). Dance and drama therapies stimulate creativity, enhance patient well-being. *Brown University Long-Term Care Letter, 7*(14), 5–6.

Kreitzer, M. J., & Snyder, M. (2002). Healing the heart: Integrating complementary therapies and healing practices into the care of cardiovascular patients. *Progress in Cardiovascular Nursing, 17*(2), 73–84.

Lambert, R. B., & Lambert, N. K. (1995). The effects of humor on secretory immunoglobulin A levels in school-aged children. *Pediatric Nursing, 21*(1), 16–19.

Lan, C., Lai, J. S., & Chen, S. Y. (1998). 12-month tai chi training in the elderly: Its effects on health fitness. *Medical Science and Sports Exercise, 30*, 345–351.

Little, C. V., Parsons, T., & Logan, S. (2002). Herbal therapy for treating osteoarthritis (Cochrane Review). In: The Cochrane Library, Issue 2. Oxford: Update Software.

McCloskey, J. C., & Bulechek, G. M. (1996). *Nursing interventions classification* (NIC) (2nd ed.). St. Louis: Mosby.

McCloskey, J. C., & Bulechek, G. M. (2000). *Nursing interventions classification* (NIC) (3rd ed.). St. Louis: Mosby.

Miles, M. (1992). Asclepius and the muses: Arts in the hospital environment. *International Journal of Arts and Medicine, 1*(2), 26–29.

Miller, J. F. (2000). *Coping with chronic illness: Overcoming powerlessness.* Philadelphia: FA Davis.

Mother Teresa. (1998). On prayer. In D. Salwak (Ed.), *The power of prayer* (pp. 3–11). New York: MJF Books.

Mramor, K. M. (2001). Music therapy with persons who are indigent and terminally ill. *Journal of Palliative Care, 17*(3), 182–186.

Murray, M. E., & Atkinson, L. D. (2000). *Understanding the nursing process in a changing health care environment* (6th ed.). St. Louis: McGraw-Hill.

Murrock, C. J. (2002). The effects of music on the rate of perceived exertion and general mood among coronary artery bypass graft patients enrolled in cardiac rehabilitation phase II. *Rehabilitation Nursing, 27*(6), 227–231.

National Association for Drama Therapy. (n.d.). *Drama therapy* (pp. 1–3). Available at: http://www.ncata.com/drama.html. Accessed March 1, 2001.

Peters, R. M. (1999). The effectiveness of therapeutic touch: A meta-analytic review. *Nursing Science Quarterly, 12*(1), 56–61.

Pratt, R. R. (1992). Healing and art. *International Journal of Arts Medicine, 1*(2), 3.

Province, M. A., Hadley, E. C., & Hornbrook M. C. (1995). The effects of exercise on falls in elderly patients. *Journal of the American Medical Association, 273*, 1341–1347.

Raymond, L. (2001). How to chart for peer review. *RN, 64*(6), 67–68, 70.

Raymond, L. (2002). Documenting for "PROs." *Nursing 2002, 32*(3), 50–53.

Rodden, C., & Bell, M. (2002). Record keeping: Developing good practice. *Nursing Standard, 17*(1), 40–42.

Ross, M. C., Bohannon, A. S., & Davis, D. C. (1999). The effects of a short-term exercise program on movement, pain, and mood in the elderly. *Journal of Holistic Nursing, 17*, 139–147.

Schlintz, V. (2001). Keeping a prayer journal. *Journal of Christian Nursing, 18*(3), 32–33.

Smolen, D., Topp, R., & Singer, L. (2002). The effect of self-selected music during colonoscopy on anxiety, heart rate, and blood pressure. *Applied Nursing Research, 15*(3), 126–136.

Spence, L. J., & Kaiser, L. (2002). Companion animals and adaptation in chronically ill children. *Western Journal of Nursing Research, 24*(6), 639–656.

Standley, J. M. (2002). A meta-analysis of the efficacy of music therapy for premature infants. *Journal of Pediatric Nursing: Nursing Care of Children and Families, 17*(2), 107–113.

Sterritt, P. F., & Pokorny, M. E. (1994). Art activities for patients with Alzheimer's and related disorders. *Geriatric Nursing, 15*(3), 155–159.

Stevens, T. (n.d.). *What is HIPAA?* Available at: http://www.hipaaplus.com/abouthipaa.htm. Accessed January 14, 2003.

Sullivan, M. J. (2000). Integrative medicine: Making it work for you. *Emergency Medicine, 32*(10), 76–83.

Tingle, J. (1998). Nurses must improve their record keeping skills. *British Journal of Nursing, 7*(5), 245.

Trieschmann, R. B. (2001). Spirituality and energy medicine. *Journal of Rehabilitation, 67*(1), 26–32.

United States Department of Health and Human Services. (2002, October 16). *The Health Insurance Portability and Accountability Act of 1996* (HIPAA). Available at: http://www.cms.hhs.gove/hipaa/. Accessed January 14, 2003.

Wangerin, W. (1996). *Whole prayer: Speaking and listening to God*. Grand Rapids, MI: Zondervan.

Williamson, M. (1998). Ladders to God. In D. Salwak (Ed.), *The power of prayer* (pp. 21–25). New York: MJF Books.

Winstead-Fry, P., & Kijek, J. (1999). An integrative review and meta-analysis of therapeutic touch research. *Alternative Therapies, 5*(6), 58–67.

Woodham, A., & Peters, D. (1997). *Encyclopedia of healing therapies*. London: Dorling Kindersley.

Wu, W., Bandilla, E., & Iccone, D. (1999). Effects of qigong on late-stage complex regional pain syndrome. *Alternative Therapies, 5,* 45–54.

Wyatt, G. K., Friedman, L. L., Given, C. W., Given, B. A., & Beckrow, K. C. (1999). Complementary therapy use among older cancer patients. *Cancer Practice: A Multidisciplinary Journal of Cancer Care, 7*(3), 136–144.

Yocum, R. F. (2002). Documenting for quality patient care. *Nursing2002, 32*(8), 58–64.

Recommended Readings

Broten, P. J. (1997). Spiritual care documentation: Where is it? *Journal of Christian Nursing, 14*(2), 29–31.

Creative Arts Therapies Concordia University Montreal. (1999). *What is drama therapy?* Available at: http://www-fofa.concordia.ca/art-therapy/whatd.html. Accessed March 1, 2001.

Resources

American Academy of Medical Acupuncture (AAMA)
4929 Wilshire Boulevard, Suite 428, Los Angeles, CA 90010
Phone: (323) 937-5514
http://www.medicalacupuncture.org/index.html

American Art Therapy Association
1202 Allanson Road, Mundelein, IL 60060-3808
Phone: (888) 290-0878 or (847) 949-6064
Fax: (847) 566-4580
http://www.arttherapy.org
Information on art therapy.

American Massage Therapy Association
820 Davis Street, Suite 100, Evanston, IL 60201-4444
Phone: (847) 864-0123
Fax: (847) 864-1178
http://www.amtamassage.org
Maintains referral information.

American Music Therapy Association
8455 Colesville Road, Suite 1000, Silver Spring, MD 20910
Phone: (301) 589-3300
Fax: (301) 589-5175
http://www.musictherapy.org

Council of Acupuncture and Oriental Medicine Associations
1217 Washington Street, Calistoga, CA 94515
Phone: (707) 942-9380
Fax: (707) 942-8242
http://www.acucouncil.org/
Maintains a wealth of information and resources for the public related to acupuncture.

Integrative Medicine
A.D.A.M., Inc.
1600 Riveredge Parkway, Suite 100, Atlanta, GA 30328
Phone: (770) 980-0888
Fax: (770) 955-2326
http://www.onemedicine.com
Information on alternative therapies.

John Templeton Foundation Spirituality and Health Programs
P.O. Box 8322, Radnor, PA 19087-8322
Phone: (610) 687-8942
Fax: (610) 687-8961
http://www.templeton.org/spirituality.asp
Maintains a prayer study archive in which selected scholarly research findings are presented, along with articles from the popular press related to prayer and health.

The National Association for Drama Therapy, Inc.
5505 Connecticut Avenue, NW, Suite 280, Washington, DC 20015
Phone: (202) 966-7409
Fax: (202) 966-2283
http://www.nadt.org/
Basic information on drama therapy.

National Center for Complementary and Alternative Medicine (NCCAM)
National Institutes of Health
Department of Health and Human Services, Bethesda, MD 20892
http://nccam.nih.gov/
The official site for the National Center of Complementary and Alternative Medicine; connects consumers with the most current and reliable information on CAM.

North American Riding for the Handicapped Association (NARHA)
P.O. Box 33150, Denver, CO 80233
Phone: (303) 452-1212; (800) 369-RIDE (7433)
Fax: (303) 252-4610
http://www.narha.org
Information on therapeutic riding.

Therapet Animal Assisted Therapy Foundation
PO Box 698, Troup, TX 75789
http://therapet.com
A non-profit organization whose mission is to facilitate the use of animals in the healing and rehabilitation of acute and chronically ill individuals.

Touch Research Institutes
University of Miami School of Medicine
Mailman Center for Child Development, P.O. Box 016820, 1601 NW 12th Avenue, 7th Floor, Suite 7037, Miami FL 33101
Phone: (305) 243-6781
http://www.miami.edu/touch-research
Conducts research on the sense of touch.

Yoga Directory
http://www.yogadirectory.com/
Information on yoga.

16

Collaboration in Spiritual Care

Nancy Habermeier

At the end of this chapter, the reader will be able to:
- Define collaboration.
- List the five gifts of collaboration.
- Discuss the benefits of collaboration when caring for a client.
- Identify members of the team who provide spiritual care.
- Recognize opportunities to enhance collaboration among health care professionals, clergy, and others within health care systems, communities of faith, and the community.
- Describe features and benefits of team ministry.

KEY TERMS

collaboration
five gifts of collaboration
team ministry
whole person care

Whole person care involves caring for the entire person—body, mind, and spirit—and presents a challenge that nurses are acutely aware of in daily practice. Because no single person can serve all the various dimensions that can be addressed to improve a client's quality of life, collaboration of people from different disciplines is essential. Regardless of the discipline, the spiritual dimension is woven throughout the care provided. This chapter discusses how collaboration contributes to spiritual care.

COLLABORATION

Collaboration can be defined as teamwork, partnership, group effort, alliance, and relationship. Collaboration can be limited to interactions between nurse and client, nurse and nurse, or nurse and another professional. Collaboration also can be interdisciplinary, involving several people with expertise in various areas. "It is unlikely that any single professional possesses the expertise required in all dimensions. It is likely, however, that the synergy produced by all can result in successful outcomes" (Cary, 1996, p. 368). Nurses and health care providers collaborate to promote the optimal well-being of clients and families by using every resource to accomplish goals. Synergistic relationships are essential in nursing, especially in parish nursing, where a nurse is in the trenches with only the allies of the community. Case Study 16.1 shows basic collaboration in the care of a family in need; in the situation, caregivers used synergistic relationships to work toward a common positive goal.

The family in Case Study 16.1 was perhaps entrenched in American "individualism." "Americans are swift defenders of individual interest, fanatical in protection of individual liberty and rights, prickly about privacy, and unaware of their neighbors and the deep streams of society that flow through their lives" (Newton, 1989, p. 47). While protecting their own interests, the family in Case Study 16.1 initially forgot how to ask for help. But when the family members reached out to others and became team players, their goals were met. Through interdisciplinary collaboration, Honora never had to leave her familiar home, and many people shared the burden of caring for her.

The Five Gifts of Collaboration

Because collaboration is vital as nurses assist patients to achieve their best potential and to maintain quality of life, developing "the gifts" of good collaboration is important. The **five gifts of collaboration** are collaborating with respect, showing positive regard for others, setting clear goals, listening, and being dedicated to caring for the whole person (Kelley, 1994). Approaching opportunities for collaboration with these gifts enhances synergistic relationships. Positive outcomes, such as decreased anxiety for the client or increased peace of mind for the family member, can result when col-

---

CASE STUDY 16.1

Honora, 98 years old, lived four houses away from her son and daughter-in-law. She was well acquainted with her home, having lived there since her 20s. Being in a familiar environment was important to her because she was nearly blind and had great difficulty hearing. She could differentiate light from dark and wore a receiver around her neck to amplify sound. Bert, her son, was 80 years old and had cared for Honora for the past 40 years. His life revolved around her care; he brought her three daily meals, fixing a portion for her each time he and his wife cooked, and he made sure that Honora was safe. She was able to live comfortably at home because of the familiarity with her surroundings.

However, Bert was bitter. He had expected things to be different. Honora was dominating his life. His wife, Beatrice, felt similarly, and also resented the relationship between Bert and Honora. Day in and day out, Honora was cared for and safe, refusing to be moved.

Honora, Bert, and Beatrice were members of the local Lutheran church. Over the years, pastors came and went, but the situation with Honora, Bert, and Beatrice remained the same. When a pastor would suggest another care option, Honora would refuse. Many years passed. Honora became home-bound and received communion at home monthly.

The Lutheran church grew and flourished, eventually beginning a parish nurse program. One of the first people the pastor referred to the parish nurse was Honora. Because Bert did not like strangers to visit Honora, the parish nurse did not do so. Nevertheless, the parish nurse began a relationship with Beatrice, who found comfort in visiting the parish nurse when she volunteered at the church. With the parish nurse, Beatrice first shared issues surrounding various ailments that she had. She eventually started to reveal the feelings that she had been hiding about Bert and Honora. Beatrice felt trapped. She wished that Honora would move to a retirement facility not only for own good, but for Beatrice's sanity as well. What could she do?

After 3 years of this friendship between the parish nurse and Beatrice, Honora began to weaken. Beatrice had a plan. She would tell her husband about the parish nurse and try to persuade him to have the parish nurse visit Honora. As Honora's health failed, Bert eventually agreed to the plan.

The parish nurse met Bert and Honora at Honora's home. The parish nurse assessed Honora, finding her weak, but otherwise in good health. Honora could ambulate and find her way around the house, using various markers that she had devised. Honora stated that she was too weak to bathe herself, and this was evident to the parish nurse.

In consultation with Honora's physician, the parish nurse arranged for a home health nurse to bathe Honora once a week. While there, the home health nurse also visited with Honora, singing hymns to her. The parish nurse arranged for Honora to visit the physician, and testing revealed that Honora had terminal metastatic cancer. Honora refused treatment because

(Case Study continues on page 280)

CASE STUDY 16.1 (continued)

she desired to stay in her home. The parish nurse visited each week to assess Honora's health status and pray with her, keeping the physician and pastor informed.

Four weeks later, Honora showed much deterioration. She was no longer able to go up the two flights of stairs to bathe or get to her bedroom; she stayed on the couch most of the time. The parish nurse visited Honora more regularly. Recognizing that Honora's health was deteriorating, the parish nurse arranged a call from the pastor. More care was needed the next week, when Honora did not go up the stairs at all. She did not finish meals and became incontinent. The parish nurse phoned the physician and arranged for a visit from a hospice care representative.

The next day, a hospice nurse arrived to assess Honora. The parish nurse, Bert, and pastor met with the hospice nurse to discuss Honora's care. A hospital bed was ordered and would be delivered the next day.

The next morning came, and the parish nurse visited early. She braided Honora's hair, positioned her on her couch, and prepared her for the day. She sang to Honora, shared familiar words of faith, prayed with her, and blessed her.

Honora died that afternoon, 15 minutes after being placed in the hospital bed. Two weeks later, Bert died of a heart attack at home. The story does not end here but continues in Case Study 16.2.

laboration is done with respect for the whole person. Approaching each opportunity to collaborate with respect, positive regard, clear goal setting, listening, and dedication is vital to the success of the interaction.

Respect. Respect is showing consideration to a team member and valuing his or her skilled input (Kelley, 1994). Providing positive feedback of appreciation enhances communication and the level of teamwork. When providing spiritual care, it is important for nurses and other professionals to respect the client's religious beliefs and practices and not force their own religious views on another.

Positive Regard for Others. Unconditional positive regard for clients and other team members facilitates growth and change (Rogers, 1957). Bringing this aspect to the forum of collaboration assists with the process. Although disagreement over some points is expected, team players must value the personhood of team members to foster collaborative experiences that result in positive outcomes.

Clear Goals. When what needs to be accomplished is not clearly identified, team members working to their own ends clutter the system (Kelley, 1994). Identifying clear, concise outcomes propels the team to value the task at hand together. When disagreement occurs, it can be helpful to remind team members that they are all there to contribute toward meeting a common goal that is in the client's best interest.

Listening. If all team members had the tool of listening, many quarrels could be avoided (Kelley, 1994). When a team member is talking, all other team members should be listening, not formulating their next move. Good listening facilitates productive interactions. Although pressed for time, professionals should allow themselves the freedom to slow down during collaborative encounters to clearly understand the message and work together for the best positive outcome.

Dedication to Caring for the Whole Person. In life, many individuals come to the collaborative process with their own agendas. Although different specialists need to accomplish different things, none of them should lose sight of the goals of the client (Kelley, 1994). Acknowledging the dynamic state of health and the many factors involved in achieving the highest quality of life for the individual is an unspoken but overarching goal of the process.

Implications for Nursing

When collaborating with others, the nurse benefits from a stronger network in which to function and a larger team that cares for the person in need. "Skills gained from collaborating within nursing can be readily transferred to interdisciplinary problem-solving situations" (Wywialowski, 1995, p. 328).

The nursing role requires nurses to be strong team members with good leadership skills to direct the progress toward the goals. "Outstanding results cannot be forced out of people. They occur only when individuals collaborate under a leader's stimulation and inspiration in striving toward a worthy common goal" (Engstrom, 1976, p. 20).

MEMBERS OF THE "TEAM"

Collaboration occurs with many team players. Coming from a variety of settings, team players are diverse in their education, training, and expertise.

Health Care Settings

In health care settings, many team players possess professional skills that can provide comprehensive care to a client. Working together is necessary as people bring their talents and abilities to address client needs. In the health care system, collaboration among nurses, physicians, discharge planners, social workers, chaplains, food service staff members, pharmacists, various therapists, laboratory technicians, and housekeeping and maintenance staff is vital to providing excellent client care. But when considering spiritual care for whole person health, the team extends beyond the health care system.

Communities of Faith

The church or faith tradition of the client is paramount when providing spiritual care. Historically, the church has been the entity to care for those with physical, psychological, and spiritual needs and has addressed the complete needs of a person. Within the faith community are many who have knowledge of local agencies and services available to the client.

Clergy
✛ ✪ Roles within the Judeo-Christian religions can include clergy, commonly known as priests, ministers, rabbis, or pastors. Some clergy have an undergraduate degree and 4 years of seminary or religious teaching. Others become ordained in their church without formal education. Clergy are directly responsible for preaching of the Word, administering sacraments, and performing rituals. Clergy also perform pastoral care, that is, care for a person who is suffering or in crisis.

Deaconesses
✛ Clergy may have a staff member who is responsible for human care needs. For instance, in the Lutheran tradition, a deaconess is prepared to teach and care for people in the congregation and community. Becoming a deaconess typically requires undergraduate training and 1 year of field work. Florence Nightingale was formally trained as a deaconess in Kaiserwerth, Germany; at that time, deaconess training encompassed two tracks: nursing and teaching.

Nuns and Brothers
✛ In the Catholic faith, nuns and brothers are not only involved in ministry, but also may be teachers, nurses, or administrators. Because of their involvement in these professions, many nuns and brothers will have graduate education beyond their baccalaureate degree. Although it is becoming less common, many of these people reside in the facility where they work, such as a nursing home or high school. Because they can visit sick members of their parish, nuns and brothers may be a member of the team.

Parish Nurses
The role of the parish nurse draws from the deaconess tradition. Although modern medicine has led nursing away from its Judeo-Christian roots, parish nursing brings whole person care back to the congregation. A parish nurse does not perform hands-on nursing but functions in the following seven roles (Solari-Twadell, 1999):

- Integrator of faith and health
- Health educator
- Personal health counselor
- Referral source
- Facilitator of volunteers
- Developer of support groups
- Health advocate

The parish nurse focuses on health promotion and early detection of disease and facilitates long-term care for members of the faith community.

Deacons
✛ Many faiths have individuals known as deacons, but the role the deacon has in the church varies among faiths. In the Catholic church, deacons assist with mass. In some Protestant faiths, deacons are church leaders who oversee the management of church affairs. As part of their ministry, some deacons may call upon the sick.

Lay Ministers and Workers
✛ Lay ministers and lay workers are persons who serve in various areas of ministry. A lay worker may focus on social ministry, evangelism, teaching, senior adults, or

other areas. The lay worker comes with the ability to operate a ministry with or without specific training. In Christianity, Stephen Ministers are lay workers who have received special training to assist others.

Community

Within the community, many agencies operate to serve needs. Nurses need to be aware of the services available within their communities because collaboration with such agencies may be needed to meet client goals.

The local township may have a general assistance office to assist people with public assistance forms and filing, food pantry resources, utilities (with qualifying circumstances), and advocacy in crisis. The county health department may have a social services division in which a case worker can assess the situation and coordinate services as available. Most county health departments offer immunizations free or at reduced costs. Because these county health departments are responsible for monitoring for communicable diseases, individuals also can receive tuberculosis screening and other related serves there.

Various agencies exist to serve specific needs. A local agency that serves refugees, providing basic needs and English language services, can be an ally in providing care for immigrants. Charities run by specific religious groups and organizations specialize in collaborating to provide care for an individual. The YMCA and similar organizations can provide after-school care and places for people to exercise.

Professionals in counseling agencies and schools are valuable partners. Clinical pastoral counselors, licensed social workers, teachers, psychologists, and psychiatrists each have a unique role in caring for the whole person because empowering and building up the person in need are required for future success.

Promoting whole person health can also include collaboration among health care professionals from a variety of settings. Meeting patient goals may require collaboration among physician office staff, hospice personnel, drug store pharmacists, and medical supply company representatives.

COLLABORATION IN HEALTH CARE SETTINGS

Through the gifts of collaboration, many people were able to provide spiritual care to promote peace and comfort for the family in Case Study 16.2. Nurses, clergy, and physicians all contributed to meeting that goal. The ministry of presence was the most important tool. They demonstrated respect for family wishes by asking permission to call the pastor. The chaplain showed positive regard for others by recognizing that the individuals present were addressing matters. Although the team did not discuss or write down formal goals, there was an unspoken understanding that the goal was to support the family during this time. By using their presence through listening, team members provided spiritual care to family members. Although team members may have had other things to do, all remained with the family because they were dedicated to caring for the whole person.

Good care depends on the contributions and interactions of various providers (Collaboration and independent practice, 1998). Care systems in the United States are complex and dynamic. Collaboration can make efficient use of the resources of these systems, thereby improving the quality of care clients receive.

CASE STUDY 16.2

Honora had been in the hospital only when she gave birth, but her daughter-in-law, Beatrice, was different. Beatrice had approached the parish nurse regarding her ailments, some of which involved minor surgeries. About 2 months after the deaths of Honora and Bert, Beatrice became ill. When conducting hospital visits, the parish nurse found a family member in the waiting room of the intensive care unit. Beatrice underwent another operation. While the parish nurse was visiting with the family member, the physician came into the waiting room and informed them the surgery was not going well. The physician left, and a nurse and nursing student came to stay in the waiting room. The relative gave permission for the parish nurse to call the pastor. A chaplain stopped by, but upon observing the situation was under control, she excused herself. The family, pastor, parish nurse, nurse, and nursing student waited for news. When word arrived that Beatrice had died, the pastor accompanied the family to talk with the physician and say goodbye to Beatrice.

COLLABORATION IN CONGREGATIONS

The team that functions to provide spiritual care for an individual within a congregation works on many levels. The team includes all staff (support staff, office staff, lay workers, pastors, counselors), volunteers, and others working together to provide a person with holistic care.

Team ministry can be defined as "a group of two or more professionally trained lay or ordained ministers who choose to approach the parish they serve with an explicit commitment to shared responsibility and mutual support. They dedicate themselves not only to the work but to the development of the team" (Kelley, 1994, p. 118).

When caring for Mary in Case Study 16.3, the members of the church provided holistic care through collaboration. The team demonstrated respect for Mary by not judging her by her clothing. Positive regard for others was evident in how the parish nurse referred Mary to individuals recognized for their unique abilities to assist Mary. The team met clearly defined goals to find Mary and her husband financial and health care assistance, while ministering to their spiritual distress. By listening carefully, the parish nurse was able to hear Mary's distress. As expected, team members ministered to Mary's spiritual needs, the parish nurse by praying and laying on of hands, and the lay minister by inviting Mary to a parish event. Through dedication to caring for the whole person, members collaborated to address the economic, mental health, and physical health needs of Mary and her husband.

COLLABORATION IN ADVANCED PRACTICE NURSING

Although the word "collaboration" within nursing should be seen as an opportunity to work together for problem solving and achieving client goals, the word "collabo-

CASE STUDY 16.3

Mary came to the church seeking financial assistance with rent. Her husband was not working many hours, and she was concerned that he might have Alzheimer's disease. She and her husband were longtime members of the parish who had not attended mass in the past 2 years. Desperate, Mary called the church, and the parish nurse agreed to meet with her to discuss her financial needs.

Upon meeting with Mary, the parish nurse conducted an assessment of Mary's finances. This discussion led to questions about prescription costs, such as "What medications do you take?" and "When was the last time you and your husband had a physical examination?" This discussion revealed Mary's thyroid deficiency, her husband's lack of a physician, and their medication side effects. During the final half of the meeting, the parish nurse and Mary talked about Mary's feelings of inadequacy to be present in God's house. Mary felt ashamed of her choices. She also indicated that she did not have an overcoat or a dress. The parish nurse placed her hands on Mary and prayed for Mary's healing and peace.

Collaborating with the local township's general assistance office, the parish nurse helped obtain rent money for Mary that month. The parish nurse notified the lay minister in charge of senior ministry that the couple would appreciate an invitation to an event. The nurse made referrals to counselors and connected with the members of the congregation who worked in the areas of finance and personal counseling. The parish nurse collaborated with church resale shop volunteers, and Mary was able to select clothing for herself appropriate to wear to church.

The following week Mary's husband saw a physician and began treatment for depression. Mary and her husband began attending mass together. They began to receive healing in their relationship with each other and in their faith life.

ration" within advanced practice nursing is a hotly debated topic because it calls into question the independence of advanced practice nurses in their individual fields of practice. The leaders of the American Nurses Association (ANA) and the American Medical Association (AMA) arrived at a definition of collaboration:

> Collaboration is the process whereby physicians and nurses plan and practice together as colleagues, working interdependently within the boundaries of their scopes of practice with shared values and mutual acknowledgment and respect for each other's contribution to care for individuals, their families, and their communities. *Collaboration and independent practice, 1998, p. 7.*

Although the ANA Board of Directors adopted this definition of collaboration in 1994, the AMA has yet to adopt it.

Differences exist within state practice acts with regard to the legal definition of collaboration; virtually every state has a variation, defining collaboration in the con-

PERSONAL REFLECTIONS

- When working within team structures, where do you find your thoughts lie?
- Which gift of collaboration is your greatest strength? Which gift of collaboration is your greatest challenge?
- Assess your community regularly. Are you familiar with the local health and social agencies that can work with you? With whom do you collaborate daily? Reflect on positive outcomes.
- In view of the legal aspects of collaboration, how can skills we use positively affect our working relationships? What personal feelings hold back your ability to network and be a team player? Where do you draw your strength when caring for a client with complex needs?

CASE STUDY 16.4

Helen, a hospital nurse, is preparing to discharge Jay, a single man who has been in the hospital after a head injury and subsequent short-term rehabilitation. Jay has had no income for his hospital stay of 6 weeks and is facing eviction from his apartment. Before his accident, Jay worked in a warehouse stocking supplies. Jay lives in a local community and sometimes attends a local synagogue. His family lives out of state. Jay calls himself a "loner."

Critical Thinking
- What community resources are open to the nurse to assist Jay with his discharge?
- What in-house options are available?
- What skills will be particularly important in this case?
- What key aspects would you keep in mind as you are discharging Jay?

text of supervision of duties. Please refer to annual updates of nurse practitioner legislation for discussion of these issues.

Key Points
- Collaboration involves teamwork as members work toward a common goal.
- Increased peace of mind and decreased anxiety are benefits to clients receiving spiritual care.
- The five gifts of collaboration are respect, positive regard for others, setting clear goals, listening, and dedication to whole-person care.
- The interdisciplinary team in the health care setting can be composed of nurses, physicians, social workers, and others.
- Team ministry involves collaboration among parish nurses, pastors, support staff, office staff, lay workers, counselors, and volunteers.
- Collaboration in advanced practice nursing can have unique definitions related to legal scope of practice.

References

Cary, A. H. (1996). Case management. In M. Stanhope & J. Lancaster (Eds.), *Community health nursing* (4th ed.). St. Louis: Mosby.

Collaboration and independent practice: Ongoing issues for nursing. (1998). *Nursing Trends & Issues, 3*(5). Retrieved September 14, 2003, from http://www.nursingworld.org/readroom/nti/9805nti.htm.

Engstrom, T. W. (1976). *The making of a Christian leader.* Grand Rapids, MI: Zondervan Publishing House.

Hawkins, J. W., Veeder, N. W., & Pearce, C. W. (1998). *Nurse–social worker collaboration.* New York: Springer.

Kelley, J.T. (1994). Five group dynamics in team ministry. *Journal of Pastoral Care, 48,* 118–130.

Newton, L. H. (1989). *Ethics in America: Study guide.* Corporation for Public Broadcasting and Columbia University Seminars on Media and Society. Englewood Cliffs, NJ: Prentice-Hall.

Rogers, C. R. (1957). The necessary and sufficient conditions of therapeutic personality change. *Journal of Consulting Psychology, 2*(21), 96.

Solari-Twadell, P. A. (1999). The emerging practice of parish nursing. In P. A. Solari-Twadell and M. A. McDermott (Eds.), *Parish nursing: Promoting whole person health within faith communities.* Thousand Oaks, CA: Sage.

Wywialowski, E. (1995). Communicating and collaborating. In P. S. Yoder Wise (Ed.), *Leading and managing in nursing.* St. Louis: Mosby.

Recommended Readings

Maslow, A. H. (1998). *Maslow on management.* With Deborah Stephens and Gary Heil. New York: John Wiley & Sons.

Stuart, G. W., & Sundeen, S. J. (1995). *Principles and practice of psychiatric nursing* (5th ed.). St. Louis: Mosby.

17

*E*thical Issues in Spiritual Care

Marie T. Cahn

LEARNING OBJECTIVES

At the end of this chapter, the reader will be able to:
- Understand the relative nature of ethics and spirituality.
- Explain how spiritual care relates to holistic nursing practice.
- Relate spiritual care to the *Code of Ethics for Nurses.*

autonomy   ethics
beneficence   justice
Categorical Imperatives   nonmalfeasance
character   teleology
Code of Ethics for Nurses   values
deontology

T hree features are certain to accompany any discussion of the ethics of spiritual care: confusion, complexity, and controversy. Those who attempt to practice spiritual care are likely to face the same challenges. Confusion, complexity, and controversy often are related and have a negative connotation in everyday encounters. However, in the context of ethics and spiritual care, these elements are constructive, providing that nurses meet them head-on and do not attempt to minimize them. If all of life's happenings and events were uncomplicated, and we all agreed on everything, things might be more pleasant, and we could live our lives being complacent and satisfied with each other. That we are spared complacency and satisfaction is most fortunate because without some degree of confusion, complexity, and controversy, nurses could not grow as people or professionals.

As thinking beings, we have a desire for some degree of clarity and order and a need to make sense of the world. When we are confused, we are forced to pull an issue or an idea apart and examine other sides of it because we enjoy order. Similarly, when complexity confronts us, we are forced to analyze the event or idea because our minds demand some degree of understanding. Inevitably, the analysis and examination of the complex events that confuse us lead to controversy because the result of the analysis and examination is quite different for each of us. So, it is in confusion that we can begin to see things clearly; it is in complexity that we are able to sort things out; and it is in controversy that we come together.

To that end, this chapter addresses and clarifies three broad issues:

- The confusion about the relationship of ethics and spirituality that is brought about in part because both are sometimes marginally related to religious beliefs
- The complexity that arises because people bring different concepts of ethics and spirituality and different sources of authority to every situation
- The controversies that arise between and among caregivers, agencies, and patients as they meet in relationships with their differing concepts of ethics and spirituality and different sources of authority

The confusion regarding the concepts of ethics and spirituality arises because both involve processes that are internal to a person and may be related to religious orientation. That means that we cannot observe them as we do physiologic processes or get at them in the same way we do with psychological processes, which have been studied and classified. To clear some of the confusion, a comparison of the two concepts follows. Because the focus of this text and chapter is practice, the comparison uses several criteria that provide an empirical focus on the concepts. It is beyond the scope of this chapter to define ethics or spirituality; others have taken on that task with at least a modicum of success. The purpose of this brief comparison is simply to look at the concepts as they exist empirically and see how they are alike and different. The comparison should provide a working knowledge of the two concepts that is sufficient to assist beginning practitioners in their encounters with patients and to give support to more experienced practitioners who find themselves confronted with the need for a better understanding of the concepts. The criteria used in the comparison are: purpose/activity, character, values, and theoretical framework (Table 17.1).

ETHICS

This chapter considers the concept of ethics as it relates to professional practice. In that sense, and in its simplest form, **ethics** is what we ought or ought not do to, for, or with patients when we face situations of moral conflict.

Purpose/Activity

The purpose of ethics in practice is to facilitate decision making and to promote actions or ethical acts that involve others in society. For nurses, those "others" are usually patients, but ethical decision making in practice also frequently involves people such as family members, significant others, physicians, other nurses, and agency staff. Very significantly and very often, the agency itself, in the form of policies and

TABLE 17.1   Comparison of Ethics and Spirituality

Characteristic	Ethics	Spirituality
Purpose/activity	To act in society	To be
	Relates to "oughts" and "ought nots," rights and wrongs	Gives meaning to the individual
		Inherent in the person, not necessarily situation related
	Enables decisions that involve others	May or may not determine activity
	Responsive to situations	
	Determines activity	
Character	Cognitive and rational, therefore explicable and open to question	Not cognitive, therefore not easily articulated or open to question
Values	Established ethical principles	No established principles
	Not always dependent on higher power	Virtually always related to a higher power in the form of an entity, object, or abstract concept
Framework	Established	Not established

procedures, becomes part of the ethical decision-making process. What occurs in many instances of decision making for nurses is that the nurse can determine the "right" or ethical thing to do in a given situation but cannot do that particular thing because of external constraints, such as hospital policy or physician orders. Although the intended result of the ethical thought process is action, occasionally the end result is only the decision to act because the ability to carry out the act is constrained in some way. Jameton (1984) refers to those moments as situations of "moral distress," for it is at those times that nurses may despair. He believes that most ethical problems nurses face are not true moral dilemmas, which occur when individuals have to choose between two or more undesirable courses of action.

Character

As discussed, ethics involves a decision, and then, ideally, an action. Therefore, because of the decision-making part involved in the process, ethics is thoughtful or cognitive. It is deliberate and, it is hoped, rational. Whatever is cognitive and rational is, by definition, also explicable. Therefore, ethics is explicable and, if given the opportunity, nurses should be able to explain their ethical thinking process so that others will understand it. The cognitive nature of ethical decision making also leaves ethical judgments open to scrutiny, discussion, and revision.

Values

Because the ethical decision-making process is cognitive, it relies on established standards or principles, which may be thought of as the underlying values of ethical thought. Taken together, those principles constitute the theoretical frameworks of ethics. The most popular and commonly applied ethical frameworks rely on certain principles that relate to each other within the framework or theory. The most established principles in bioethics are autonomy, beneficence, nonmalfeasance, and justice, which underlie deontological theory, and "the greatest happiness principle," which is basic to teleological theory. Those who explore other theoretical ethical approaches will find other principles underpinning their ways of thinking. Ethical thought often relates in some ways to religious or spiritual thought, either because of what the nurse brings to the process or because of the theory itself. However, many ethical ways of thinking do not involve a higher power. That reality is significant in a discussion of ethics and spirituality.

Theoretical Framework

As established, ethical thinking is cognitive and rational, so it occurs within a logical, organized framework. Each ethical framework has its own set of principles or concepts that relate to one another in different ways. This chapter examines the two most commonly used frameworks: deontology and teleology (Table 17.2).

Deontology

Other terms for **deontology** found in the literature are *rule ethics, duty ethics, formalism,* or *Kantian ethics.* The latter takes its name from Immanuel Kant (1724–1804), the originator of deontological theory (Bandman & Bandman, 2001; Beauchamp & Childress, 2001). Deontological ethics are duty based, and their goal is to act out of respect

TABLE 17.2   Comparison of Ethical Frameworks

Framework	Synopsis	Process
Deontology *Originator:* Immanuel Kant *Other names:* Kantian ethic; duty ethic; rule ethic; formalism *Root of word:* Greek *deon, deont-*, obligation, necessity	Concerned with duties and rights of individuals. An act is moral if it originates from "good will," which comes from a sense of duty, not just inclination. One acts out of respect for the moral law—what ought to be done, not what one desires to do. Emphasis is on principles, not consequences (not considered).	Identify the principles involved in the ethical dilemma and weigh them against one another, using the deontological framework. Use the categorical imperatives to test the proposed action.
Teleology *Originators:* Jeremy Bentham, John Stuart Mill *Other names:* Consequentialism; utilitarianism (most common)—various forms include act-utilitarian, situation-utilitarian *Root of word:* Greek *telos-*, end, result	All action should be directed toward achieving the greatest happiness for the greatest number of people. Good is happiness; what is right promotes good. Actions are right in proportion to the happiness they produce and wrong if they produce unhappiness. Framework looks at consequences or results of an action and does not consider feelings, intentions, social norms, or ethical codes.	Identify the community of concern and assign values of happiness for the proposed action. Realize that consequences and happiness values may not be accurate.

for the moral law, rather than out of desire. In other words, the deontologist acts on principle and has little or no concern for the results or consequences of those actions. The assumption of deontology is that if one acts based on principles that are good and right, the result of such principled actions also will be good and right. The decision-making process for the deontologist consists of weighing and balancing four basic principles: autonomy, beneficence, nonmalfeasance, and justice.

- **Autonomy** relates to personal liberty and means free choice of action by a person based on due consideration of the action taken. That means that the person must be fully informed in relation to his or her decision. By acting ethically to uphold autonomy, one cannot help but respect the worth and dignity of the person.
- **Beneficence** means to take actions to benefit others, to do good, and to prevent harm. It is active, meaning that the ethical person actually engages in doing good works or in preventing or stopping harm.
- **Nonmalfeasance** means to refrain from doing harm, with harm being physical, mental, or spiritual, but also extending to reputation and property in the broadest sense. Although related to beneficence, nonmalfeasance is passive, meaning that the ethical person refrains from engaging in harmful acts.
- **Justice** has several meanings, but its bioethical connotation most commonly relates to fairness or what a person deserves or is owed on a social level. It is related to the appropriate distribution of social benefits and burdens.

When facing an ethical situation, the deontological person uses his or her understanding of the principles and weighs them against one another systematically to make ethical judgments for each alternative. When the judgment or decision is made, the final test is in statements that Kant called **Categorical Imperatives**, which involve the "oughts and shoulds" of decisions made on principle. Three categorical imperatives, pertinent to nursing practice and worded as common questions, are:

- ✚ *Will I be treating this person the way I think I ought to be treated?* Many readers will recognize this as the Golden Rule of Christianity.
- *What would happen if everyone in a similar situation acted as I am about to act?* Thinking this way generalizes the ethical action so it is not situational but universal. Universal judgments are more useful because they can be used in future encounters of a similar nature.
- ✚ *Am I about to treat this person as an end in himself or herself or as a means to someone else's end?* Asking this question focuses the action on the person involved, ensuring respect for that person's autonomy. For instance, a Christian nurse may consider that spiritual care involves trying to "save" a dying patient by having the patient convert to Christianity. This proselytizing behavior to meet personal religious desires, rather than respecting the patient's right to religious freedom, uses the patient as a means to the nurse's end.

The Categorical Imperatives also may be useful after a decision is made, an action is taken, and the fallout has occurred. The Imperatives serve as an evaluation tool for the decision made and for future decisions.

A limitation of deontological decision making is that although the person may act according to the rule, the outcome of the action may not always be desirable. For example, although truth telling may be considered an imperative, there may be rare circumstances when the nurse may not desire or be obligated to reveal information.

For instance, if parents suspected of child abuse inquire as to who reported them to the authorities, the deontological view may argue that the nurse would need to admit making the report. However, the current process of dealing with child abuse protects the identity of mandated reporters.

Teleology

Teleology or consequentialism is a grouping of frameworks largely attributed to the thoughts and writings of Jeremy Bentham (1748–1832) and John Stuart Mill (1806–1873). The best known of these frameworks is **utilitarianism**. The consequentialist, as the name implies, is concerned with results or consequences of his acts. More than that, one major principle guides the ethical decision making: "the greatest good (or happiness) principle." With teleology, what is most important in an ethical decision is that the actions result in the greatest good for the greatest number of people. The assumption is that good is happiness and what is right promotes good. To be a consequentialist, one has to do a sort of math that relates to the outcomes of the decision and all those involved in it. To arrive at a determination of the greatest happiness for the greatest number, the ethical agent identifies the community of interest and actually calculates a happiness quotient for each person in the situation for each alternative. The highest happiness value is the right decision.

For everyday use, consequential theory has two major flaws. First, one must be able to predict consequences accurately, and second, one must be able to estimate accurately the happiness value those consequences will bring to each person in the community of interest. Both are difficult to do, although being a professional with knowledge of health care outcomes helps, as does knowing the participants involved (a luxury in today's health care system). An ethical problem in the teleological approach for nurses is that in the original theory, it is very clear that in the calculation for happiness, each person counts as one person, and no person counts as more than one. This poses an inherent conflict for nurses because the *Code of Ethics for Nurses* (American Nurses Association, 2001) makes it clear that the nurse's first and primary obligation is to the patient, and not to others.

The difference between the two frameworks is obvious. In deontology, the emphasis is on principles and the good will of the moral agent. Consequences are not even considered in the process. Contrast that with teleological thinking, in which one looks at consequences or results of an action and considers only the good or the happiness of the people involved, and nothing more.

Virtually no one is pure in ethical thinking. In other words, probably few people think exclusively about duty or consequences when facing an ethical situation that requires a decision. People tend to do both. This is particularly true in the United States, where diversity of thinking and religious beliefs is common. It may be less true in countries or regions where the government is closely connected to a fundamental form of a particular religion or philosophy or where people are more homogeneous in their thinking and actions because of truly held beliefs, indoctrination, or fear of reprisal. It should also be noted that the underpinnings of deontological thinking—autonomy, beneficence, nonmalfeasance, and justice—are universal but may have very different meanings in other cultures or in the aforementioned cadres of fundamentalism. What did "autonomy" (for all, but especially for women) mean in the Afghanistan of the Taliban? What does "justice" mean in Iraq, Israel, and Palestine?

SPIRITUALITY

The concept of **spirituality** is integral to the practice of nursing. Beginning with Florence Nightingale, nurses have been trying to get at its meaning, most recently with formal attempts at concept analysis (Emblen, 1992; Goldberg, 1998; McIntyre, 2000). That academic activity has produced many definitions or conceptualizations of spirituality. The chapter explores the term as it relates to professional practice.

When spirituality is used in practice, it generally refers to the person's own perception of it, and not to a well-defined entity or idea. To compare spirituality and ethics, we will use the same criteria of purpose/activity, character, values, and theoretical framework.

Purpose/Activity

It is difficult to say that spirituality actually has a purpose; however, examining the question of purpose serves to emphasize how spirituality differs from ethics. If pressed, one could say that the purpose of spirituality is for the individual "to be." Spirituality is native and intrinsic to the person and gives meaning to his or her existence. It is not situational, although certain events, either positive or negative, certainly can trigger the sense, perception, or awareness of it. That fact is significant in a discussion relating to spirituality and nursing care because illness or injury can be and often is a trigger event. Spiritual awareness does not necessarily lead to or determine activity, but it is certainly possible that some sort of activity, such as prayer, meditation, or ritual, will follow the awareness. On a larger scale, the person might make a behavior change in himself or herself or in his or her relationships with others.

Character

Spirituality is not cognitive. For that reason, most people cannot easily articulate their own sense of spirituality. Although spirituality can be difficult for patients to explain, spirituality is not open to question by others. That certainly is not to say that nurses should ignore it or not attempt to learn more about the spirituality of people in their care. Rather, it means that the nurse can only attempt to understand it and must rely on each person's articulation of it. Most certainly, nurses cannot stand in judgment of a person's spirituality.

Values

Spirituality is virtually always related to a higher power. That higher power may be an entity, object, or abstract concept. Typically, a higher power is one or more of the various deity or god forms held by humans, especially religious humans. However, it is possible that the higher power has nothing to do with God, gods, or religion. The sense of spirit in a person may arise, and in some instances does arise, from nature, art, cosmic bodies, or energy fields. The possibilities are as endless as human beings' abilities to conjure and relate to entities, objects, or abstractions outside themselves. Examples can be found among various cultures and religions. Alaskan Natives, Presbyterians, and Hindus are all spiritual groups that relate to a higher power or powers. The seminal differences among their spiritual beginnings are in the actual or perceived nature of that higher power.

Theoretical Framework

In keeping with the variable nature of spirituality, a person's sense of spirituality is not necessarily confined to any established framework, although it may be. When spirituality arises from religious belief, which is quite common, it probably fits into a creed or framework. However, its existence for the person is a matter of faith and therefore highly individualized. Thus, an understanding of the associated creed or framework can help the nurse to understand the person's spirituality, although the nurse may never really fully grasp it because of individual variations. For instance, several Catholics may hold the same set of core beliefs. Nevertheless, each Catholic's sense of the spiritual will vary based on his or her closeness with nature, particular life experiences, and other factors. All of them consider themselves Catholics because of their religious beliefs, but the spirituality of each encompasses something different.

ETHICS AND SPIRITUALITY

Although ethics and spirituality are separate and different entities by several criteria, they are often related, usually quite closely. For the nursing profession, the common unifier of ethics and spirituality is the *Code of Ethics for Nurses* (American Nurses Association, 2001). The Code strongly exhibits all the principles used in deontological thinking. Although The Code is best known as an ethical document, it relates to spirituality in that it requires nurses, as ethical practitioners, to value and show consideration for every facet and dimension of all patients entrusted to their care. The Code articulates the ethical relationship of patients and nurses and clarifies their collective position.

A very careful reading of The Code is not necessary to realize how strongly grounded it is in autonomy. The first provision is "The nurse, in all professional relationships, practices with compassion and respect for inherent dignity, worth and uniqueness of every individual, unrestricted by considerations of social or economic status, personal attributes, or the nature of health problems" (American Nurses Association, 2001). In that one statement, The Code demands that the nurse attend to every aspect, facet, and characteristic of every patient, which include spiritual beliefs and practices.

Complexity in the provision of spiritual care occurs partially because people have highly individual views of spirituality and spiritual practices that arise from different sources of authority. People are all different in many ways, but the greatest and hardest-to-grasp differences among us probably occur in individual concepts of own spirituality. As the essence of the individual, spirituality is so highly personal and intangible that it can be difficult or impossible to articulate. At times, people are aware of their spirituality, or at least pieces of it. At other times, for many people, spirituality is just something that is with them, as background music might be, ebbing and flowing through their consciousness and daily lives. Spirituality is native and intrinsic to the person and gives meaning to his or her existence. Each person experiences spirituality through his or her own eyes, with individual interpretations and understandings, based on life experiences. Although some people share some events, spaces, niches, and even common beliefs, they do not share a being, an essence, a spirituality. Thus, any interaction or transaction among people based on assumptions of the specifics of spirituality is going to result in a missed understanding of the nature of the spirituality, which is so complex. There is really nothing to be done about it. Like spirituality itself, the situation just "is." That does not mean nurses can ignore the need for holistic care in their interactions with patients. It means that they must attempt to get at spiritual meaning by other, more tangible, means. A good way to start is to establish the stated source or sources of the person's spirituality.

Religion is probably the most common and likely source. Because spirituality tends to be related to a higher power, and definitions of religion include some notion of a belief in and reverence for a supernatural power or powers, it follows that the two are often related and may even be lumped together. Religion is broader in scope than spirituality because it also involves belief in a creator and ruler or governor of the universe, and is generally accompanied by doctrines and precepts. However, as already stated, religious beliefs are only one source of the spiritual. The person whose sense of spirit is related to energy fields, rainbows, or rocks has spirituality as real as the person who derives spirituality from Christianity or Buddhism.

There are as many sources of spirituality as there are people; in health care, those people and sources all come together frequently and with intensity. It is natural for one's spirituality to come to the fore in times of fear, vulnerability, pain, or any one of the great assortment of human emotions that accompany illness. Physical illness is an assault on the body—it is at such times that people may feel threatened to the core of their being, soul, and spirit. If one accepts that the purpose of spirituality is for a person "to be" and that its presence gives meaning to the person's existence, it follows that in times of illness, when the person's very being and existence may be threatened, his or her spirituality will leap to the forefront with intensity. It is at those moments that patients often enter into existential crises. They may question their lives, their place in the world, their reason for being, and their very existence. They may take a new look at the world as they assume a new identity within that world and try to make sense of the world's absurdity, capriciousness, and vagaries. They may question the source of their spiritual authority, or they may cling desperately to it. The important point is that people in extreme situations search and reach. They search inwardly and outwardly. To make sense of loss, suffering, uncertainty, and sometimes, death, they reach for what is inside and what gives them being and meaning—their spirituality. They also reach out for the source of that spirituality. Nurses do not understand the patient's spirituality exactly as the patient does, but they know such reach is occurring. They know that they have an ethical obligation to attend to it—an obligation to help people in their reaching.

It seems unfortunate that such a personal, harmless, and human characteristic should cause trouble in times of trouble, but it does. Spirituality and its manifestations or associated actions can be the source of great controversy among and between patients, their families, and their health care providers. There can be disagreements between and among families and patients, patients and agencies, caregivers and patients, or any combination thereof. Nurses are often in the middle of such controversies.

What happens when the fulfillment or realization of a person's sense of spirituality depends on a certain event, such as a ritual dance, lighted candles, or visits from the youngest descendant (e.g., child, grandchild, great-grandchild), and hospital policy forbids it? What should the nurse do when he or she discovers that lesions on a patient's skin are new and result from certain religious/spiritual practices? What can be done when a dying person wants to meditate on some unknown cosmic being who she believes will take her away, and asks her nurse, who strongly opposes such beliefs, to hold her hand while she meditates and waits?

When such spiritual controversies arise, nurses have at least three things to inform and assist them: the *Code of Ethics for Nurses*, the ability to assess, and their own ethical reasoning. The Code is commonly shared among all nurses. Assessment and ethical reasoning, although universal in nursing, are more individual because of varying knowledge and skill levels.

The Code informs nurses that they must attend to every aspect, facet, and characteristic of every patient. It demands that they do no harm and not abandon the patient. When confronting a difficult situation involving spirituality, nurses must work within those parameters. They must treat every patient holistically and consider his or her spiritual needs. They must attempt to not do harm, although this principle poses difficulty in practice, frequently in the form of cost benefits. For example, nurses frequently cite the lack of time resulting from low staffing ratios (a cost-saving measure) as a barrier to incorporating spiritual care (see Chapter 18). Failure to overcome this barrier may result in nursing care that is not holistic in nature, thereby resulting in harm to the patient's personal integrity. The important thing is that nurses weigh situations and their own actions to determine the harm or benefit or even happiness they will bring to the patient, which is part of the ethical reasoning process, and act accordingly. Most importantly, they cannot abandon the patient, physically, emotionally, or psychologically. If their own religion, ethic, or sense of spirit will not allow them to sit with a patient who is meditating on an ancestor or an unfamiliar god, nurses must find alternatives to accommodate the patient's needs.

Assessment is within the abilities of every nurse; many consider it the cornerstone of the nursing process. Spiritual assessment should be part of every assessment done by every nurse (see Chapter 14). The frequency of and degree to which it is done will necessarily vary for several reasons, including the context of care and the skill of the nurse. Agencies vary in their interest in the spiritual care of patients and in the degree to which they support it. Spiritual care is far more likely to be supported in religious institutions, but then, the breadth and scope of that interest will vary according to the particular denomination or source of authority. The same is true of religious nurses. In addition, the skills of nurses will vary, as will their level of comfort with spiritual care. Many assessment tools are available that nurses can use to formally assess the spiritual dimension of patients (see Chapter 14). Such tools can provide comfort for nurses who are not confident in their skills and guidance for those who are not sure how or where to start.

Ethical reasoning, like assessment, is highly individual. Some people are more or less skilled at it than others. It would seem that ethical reasoning related to spirituality would be no different from ethical reasoning in any other situation. That is partially true because the same cognitive skills and reasoning abilities are involved. However, there is a difference in that the religious, emotional, and psychological investment on the nurse's part is often much greater in an ethical situation relating to the spiritual. That is especially true when the ethical framework out of which the nurse reasons and acts is strongly grounded in a rigid and unyielding religious perspective. Nurses who are so encumbered have no less an obligation to follow The Code, which means they must attend to and not abandon the spiritual needs of patients. As in any other practice situation of conscientious objection, they must simply find another way to fulfill the obligation.

🖋 ✚ The Native American client in Oklahoma who has just received a diagnosis of a life-threatening disorder, and who is in the care of a Roman Catholic nurse born and raised in New York City and a New Age physician from Arizona, has a spiritual sense and being unknown to both health care providers in any tangible way. Neither of them can get into the patient's psyche and soul and truly know what it means to that patient to be alone in a room, in pain, in fear, and longing for the people and places that provide the source of his spirituality—his sense of being and his comfort. The best they can do is to try to develop a cognitive understanding of his cultural mores, beliefs, and customs. Doing so will get them halfway to the place where they can assess his spirituality. Nurses have an obligation to provide the best, most holistic care possible. That means going outside themselves and their own truly held beliefs.

The ethical obligations are clear. If nurses claim to give holistic care, they must try to understand the nature of their patients' spirituality. More concretely, they cannot take a cookie cutter approach and assume that because someone belongs to a particular religious group, the person's sense of spirituality corresponds exactly with a textbook or stereotyped representation of that particular religion. Nurses are obligated to assess for the spiritual to clarify its nature. Then, they are obligated to follow through on the care related to the patient's spiritual needs. If they cannot provide the assessment and care themselves, they must find a person who will be able to do so. To do less is to abandon a person who might benefit from the intervention. To do less is to not respect the inherent dignity, worth, and uniqueness of the person and to not provide holistic nursing care.

PERSONAL REFLECTIONS

- What characteristics do you have that enable you to provide good spiritual care?
- What barriers to providing good spiritual care do you see in yourself?
- Try to explain your own sense of spirituality to someone who does not know you very well.
- Do nurses generally provide spiritual care at the same level and intensity as they do physiologic care?
- What would happen to health care if every nurse made a concerted effort to provide spiritual care to every patient he or she encountered?
- Would attitudes change?
- Would patient outcomes change?
- Would our practice ethic change?

CASE STUDY 17.1

Hosea is the nurse caring for a female patient, Rita. Rita believes that she must have her blood transfused to cure her illness. She was hospitalized for what the chart records as "attempted suicide" for slicing her forearms to drain some of her blood. She was placed on suicide watch in the locked unit of a psychiatric hospital near her home. Rita tells Hosea that she is convinced an evil spirit is inside of her; it entered when she had an illegal abortion a few months ago. Rita believes that if she just had a blood transfusion, her body would be cleansed, and the evil would leave her, allowing her to return to a normal life. She tries to explain that this is related to her religious beliefs rooted in Voodoo.

Hosea reviews the chart and finds that Rita has no prior record of physical or mental problems. Rita's sessions with the psychiatrist and treatment with traditional medications seem to have little or no effect. Rita's physical condition begins to deteriorate. Hosea is conflicted about how to handle Rita's repeated requests for a blood transfusion. Rita remains convinced that the transfusion is the only cure for her problem.

Critical Thinking
- What options are open to Hosea?
- What ethical principles may be in conflict in this situation? Is there an ethical dilemma? If so, what is it?
- If Hosea used the deontological approach to Rita's case, what would be the outcome?
- What if Hosea used the teleological approach?
- How can Hosea provide spiritual care to this patient? Should he ask any other questions of her?
- What would be the ideal resolution to this case?

Key Points
- The confusion about the relationship between ethics and spirituality is brought about in part because both can be related to religious beliefs.
- Ethics is what we ought or ought not do to, for, or with patients when we face situations of moral conflict. The purpose of ethics in practice is to facilitate decision making and to promote actions or ethical acts that involve others in society.
- The most established principles in bioethics are autonomy, beneficence, non-malfeasance, and justice, which underlie deontological theory.
- "The greatest happiness principle" is basic to teleological theory.
- For the nursing profession, the common unifier of ethics and spirituality is the *Code of Ethics for Nurses*. The Code articulates the ethical relationship of patients and nurses and clarifies their collective position.
- The *Code of Ethics for Nurses* relates to spirituality in that it requires nurses, as ethical practitioners, to value and show consideration for every facet and dimension of all patients entrusted to their care.

References

American Nurses Association. (2001). *Code of ethics for nurses with interpretive statements*. Available at: http://www.nursingworld.org/ethics/code/ethicscode150.htm. Accessed August 3, 2002.

Bandman, E. L., & Bandman, B. (2001). *Nursing ethics through the life span* (4th ed.). Upper Saddle River, NJ: Prentice Hall.

Beauchamp, T. L., & Childress, J. F. (2001). *Principles of biomedical ethics* (5th ed.). Oxford: Oxford University Press.

Emblen, J. D. (1992). Religion and spirituality defined according to current use in nursing literature. *Journal of Professional Nursing, 8*(1), 41–47.

Goldberg, B. (1998). Connection: An exploration of spirituality in nursing care. *Journal of Advanced Nursing, 27*(4), 836–842.

Jameton, A. (1984). Death, pain, and suffering. In E. H. Author (Ed.), *Nursing practice: The ethical issues* (pp. 221–243). Englewood Cliffs, NJ: Prentice Hall.

McIntyre, T. L. (2000). *An analysis of the concept of spirituality*. Unpublished manuscript, Purdue University Calumet, Hammond, IN.

Recommended Readings

Johnson, E. (1998). Integrating healthcare and spirituality: Considerations for ethical and cultural sensitivity. *Maryland Nurse, 17*(5). Available at: http://FirstSearch.oclc.org. Accessed November 3, 2002.

McSherry, W. (1998). Nurses' perceptions of spirituality and spiritual care. *Nursing Standard, 13*(4), 36–40.

McSherry, W., & Draper, P. (1998). The debates emerging from the literature surrounding the concept of spirituality as applied to nursing. *Journal of Advanced Nursing, 27*, 683–691.

O'Brien, M. E. (1999). *Spirituality in nursing: Standing on holy ground*. Sudbury, MA: Jones and Bartlett.

Oldnall, A. (1996). A critical analysis of nursing: Meeting the spiritual needs of patients. *Journal of Advanced Nursing, 23*(1), 138–144.

Wright, K. B. (1998). Professional, ethical, and legal implications for spiritual care in nursing. *Image: The Journal of Nursing Scholarship, 30*, 81–83.

18

Nursing Research About Spirituality and Health

Nola A. Schmidt

At the end of this chapter, the reader will be able to:

- Discuss the importance of research in spirituality and health to the discipline of nursing.
- Identify nursing theories that include the concept of spirituality.
- List instruments that nursing researchers commonly use to measure spirituality.
- Describe recent findings of nursing research about spirituality and health.
- Identify areas for future nursing research regarding the relationship between spirituality and health.

ethnography
God Locus of Health Control Scale
 (GLHCS)
grounded theory
phenomenology
qualitative research methods
quantitative research methods
self-reliance

Self-transcendence Scale (STS)
Spiritual Care Practice Questionnaire
 (SCP)
Spiritual Health Inventory (SHI)
Spiritual Involvement and Beliefs Scale
 (SIBS)
Spiritual Perspective Scale (SPS)
Spiritual Well-Being Scale (SWBS)

Because nursing is a science, it is imperative that spiritual care in nursing practice be based on knowledge from evidence. Evidence has many sources: tradition, intuition, trial and error, authority, personal experience, and common sense. Research is also a way of acquiring evidence about nursing, and in scientific communities research is thought to be the most reliable source of knowledge.

The purpose of this chapter is to provide an introduction to the body of nursing research about spirituality and health. After briefly discussing why nurses should be involved in researching spirituality and health, this chapter identifies some instruments commonly used in nursing research to measure spirituality and summarizes the findings of select recent nursing studies involving spirituality and health.

SHOULD NURSES PERFORM RESEARCH ABOUT SPIRITUALITY?

If nurses assume human beings to be biopsychosocial and spiritual beings, then it follows that nursing research should be involved in describing the relationship of the spiritual dimension of human beings to health. Nurses would not think twice about studying the physical effects of a nursing intervention, the psychological effects of an illness, or the social aspects of a community health education program. So, why are nurses hesitant to study the spiritual aspects of health?

Perhaps the hesitancy to study spirituality exists because, at first glance, it may seem odd to talk about research and spirituality. One might think it impertinent for human beings to think that they can "research" spirituality. After all, would that not be studying God? Is it appropriate to mix science with the sacred?

The purpose of nursing research related to the study of spirituality and health is not to study God. It is to study human beings. Through research, nurses aim to describe, explain, and predict how beliefs in a higher power, religious practices, or interactions with members of faith communities affect the health of individuals. Furthermore, nursing research can study the effects of spirituality on health or the meanings people give spirituality during health or illness.

Some nursing theorists discuss spirituality or related concepts in their theories; thus, nursing research about spirituality is relevant from a theoretical perspective. Theories are fundamental to the scientific discipline of nursing. Nurses can use theories to guide research. They also can derive research designs from theories for the purpose of testing the theories. Findings from research can allow researchers to support or alter current theories or to build new theories.

For some nursing theorists, spirituality is encompassed in theoretical underpinnings. Nightingale (1969) proposed that nursing was a process that manifested the presence of the Creator in the world. In her transpersonal theory of caring, Watson (1999) built on Nightingale's philosophical notions, viewing the person as spirit, the soul as sacred energy, and the body as an instrument of the soul. When viewing human beings as persons, Orem (2001) linked spiritual experiences with a state of well-being, that is, the perceived condition of personal existence.

Other theorists have specified spirituality as a concept in their theories. Neuman (1995) suggested that spirituality, as a client variable, moves the client system toward well-being through spiritual energy. Roy and Andrews (1999) described spirituality within the self-concept mode of a person as an adaptive system. Leininger's (1991) sunrise model specifies religion as a factor that gives meaning to a cultural group. Although Rogers' (1992) science of unitary human beings does not specifically mention spirituality as a concept, several authors have proposed middle-range theories of spirituality (Malinski, 1994; Smith, 1994) and self-transcendence (Coward & Reed, 1996; Reed, 1991c, 1992) based on Rogers' work. The theoretical works by Parse (1981, 1995) on co-transcending and Newman (1994) on expanding consciousness also reflect notions of spirituality. Given the inclusion of spirituality in various nursing theories, it is reasonable for nurses to study spirituality to increase their understanding of nursing.

Using knowledge about spirituality generated from nursing research can positively inform practice. Unfortunately, if nurses continue to overlook the spiritual dimension of clients and the relationship of the spiritual dimension to health, they are doing a disservice to clients and the discipline of nursing. Because nurses are obligated to perform safe and effective nursing care, it follows that nurses must continue to inquire about the relationships between spirituality and health. Nurses must overcome their hesitancy to study spirituality or implement spiritual care, especially because spirituality is at the very core of human existence.

MEASURING SPIRITUALITY IN RESEARCH

Because spirituality is an abstract concept and not directly observable, its measurement depends primarily on how it is defined. A good researcher works hard to ensure that what he or she is measuring accurately reflects the concept guiding the study. He or she begins with a conceptual definition of spirituality (e.g., the core of one's being). Next, the researcher must create what is known as an empirical definition, that is, a definition whereby the concept can be measured. For instance, an empirical definition of spirituality may be the score received on the Spiritual Well-Being Scale.

Quantitative Research

Quantitative research methods use numbers to measure variables. Experiments, quasi-experiments, correlational designs, and descriptive surveys are examples of quantitative designs. Findings are usually reported by using statistics.

For quantitative designs, various instruments are available to measure spirituality and related concepts, such as transcendence, religious belief, religiosity, and religious activity. It has been reported that the first two volumes of the *Compendium of Spirituality and Religiosity Measures* contains 126 scales (Mackenzie, Rajagopal, Meilbohm, & Lavizzo-Mourey, 2000). Ellerhorst-Ryan (1997) identified four concepts typically measured by instruments: spiritual needs, spiritual well-being, spiritual coping, and religious orientation. Concepts such as hope, meaning and purpose in life, love and relatedness, and forgiveness were identified as "singular concepts of spiritual need" (Ellerhorst-Ryan, p. 205).

Another issue that requires consideration is the ambiguity between spiritual and psychological domains. For instance, coping can be considered both from spiritual and psychological aspects. If researchers wish to study spiritual coping, they would need to carefully examine items on the instruments to be sure the items are about spiritual coping and not psychological coping (Ellerhorst-Ryan, 1997). By looking at the types of questions on the instrument, the researcher would need to evaluate whether questions are measuring spiritual or psychological aspects. For instance, the question "Does your belief in a higher being help you to cope with your illness?" is an example of an item related to spirituality. However, the question, "Do you find talking with others to be helpful when coping with your illness?" is an ambiguous question. A response to this question fails to capture whether talking with others includes spiritual leaders or God. Thus, the question in this format inquires about only psychological coping. The question could be adapted to look at spiritual coping by rephrasing it to "Do you find talking about your religious and spiritual beliefs helpful when coping with your illness?"

In many studies, researchers collect information about the religious affiliations of individuals, which they use only to describe the sample. Other times, they use religious affiliation as a study variable in an attempt to identify correlations with other study variables. The use of religious affiliation as a measure of spirituality is limited because spirituality can encompass much more than religious affiliation. Likewise, when taking a patient history, inquiring only about patients' religious affiliation hardly does justice in describing their spirituality. Future researchers need to be aware that religious affiliation is a related, but not a comprehensive, measure of spirituality.

The **Spiritual Well-Being Scale (SWBS)** is designed to measure both horizontal and vertical dimensions of spiritual well-being using a Likert-type scale (Ellerhorst-Ryan, 1997; Paloutzian & Ellison, 1982). The vertical dimension, measured by the Religious Well-Being (RWB) subscale, refers to the sense of well-being in the relationship with God. An example of an item representing the vertical dimension is "I have a personally meaningful relationship with God." The Existential Well-Being (EWB) subscale, representing the horizontal dimension of spiritual well-being, measures a person's sense of purpose in and satisfaction with life. "I believe that there is a purpose for my life" is an item from the EWB subscale. In all, the SWBS contains 20 items. Although the instrument has demonstrated face validity and reliability, the authors have indicated the instrument may be biased toward a Judeo-Christian perspective.

The **Spiritual Health Inventory (SHI)** measures four aspects of spiritual health: satisfactorily meeting spiritual needs for self-acceptance; a trusting relationship with self based on a sense of life meaning and purpose; having relationships characterized by unconditional love, trust, and forgiveness with others or a supreme being; and hope (Highfield, 1992). The SHI asks takers to rank 31 items on a 1-to-5 Likert-type scale, with higher scores indicating higher levels of spiritual health (Ellerhorst-Ryan, 1997). This instrument has demonstrated acceptable validity and reliability, with more than 70% of the variance accounted for by the aspects of spiritual needs for self-acceptance, relationships, and hope.

The **Spiritual Perspective Scale (SPS)** measures a person's perceptions of the extent to which spirituality permeates his or her life as well as his or her engagement in spiritually related interactions. One of the ten items is "In talking with your family or friends, how often do you mention spiritual matters?" Respondents rate each item on a scale of 1 to 6, and a mean, or average, score for all ten items is calculated. Higher mean scores indicate a greater spiritual perspective for this instrument with demonstrated reliability and validity (Ellerhorst-Ryan, 1997; Reed, 1987).

The recently developed **Spiritual Involvement and Beliefs Scale (SIBS)** (Hatch, Burg, Naberhause, & Hellmich, 1998) was designed to measure actions and beliefs. This instrument attempts to avoid bias by broadening the scope and using terms that avoid cultural-religious bias (Hatch et al., 1998; Vance, 2001). Scores, a sum of the item ratings, can range from 24 to 130, with high scores representing a very spiritually minded person. Initial validity and reliability for this instrument is strong.

The **God Locus of Health Control Scale (GLHCS)** (Wallston et al., 1999) measures "the degree to which one believes that God has ultimate control over health" (Kinney, Emery, Dudley, & Croyle, 2002, p. 836). The GLHCS derives from the locus of control theory, which suggests that people with an internal locus of control believe that they have control over situations and outcomes. People with an external locus of control believe that other forces, such as God, have control over situations and outcomes. Theorists have hypothesized that people with an external locus of control will seek less screening and treatment because of their complete reliance on God (Kinney et al.; Sowell et al., 1997; Woodard & Sowell, 2001). The six items and responses range from 1 (strongly agree) to 6 (strongly disagree) (Kinney et al.). Responses are totaled, with high scores indicating a strong belief in God as locus of control. Acceptable reliability of the instrument has been demonstrated.

Self-transcendence is a frequently studied concept related to spirituality. "Self-transcendence refers to the person's capacity to expand self-boundaries intrapersonally, interpersonally, and transpersonally, to acquire a perspective that exceeds ordinary boundaries or limits" (Ellermann & Reed, 2001, p. 699). The **Self-Transcendence Scale (STS)** has 15 items that use a 4-point Likert-type scale, with 1 indicating "not at all" and 4 indicating "very much." Although the reliability of the STS has been acceptable, the instrument was designed to measure characteristics associated with later life, and thus may be less reliable with younger people.

Instruments designed specifically to measure the perceptions of nurses are also available. Vance (2001) developed the **Spiritual Care Practice Questionnaire (SCP)** to measure the spiritual care practices of nurses. Part I of the SCP focuses on nursing process by measuring the frequency of assessment and intervention. Respondents rate nine items on a 1-to-5 Likert-type scale. Part II of the SCP assesses barriers to providing spiritual care, asking nurses to agree or disagree that the item is a barrier to providing spiritual care. Content validity and reliability were acceptable; however, additional testing of this instrument is indicated.

Qualitative Research

Many nursing studies about spirituality use **qualitative research methods,** rather than quantitative designs. Because qualitative studies use words, rather than numbers, data collection usually is through semistructured interview guides containing open-ended questions. Observation is another method of data collection. Typically, qualitative researchers constantly compare transcripts from tape-recorded interviews to find patterns. They report findings from qualitative studies as themes or categories, which they sometimes use to formulate a theory about the phenomenon of interest. Because it is generally accepted that spirituality is a personal experience, qualitative designs may be more appropriate; quantitative instruments may not capture the personal experience of spirituality (Malinski, 2002). Furthermore, it is not surprising that nursing theories by Parse, Newman, Rogers, and Watson, all involving spirituality, are amenable to the qualitative approach.

Various approaches to qualitative research are distinguished by their philosophical underpinnings and purpose. **Ethnography**, which is commonly associated with Leininger's (1991) theory of culture care, aims to describe the lifeways and patterns phenomenon within the context of culture. In using ethnography, the researcher might be interested in understanding how people in a certain culture perceive spirituality. **Grounded theory** uses constant comparison (Glaser & Strauss, 1967) to create a theoretical construct about a process. A researcher might use this method to develop a theory about spiritual coping by parents after the death of a child. **Phenomenology**, through accounts of the lived experience of people, allows researchers to describe the essence or meaning of a phenomenon. The question "What is the lived experience of waiting for a liver transplant?" might be answered using the phenomenological approach.

NURSING RESEARCH FINDINGS REGARDING SPIRITUALITY AND HEALTH

Interest in the study of spirituality and health is increasing, with more studies being conducted in recent years. In a survey of spiritual and religious variables, 17% of all research studies published in three major oncology nursing journals between 1990 and 1999 included some aspect of spirituality or religion (Flannelly, Flannelly, & Weaver, 2002). In two major gerontological journals published between 1991 and 1997, 7.7% of the research articles mentioned spirituality (Weaver, Flannelly, & Flannelly, 2001). Both studies noted that the percentage of qualitative studies was greater than the percentage of quantitative studies (Flannelly et al.; Weaver et al.). Mental health nursing journals have reported a rate of 10% (Flannelly et al.). Similar studies conducted with mental health psychology journals and medical journals found 1% to 4% of the research articles included spiritual or religious variables (Flannelly et al.). When compared with other disciplines, nursing is making significant contributions to the understanding of spirituality and health.

The diversity of nursing research as it relates to spirituality is noticeable. The following section provides a snapshot of nursing research about spirituality using a selection of recent studies (Table 18.1). Readers interested in learning more about research involving spirituality and health can study the nursing literature or examine the disciplines of medicine, psychology, sociology, social work, and anthropology (see recommended readings at end of chapter).

Spirituality and Healthy Adults

Research findings have indicated that spirituality is related to a sense of well-being in older adults. One study showed that older adults believe a higher power supports

(*text continues on page 314*)

(continued)

TABLE 18.1 Summary of Select Nursing Studies About Spirituality

Citation	Purpose	Sample	Design and Theoretical Framework	Variable Measures	Findings
Ellermann & Reed (2001)	Examined the relationship of transcendence to depression; also examined relationships among parenting, acceptance, and spirituality with main study variables	Convenience sample of 133 healthy adults, ages 25–64 yr, obtained from a shopping mall located in the southwest United States	Descriptive, correlational, cross-sectional Grouped by age: 25–44 yr 45–64 yr Reed's theory of self-transcendence	Self-Transcendence Scale (STS) Center for Epidemiological Studies Depression Scale Demographic and Health Related Questionnaire	Younger group scored significantly higher on depression scale. Significant negative relationship between self-transcendence and depression. No significant relationship between spirituality and depression. Spirituality positively related to self-transcendence.
Halstead & Hull (2001)	Examined the process of spiritual development in women with cancer	Purposive sample of 10 Caucasian women, ages 45–70 yr, within 5 yr of diagnosis of non-Hodgkin's lymphoma, breast cancer, or ovarian cancer who were not receiving treatment	Grounded theory	Two semi-structured interviews with each participant	Major theme for women was "struggling with paradoxes," with three phases: (1) deciphering the meaning of cancer for me, (2) realizing human limitations, and (3) learning to live with uncertainty. The women were able to find meaning in their belief system; however, that meaning was challenged by cancer diagnosis. Women sought to be connected to God.

TABLE 18.1 Summary of Select Nursing Studies About Spirituality (continued)

Citation	Purpose	Sample	Design and Theoretical Framework	Variable Measures	Findings
Johnson (2002)	Described women's perceptions about the use of humor in their care and recovery from breast cancer	Purposive sample of nine Christian women, ages 41–48 yr, who were recruited from breast cancer support groups in Texas	Descriptive, qualitative pilot Watson's theory of human caring	One semi-structured interview with each participant	Women had individual definitions of spirituality, and not all women could link humor to Christian beliefs. Themes about humor and spirituality included: humor helps me to laugh at myself land life; God has a sense of humor; humor helps me understand myself better; humor is a step to recovery; humor makes me want to help others.
Kinney, Emery, Dudley, & Croyle (2002)	Examined the relationship between beliefs about God as a controlling force in health and adherence to breast cancer screening among high-risk African-American women	Convenience sample of 52 African-American women from Louisiana with a BRCA1, ages 18–78 yr	Descriptive, correlational, cross-sectional In-person and telephone interviews Transactional Model of Stress and Coping	Self-reported adherence to age-specific screening recommendations God Locus of Health Control Scale (GLHCS) Demographics including religion and frequency of church attendance	Women older than 25 yr with high scores on the GLHCS were less likely to adhere to screening recommendations. GLHCS scores were not correlated with religion or frequency of church attendance. Presence of a primary care provider was significant influence on adherence to screening recommendations.

Lowe (2002)	Described adult Cherokee men's perceptions of self-reliance	Purposive sample of 14 Cherokee men as key informants and 12 Cherokee men and women as general informants	Ethnography	One semi-structured interview with each key informant. Observation of five key informants.	Themes of being true to oneself and being connected cut across three categories: being responsible, being disciplined, and being confident. The holistic world view of being connected to the Creator and interdependent with others was evident.
Mendelson (2002)	Described the health perceptions of Mexican-American women.	Purposive sample of 13 highly acculturated, English-speaking Mexican-American women ages 26 to 53 yr living in the southwest United States	Ethnography World Health Organization (WHO) definition of health	Two–three in-depth ethnographic interviews with each participant	Health perceptions were framed by participant's spirituality a and role as mother. Prayer and personal relationship with God had a powerful effect on health perceptions, although none found church central to religious beliefs. Relied on spirituality to maintain sense of emotional balance.
Pincharoen & Congdon (2003)	Described how spirituality helped older Thai persons maintain their health and what they valued most as they aged.	Purposive sample, using snowball approach, of nine Thai persons, ages 60–82 yr, from an urban U.S. community. Eight participants were Buddhist, recruited from a Thai Buddhist temple.	Ethnography	Two semi-structured interviews with each Thai participant, conducted in Thai language Observation at temple	Five themes emerged from the data: (1) connecting with spiritual resources for comfort and peace, (2) finding harmony through a healthy mind and body, (3) living a valuable life, (4) valuing tranquil relationship with family and friends, and (5) experiencing meaning and confidence in death. Participants used religion, sacred places, and persons to foster harmony of mind, body, and spirit.

(continued)

TABLE 18.1   Summary of Select Nursing Studies About Spirituality (continued)

Citation	Purpose	Sample	Design and Theoretical Framework	Variable Measures	Findings
Swinney, Anson-Wonkka, Maki, & Corneau (2001)	Described the health status of parishioners, identifying their health needs, risk factors, and perceived barriers to meeting those needs by performing a community assessment	421 surveys from parishioners, ages 7–90 yr, in a Catholic parish located in Massachusetts. Focus groups were also conducted.	Descriptive Healthy People 2000	Adapted questionnaire from National Parish Nurse Association Six focus group interviews	91% surveyed indicated that faith and spiritual beliefs play a role in maintaining health. 82% believed church should facilitate supportive relationships among members. 76% strongly believed that church has role in meeting health needs of parishioners. 31% turned to church for support and advice. Focus groups identified prayer and faith in God as factors that helped them remain healthy. Areas of health concerns included adolescents and elderly members, and respite care to assist caregivers. Most were supportive of parish nurse.
Thorpe & Barsky (2001)	Described how registered nurses use self-reflection to describe their need and potential for healing personally and professionally	Purposive sample of eight women, all who were registered nurses at rural and urban health care facilities in Canada	Ethnography Atkins & Murphy (1993) stages of reflection	One semi-structured interview with each participant	Three themes emerged from the data: (1) spirituality, (2) be-ing vs. do-ing, and (3) eustress vs. distress. Spirituality was defined as an inner guidance toward one's life purpose reflecting one's values and beliefs; however, spirituality also involved loss of dreams, regret, grieving, and desire for interconnectedness with others.

Vance (2001)	Examined acute care nurses' perceptions of how spirituality influences spiritual care delivery, and barriers to providing spiritual care.	Stratified random sample of 173 registered nurses, ages 20–69 yr, from a Midwestern community teaching hospital. Sample stratified on area of practice.	Descriptive, correlational, cross-sectional	Spiritual Well-Being Scale (SWBS) Spiritual Involvement and Beliefs Scale (SIBS) Spiritual Care Practice Questionnaire (SCP)	34.6% indicated that they provided spiritual care to patients at the ideal level. SWBS and SIBS scores were positively correlated with delivery of spiritual care (SCP Part I). Nurses' spirituality was not correlated with number of perceived barriers. Most common barriers were lack of time and insufficient education.
Woodard & Sowell (2001)	Described women's meaning and use of spiritual beliefs and activities in dealing with HIV/AIDS	Purposive sample of 21 women ages 24–74 yr infected with HIV, recruited from community agencies and HIV clinics in North Carolina	Grounded theory	One semi-structured interview with each participant	"God is in control" was the major theme to emerge, with four categories: (1) active faith, (2) God's presence, (3) benefits, and (4) partnership. Women engaged in praying, fasting, listening to Christian radio stations, reading the Bible, talking with God, and attending church. Women perceived modern medicine as adjunctive therapy to relationship with God.

them and that having a relationship with God forms a foundation for psychological well-being (Mackenzie et al., 2000). Burkhardt (1994) also described the spiritual development of healthy women. Other studies have found that self-transcendence is a predictor of mental health in older adults (Reed, 1986a, 1989, 1991b; Young and Reed, 1995). Another study demonstrated a positive relationship between self-transcendence and emotional well-being in middle-aged adults (Coward, 1996).

Ellermann and Reed (2001) sought to build on this knowledge in a correlational study examining the relationship of self-transcendence to depression in middle-aged adults. They selected middle-aged adults because little in the literature had been done with this age group. They obtained a convenience sample of healthy adults (n = 133) from a shopping mall in a southwest city. The number of men and women, whose ages ranged from 25 to 64 years, was nearly equal. The researchers compared scores received on the STS with scores received on the Center for Epidemiological Studies-Depression Scale (CES-D). They also compared self-transcendence variables measuring parenting, acceptance, and spirituality (as measured by the single-item question "How spiritual do you believe you are?") with CES-D scores. The researchers made comparisons for the total group, as well as for subgroups of young middle-aged adults (25 to 44 years) and older middle-aged adults (45 to 64 years). Ellermann and Reed found that in the total group and younger group, higher scores of self-transcendence were associated with lower levels of depression. No significant correlation appeared between spirituality and depression in any groups; however, spirituality was significantly correlated with self-transcendence in the total and young groups. The researchers also found that self-transcendence and acceptance explained significant variance in the total group. An incidental finding was that men and women differed. For women, spirituality and parenting were less of a resource for mental health.

Spirituality, Health, and Adults with Chronic or Terminal Illness

In nursing, one of the most researched areas of spirituality involves adults with chronic illness or at the end of life. Spirituality has emerged as a significant aspect in people with cancer (Coward, 1990, 1991, 1997; Messias, Yeager, Dibble, & Dodd, 1997; Taylor, 1993, 1995) and human immunodeficiency virus (HIV) (Coward & Lewis, 1993; Hall, 1994; Sowell, Moneyham, & Aranda-Naranjo, 1999). Hope and spirituality have been linked with positive mental health outcomes in elderly people with cancer (Fehring, Miller, & Shaw, 1997) and terminally ill adults (Hall, 1990). Studies involving people with HIV/AIDS also have shown that spiritual activities are a resource (Sowell et al., 1997, 2000) and that transcendence is an important aspect of healing (Coward, 1995; Coward & Lewis; Hall, 1998). It has been noted that terminally ill patients can have moderately high levels of well-being (Reed, 1986b) and that well-being may be positively related to spiritual perspective (Reed, 1987). Hospitalized terminally ill patients, when compared with nonterminally ill hospitalized patients, have a higher preference for direct, spiritually related nursing interventions (Reed, 1991a).

Halstead and Hull (2001) noted that with all the research involving spiritual development in women with cancer, no theory described the process of spiritual development during the cancer experience. Using grounded theory, these researchers aimed to fill this gap in knowledge by interviewing 10 women with cancer. These women, 45 to 70 years, had diagnoses of breast or ovarian cancer or non-Hodgkin's lymphoma. They were interviewed twice using semistructured interview guides that included questions such as, "What does the term *spirituality* mean to you?" and "What are some of the experiences that have shaped your spirituality?" The major theme to emerge from the data was Struggling with Paradoxes. Spiritually, the women struggled with the paradox that their meaningful belief system was being challenged by their diagnosis. Struggling with Paradoxes involves three phases: deciphering the meaning of cancer for me, realizing human limitations, and learning to live with uncertainty.

During the first phase, deciphering the meaning of cancer for me, the distress women experienced about their diagnosis affected their spirituality. Women attempted to maintain coherence by using both old and new ways. To resolve the struggles in this phase, women looked to their faith, even if their faith did not immediately bring them comfort. They reported receiving spiritual assurances from within, even though they could not explain the source of these assurances. Women attempted to remain connected to God, themselves, and others, relying on old ways, such as prayer and discussions with family. Attending support groups and healing services at church or temple became new strategies they used to maintain coherence.

Realizing human limitations, phase II, women turned to God. Some women reported struggling with faith and doubt, wondering how God could have let this happen. During this phase, connectedness became a necessity, and they enlisted help from God. Interestingly, the authors reported "that although spiritual concerns were very evident in this phase of the experience, spiritual care from a professional, such as a chaplain or clergy, was not offered to 8 of the 10 women" (Halstead & Hull, 2001, p. 1539). Although some patients described experiences in which nurses were unconcerned about or too busy to offer spiritual care and reassurances, other women indicated they found caregivers comfortable with providing spiritual care and were grateful for the assistance provided. Because women began to realize that there were no easy answers to their questions, they began to let go of their need for answers. Through reflection, support groups, prayer, and reading scripture, women were able to transition to the next phase.

In the final phase, learning to live with uncertainty, one dimension that emerged was identifying spiritual growth (Halstead & Hull, 2001). Women identified five benchmarks to arriving at their new self-defined spirituality: enhanced appreciation of life nourished their spirits; growth involved connecting with others; increased faith and trust evolved over time; growing in spiritual assurances; and prioritizing spirituality.

The researchers concluded that the women's descriptions of their spiritual experience were developmental in nature, but not necessarily age-related (Halstead & Hull, 2001). Although holding different perspectives of spirituality, the women described similar spiritual processes in response to their diagnosis.

✚ In another study of patients with cancer, Johnson (2002) described patients' perceptions about the use of humor as an element of spiritual coping. Building on the literature about healing and humor, Johnson sought to describe how nine women with breast cancer used humor to cope with their diagnosis, treatment, and life after cancer. All women were considered survivors, in that 1 year or more had passed since they completed treatment. All mothers, the women ranged in age from 41 to 48 years. All women were Christian; eight were Caucasian, and one was African-American. Three categories were identified: humor and coping; humor and nurses; and humor and spirituality. Although all the women individually defined spirituality, they looked for meaning in their lives through spirituality and humor. There were five related themes for the category of humor and spirituality. First, some women felt that "humor helped them laugh at themselves and life." Taking life less seriously helped to change their outlook. Second, some women noted, "God has a sense of humor."

Women also used humor and spirituality to "understand [themselves] better" and recognized that "humor is a step to recovery." Finally, women identified that they "want to help others" and used humor to help their families cope. Although the author noted that it was difficult to determine how humor influenced spirituality, she concluded that nurses need additional education to recognize that spirituality is an integral part of coping for breast cancer survivors.

There have been concerns raised that a strong reliance on God may make individuals, particularly African-American women (Bourjolly, 1998), less likely to seek screening and treatment (Pargament et al., 1998). Kinney and colleagues (2002) studied the relationship between beliefs about God as a controlling force in health and adherence to breast cancer screening by African-American women at high risk for breast cancer. Women (n = 52) with a breast cancer susceptibility gene 1 (BRCA1) mutation associated with increased risk for breast and ovarian cancer were surveyed either in person or over the telephone regarding their adherence to breast cancer screening recommendations based on their age. The women were residents of Louisiana; their ages ranged from 18 to 78 years; the majority (92%) had completed high school; and 42% indicated they were married. Most (69%) were Catholic, and 50% of the women indicated they attended church regularly. Women completed the God Locus of Health Control Scale (GLHCS) containing six items measuring the extent of belief that God exerts control over one's health state. They also completed the Intrusion Subscale of the Impact of Event Scale (IES) to measure cancer-specific distress. There was no significant relationship between the GLHCS score and adherence to screening recommendations in the entire sample. However, when looking at the women 25 years and older, the GLHCS was significantly correlated with adherence to the cancer breast examination and mammography, but not with self-breast examination. For the whole sample, the GLHCS was negatively correlated with age and positively correlated with marital status, although there were no significant correlations with hopelessness about cancer, religious affiliation, education, or cancer-specific distress. The presence of a primary care provider was associated with overall screening adherence, although not with breast self-examination. The researchers noted that overall the rate of adherence was low, and 100% of the women without a primary care provider reported they were not adhering to recommended screening guidelines. The researchers concluded their findings were consistent with the transactional model of stress and coping. They suggested that communication interventions used by nurses to assess spirituality and beliefs in God may have an important role in increasing cancer screening in African-American women and that additional investigation was needed.

Belief in God as a controlling force of health was central in another study involving women with HIV infection. To describe the meaning and use of spiritual beliefs and practices of women with HIV, Woodard and Sowell (2001) interviewed 21 women, ages 24 to 74 years, living in North Carolina. A semistructured interview began by asking women, "What is spirituality and what does it mean to you?" Although all the women did not have a religious affiliation, in general they all based their spirituality in a Judeo-Christian God. "God in Control," the major theme to emerge from the qualitative analysis, was the perception of the majority of the women. They believed God was in control for both majestic matters, such as healing, and mundane matters, such as getting a ride to the clinic. Women expressed that God's influence in their lives allowed them to deal with having HIV/AIDS. "God in control" had four categories: active faith, God's presence, partnership, and benefits. Praying, fasting, attending church, listening to Christian radio stations, reading the Bible, or talking with God were ways women demonstrated active faith. Through active faith, women developed daily spiritual rituals and engaged God to help them deal with life issues. God's presence was described as a living presence with whom they spoke. Although most women spoke of God's presence in a positive manner, three women expressed anger at God for their illness while acknowledging God's presence. Women described the relationship they had with God as a partnership and indicated there was a partnership between God and health care providers. They viewed physicians and medicines as serving God's purposes, and medical care was viewed as adjunctive therapy to their spiritual beliefs. Although these women had a high degree of belief in God in control, "most women believed that not taking medicine and waiting for divine healing was 'stupid'" (Woodard & Sowell, p. 243). Women also described partnerships with individuals with whom they could confide their feelings. Women perceived many benefits, such as peace, happiness, and reduced stress, from having an active spiritual life. An incidental, but important, finding was that most women worshiped in isolation because the stigma associated with HIV did "not stop at the church door" (Woodard & Sowell, p. 246), and the authors suggested that health care providers collaborate with congregations to educate individuals about HIV/AIDS. The women also revealed they believed health care providers should discuss spirituality with patients.

Spirituality, Health, and Individuals of Diverse Cultures or Faiths

Because diversity in the United States is increasing, the number of nursing studies focusing on the meanings of health and illness to people of different cultures also is increasing. As discussed in Unit II, culture and spirituality are related, so it is not surprising to find nursing studies describing both culture and spirituality. Although some of these studies specifically aim to describe spiritual beliefs of people of a particular culture, other studies uncover findings about spirituality that were not necessarily explicit in their purpose.

⬤ In an ethnographic study, Pincharoen and Congdon (2003) described spirituality as experienced by older Thai people living in the United States, focusing on how spirituality helped them maintain health and to describe what they valued most as they aged. Describing spirituality for Thai people is important because spirituality, based on religious and supernatural beliefs, is part of their daily lives. Older Thai people, 90% of whom identify themselves as Buddhist, view later life as a time to visit temple, meditate, and calm the mind. Using participant observation, one researcher visited the Buddhist temple frequently and participated in cultural activities, thereby establishing trust within the Thai Buddhist community. Using purposive sampling, nine Thai people, 60 to 82 years of age, living in an urban community were interviewed. Eight of the participants identified themselves as Buddhist, and the other participant acknowledged being Christian. They had lived in the United States from 8 to 30 years. The researchers defined spirituality as internal beliefs and what people valued most in life, based on definitions by Burkhardt and Nagai-Jacobson (2002). Because words such as "spirit" and "spirituality" in the Thai culture refer to ghosts or souls in the afterlife, the researcher avoided using these words in the semistructured interview. The interview included open-ended questions such as "Describe how you keep healthy as you age" and "Describe what is most important to you in your life at this time." Five major themes were identified: connecting with spiritual resources provided comfort and peace; finding harmony through a healthy mind and body; living a valuable life; valuing tranquil relationships with family and friends; and experiencing meaning and confidence in death. For these older Thai persons, connecting with spiritual resources included seeking religious resources, maintaining religious beliefs, and practicing religious activities and accumulating religious merit. Attending temple, practicing rituals, reading Buddhist teachings, and meditating were all activities that provided connections. Finding harmony through a healthy mind and body involved having a healthy body to complete their activities of daily living, thus leading to a healthy mind. Letting go of anger and conflicts, sustaining a body free of disease and disability, and continuing with favorite activities contributed to finding harmony. Living a valuable life was determined as participants used self-reflection to examine the past, finding meaning in their struggles and successes. Contributions to society, such as volunteering, provided participants with a sense of feeling valued and productive. By valuing tranquil relationships with family and friends, these participants hoped for a good future for their children, desired respect from their grandchildren, and preserved social relationships with friends. Viewing death as a normal part of life, participants experienced meaning and confidence in death by using their religious resources and faith. Participants reported preparing for death by accepting death as a last stage in life, but desiring a comfortable death, free of pain and discomfort. Because of their Buddhist faith, they hoped for a positive reincarnation and good destiny in their next existence. The authors concluded that for these participants, spirituality and health were integrated, coexisting in all of life, and should not be separated in health care.

Another study demonstrating the link between spirituality and health described the health perceptions of Mexican-American women (Mendelson, 2002). Because the author used the World Health Organization (WHO) definition of health as a "state of complete physical, mental, and social well-being and not merely absence of disease and infirmity" (WHO, 1978, p. 2), it is significant that spirituality emerged as a finding because spirituality is not explicit in the definition. Using ethnography, the researcher interviewed 13 Mexican-American women, ages 26 to 53 years. Although all the highly acculturated women resided permanently in the United States, three had been born in Mexico and another, born in the United States, resided in Mexico as a child. All the participants were mothers. The researchers found that "the women's stories and experiences of health perceptions arose from the context of their households and were framed by their spirituality and their experiences as children, as mothers, and as partners" (Mendelson, p. 213). Spirituality formed the frame for the women's perceptions, as they indicated that their spirituality developed over time to result in a meaningful, personal relationship with God. Many of the women incorporated their spiritual beliefs into their daily routine; however, none found church central to their religious beliefs. Generally, participants perceived health as a combination of good physical health, sound mental health, and a socially and spiritually satisfying life that exceeded the sum of these components. Health, based in relationships with family and supported by their spirituality, transcended illness. Although illness was grounded in the body, resulting in an inability to fulfill functional roles, health transcended the body as an integrated holistic experience. Participants described emotional balance as an essential component of health. Imbalance occurred when emotional and social dimensions were in turmoil, leaving women vulnerable to the development of physical ailments. Women provided three explanations for the interaction between physical and mental health: mental or emotional stress caused stress-related illness (i.e., headache); physical ailment was an indication to look deeper into life and find the problem; and mental stress caused physical deterioration until the body reached a breaking point, resulting in illness. Women reported that the power of their spirituality contributed toward maintaining or restoring emotional balance through a relationship built on prayerful dialogue with God, the Virgin of Guadalupe, and St. Francis.

⬤ For Cherokee men, spirituality is embedded in the concept of **self-reliance** (Lowe, 2002). Self-reliance, identified as the mainstay of Cherokee culture, is a way of life that influences health and helps to keep the Cherokee in balance. Lowe used ethnography to study Cherokee conceptualizations of self-reliance and how adult Cherokee men perceive, achieve, and demonstrate self-reliance. A group of male and female general informants (n = 12) were interviewed about their definition of self-reliance. The key informants (n = 14) were adult Cherokee men who had been identified by at least two general informants as being self-reliant. In-depth interviews were conducted with all the key informants, and participant observation was used with five informants to observe them during their normal daily routines. Two major themes emerged from the data. Being true to oneself, the first theme, referred to acknowledging one's heritage as Cherokee and living by the Cherokee world view. This holistic, circular world view believes that all of creation has spirit that is connected to the Creator. Maintaining balance within creation is the primary purpose for Cherokee people. The second theme, being connected, views each person as a resource within the creation who possesses gifts and talents that benefit the family, community, and tribe.

Three categories embedded in the two major themes provide meaning to Cherokee self-reliance: being responsible, being disciplined, and being confident. Being responsible concerns caring for self and others and emphasizes the interdependency of family, community, tribe, and Creator. Getting help, doing good work, being connected to others, using resources wisely, and honoring traditional ceremonies are ways Cherokee men are responsible. Being disciplined involves setting and pursuing goals, and it is acceptable that some risk for failure may be involved. When men are not disciplined, their ability to contribute to family, community, and tribe is lessened because others will then make the decisions. Being confident means having a sense of identity and self-worth, being proud of the Cherokee heritage, beliefs, and values. The Creator intends that everyone belong in the group, thereby knowing acceptance and developing self-confidence. Men are connected to the group by their gifts and talents. In general, self-reliance involves interdependence with all creation. Self-reliance is a balance of independence and interdependence, and being a part of the family, community, and tribe are valued more than the individual self. Because common health problems of Cherokee men, such as substance abuse and suicide, stem from being disconnected and independent, Lowe (2002) concluded that nurses need to assess for interdependence when caring for Cherokee clients.

✝ In another study involving Catholics in a Massachusetts parish, Swinney, Anson-Wonkka, Maki, and Corneau (2001) surveyed individuals to determine the health status of parishioners and identify the parishioners' perceived health needs and perceived barriers to meet those needs. This community assessment was initiated to assist the church in developing a health ministry in their faith community. The researchers, in conjunction with the parish health council, developed a 21-item health questionnaire that was distributed at all masses during a single weekend. Of the 800 questionnaires available, 421 surveys were returned by individuals ages 7 to 90 years. Although 34% of the parishioners indicated that they had a health problem, the majority (93%) of them indicated they were generally in good physical health. Of those surveyed, 88% indicated that they were nonsmokers, and 58% indicated they did not consume alcoholic beverages. Some (21%) respondents indicated there were members of the church who were not receiving the care they needed for their health problems. Parishioners indicated that they were aware of someone experiencing spousal abuse (7%) or child abuse (4%). When asked about the relationship between spirituality and health, 91% of the respondents indicated that faith and spiritual beliefs play a role in maintaining health and well-being, 82% believed that the church should facilitate supportive relationships among parishioners, and 76% strongly believed that the church has a role in meeting the health needs of members. Similar findings were obtained during the six focus groups, composed of 4 to 17 church members, conducted by the researchers. During the focus groups, comments indicated that prayer and faith in God helped individuals remain healthy. Focus group members were especially concerned about adolescent members (i.e., particularly risk-taking behaviors, alcohol consumption, peer pressure, and low self-esteem) and elderly members (i.e., lack of transportation, finances, extended care, medication information). Participants in the focus groups identified starting a network that could coordinate child care, deliver meals to home-bound members, visit families in crisis, provide respite care, and meet transportation needs as a strategy for improving the health of parishioners. The researchers concluded that the health needs of this faith community were comparable to the goals of Healthy People 2000.

Spirituality, Health, and Professional Nurses

Studies have been conducted with nurses and other health care professionals to describe their knowledge, attitudes, and beliefs about spirituality and health. For instance, nurses with higher scores on the Spiritual Orientation Inventory (SOI) are more likely to care for patients with AIDS and have less anxiety about death (Sherman, 1996). As described in Chapter 1, studies involving spiritual care also have been conducted.

In a descriptive, correlational study, Vance (2001) studied how nurses' attitudes toward spirituality influenced spiritual care delivery and their perceptions of barriers to providing spiritual care. A random sample of registered nurses, stratified by specialty area of practice and employed at a hospital in a large Midwestern city, participated in this study. The SWBS, the SIBS, and the SCP were mailed to 425 nurses, and 173 nurses returned the surveys. Most nurses were white (94.2%), Christian (88.4%), and female (89.6%). Vance reported that, although the nurses responding to the survey perceived themselves as highly spiritual, only 34.6% (n = 60) indicated that they provided spiritual support to their patients at or above an ideal level. Nurses with higher measures of spirituality (SWBS and SIBS) scored significantly higher in their spiritual care practices than did nurses with lower spirituality scores; however, nurses with higher measures of spirituality and nurses with lower measures of spirituality identified the same barriers. Nurses who scored higher on assessment and intervention for spiritual care identified significantly fewer barriers than did nurses with lower assessment and intervention scores. There were no significant correlations with the key measures and education, years of experience, or attendance at a religiously affiliated nursing school; however, nurses practicing in women's health scored significantly lower on delivery of spiritual care than did nurses in other areas. The five most frequently identified barriers to providing spiritual care were insufficient time (82.9%), insufficient education (64.9%), patient privacy (45.5%), lack of confidence of the nurse (35.1%), and difference in spirituality between the patient and nurse (34.7%). The author concluded that continuing education for nurses regarding spirituality may be beneficial for increasing the delivery of spiritual care.

Thorpe and Barsky (2001) applied a reflective-thinking model to explain to what extent and in what ways nurses use self-reflection to describe their need and potential for personal and professional healing. Self-reflection, according to the model, involves awareness, critical analysis, and developing a new perspective. Using purposive sampling, the researchers interviewed eight Canadian registered nurses, working as staff nurses, managers, and administrators. All were women, and they worked in both community and hospital settings and had various educational degrees. From qualitative analysis of in-depth interviews, three themes emerged: spirituality; be-ing versus do-ing; and eustress versus distress. The nurses expressed awareness about how values provided inner guidance toward one's life purpose. A new perspective of their spirituality emerged from their critical analysis of personal and professional experiences. Be-ing versus do-ing, the tension between meeting the needs of self and meeting the needs of others, was a struggle for these women as they reflected on life. They acknowledged feelings of discomfort as they tried to balance their roles, and through critical analysis the nurses were able to set priorities. Through self-reflection, the women were able to change their perspective and move from self-sacrificing behaviors related to perfectionism to a perspective that acknowledged self-worth and self-caring. The nurses were aware of both positive stress (eustress) and negative stress (distress) in their professional and personal lives. Through critical analysis, some were able to temporarily remove themselves from stressful work situations to gain new perspectives of their situations. Many used self-reflection to find a balance between eustress and distress. The researchers suggested that as nurses reflected on professional and personal experiences, they were able to identify the need for change so that healing could occur.

DIRECTIONS FOR FUTURE RESEARCH

Although nursing research has contributed significantly toward an understanding of the connections between spirituality and health, many questions remain unanswered. Much more research could be done to articulate the influence of spirituality on health and well-being. The inclusion of adolescents and children in studies would contribute significantly to an understanding of spirituality and health across the lifespan. In addition, expanding the focus of research to include patients with chronic illnesses other than cancer and HIV/AIDS is indicated. Work also can continue on refining measurement of complex concepts such as spirituality and transcendence. Using nursing theories to guide studies is imperative for building nursing knowledge. Building on the foundations of previous studies, continued research with people of different cultural or faith communities can serve not only to describe belief patterns, but also to perhaps cultivate tolerance in health care providers overwhelmed by the diversity of the population they serve. Although it is clear that people use spiritual practices to promote health or healing from illness, intervention studies to test the effects of such practices would likely be a next step. Because the provision of spiritual care involves collaboration among various disciplines (see Chapter 16), interdisciplinary research is needed. Researchers must involve those in clinical practice to identify and test strategies for overcoming barriers to providing spiritual care.

Basing nursing practice on knowledge generated from research is important for providing excellent patient care. The *Code of Ethics for Nurses* (American Nurses Association, 2001) asserts that nurses have a duty to respect the uniqueness of each patient. Nurses are also obligated to continue professional growth and advance the profession through knowledge development, dissemination, and application to practice.

It is reasonable for nurses to explore spirituality and health through research in an effort to maintain an ethical and holistic perspective when practicing nursing. Conducting future research to increase understanding of the complexity of spirituality and its relationship with health and using those findings are important ways to improve spiritual care in nursing.

PERSONAL REFLECTIONS

- Are you surprised by any of the findings from the research studies described in this chapter? Why or why not?
- How do your beliefs in God influence your health behaviors?
- What nursing research findings could you include when caring for your next client?
- Are the barriers to providing spiritual care that you encounter a symptom of your discomfort with providing spiritual care? What can you do to become more comfortable in providing spirituality care?
- What areas of spirituality and health would you like to learn more about? If you were going to do research, what would you study?

CASE STUDY 18.1

Ronnie, a nurse on an oncology unit, is caring for Ling-Chu, a 75-year-old Thai woman with breast cancer. Ling-Chu is undergoing chemotherapy and has been hospitalized for anemia and bleeding. She has lived in the United States for nearly 55 years. She is widowed and lives with Lyn, her only daughter, who has been present throughout most of the hospitalization. Her son-in-law and grandchildren visit regularly.

Ronnie notices that Ling-Chu is agitated after a visit by her adolescent grandchild. When Ronnie probes deeper, Ling-Chu states that she wishes that young people would have respect for the elderly. Ling-Chu also reveals that she misses the tranquility that comes from visiting her Buddhist temple. Later, in confidence, Lyn expresses to Ronnie that her mother's statements about being at peace with death upset her. Lyn is also upset because sometimes her mother makes jokes about chemotherapy side effects.

Critical Thinking
- What kind of horizontal and vertical relationships do older Thai adults value in later life?
- Are Ling-Chu's behaviors typical?
- What could the nurse do to address Ling-Chu's spiritual needs?
- What could the nurse do to support the family throughout this hospitalization?
- What barriers might get in the way of the nurse providing spiritual care to Ling-Chu and her family?

Key Points

- Spirituality, although universal, is experienced in a unique manner.
- Research about spirituality and health is relevant for the discipline of nursing.
- Nurse researchers use both quantitative and qualitative methods to study spirituality and health.
- There are a variety of instruments to measure spirituality available for nurse researchers.
- Many nursing theories include aspects of spirituality, and these theories can be used to guide nursing research.
- Transcendence is a relevant concept in nursing research involving spirituality and health.
- Many individuals believe that health and well-being are linked with spirituality.
- The horizontal and vertical dimensions of spirituality are evident in research findings.
- Many individuals use a variety of spiritual practices to promote health and healing during illness.
- Some individuals believe that communities of faith, in addition to addressing spiritual needs, have a role in addressing the physical and mental needs of members.
- Although some individuals have indicated that they desire spiritual care, there are barriers that prevent nurses and other health care providers from providing ideal spiritual care.
- There are many areas for additional nursing and interdisciplinary research about spirituality and health.

References

American Nurses Association. (2001). *Code of ethics for nurses with interpretive statements*. Washington, DC: Author.

Bourjolly, J. N. (1998). Differences in religiousness among black and white women with breast cancer. *Social Work in Health Care, 28*(1), 21–39.

Burkhardt, M. (1994). Becoming and connecting: Elements of spirituality for women. *Holistic Nursing Practice, 8*(4), 12–21.

Burkhardt, M. A., & Nagai-Jacobson, M. G. (2002). *Spirituality: Living our connectedness*. New York: Delmar.

Coward, D. D. (1990). The lived experience of self-transcendence in women with advanced breast cancer. *Nursing Science Quarterly, 3*(4), 162–169.

Coward, D. D. (1991). Self-transcendence and emotional well-being in women with advanced breast cancer. *Oncology Nursing Forum, 18*, 857–863.

Coward, D. D. (1995). The lived experience of self-transcendence in women with AIDS. *JOGNN, 24*, 314–318.

Coward, D. D. (1996). Self-transcendence and correlates in a healthy population. *Nursing Research, 45*, 116–121.

Coward, D. D. (1997). Constructing meaning from the experience of cancer. *Seminars in Oncology Nursing, 13*, 248–251.

Coward, D. D., & Lewis, F. (1993). The lived experience of self-transcendence in gay men with AIDS. *Oncology Nursing Forum, 20*, 1363–1369.

Coward, D. D., & Reed, P. G. (1996). Self-transcendence: A source of healing at the end of life. *Issues in Mental Health Nursing, 17*, 275–288.

Ellerhorst-Ryan, J. M. (1997). Instruments to measure aspects of spirituality. In M. Frank-Stromborg & S. J. Olsen (Eds.), *Instruments for clinical health-care research* (2nd ed.) (pp. 202–212.). Sudbury, MA: Jones & Bartlett.

Ellermann, C. R., & Reed, P. G. (2001). Self-transcendence and depression in middle-aged adults. *Western Journal of Nursing Research, 23,* 698–713.

Fehring, R., Miller, J., & Shaw, C. (1997). Spiritual well-being, religiosity, hope, depression and other mood states in elderly people coping with cancer. *Oncology Nursing Forum, 24,* 663–671.

Flannelly, L. T., Flannelly, K. J., & Weaver, A. J. (2002). Religious and spiritual variables in three major oncology nursing journals: 1990–1999. *Oncology Nursing Forum, 29,* 679–685.

Glaser, B. G., & Strauss, A. L. (1967). *The discovery of grounded theory: Strategies for qualitative research.* Hawthorne, NY: Aldine.

Hall, B. A. (1990). The struggle of the diagnosed terminally ill person to maintain hope. *Nursing Science Quarterly, 3,* 177–184.

Hall, B. A. (1994). Ways of maintaining hope in HIV disease. *Research in Nursing and Health, 17,* 283–293.

Hall, B. A. (1998). Patterns of spirituality in persons with advanced HIV disease. *Research in Nursing and Health, 21,* 145–153.

Halstead, M. T., & Hull, M. (2001). Struggling with paradoxes: The process of spiritual development in women with cancer. *Oncology Nursing Forum, 28,* 1534–1544.

Hatch, R. L., Burg, M. A., Naberhause, D. S., & Hellmich, L. K. (1998). The spiritual involvement and beliefs scale: Development and testing of a new instrument. *The Journal of Family Practice, 46,* 476–486.

Highfield, M. F. (1992). Spiritual health of oncology patients. *Cancer Nursing, 15*(1), 1.

Johnson, P. (2002). The use of humor and its influences on spirituality and coping in breast cancer survivors. *Oncology Nursing Forum, 29,* 691–695.

Kinney, A. Y, Emery, G., Dudley, W. N., & Croyle, R. T. (2002). Screening behaviors among African American women at high risk for breast cancer: Do beliefs about God matter? *Oncology Nursing Forum, 29,* 835–843.

Leininger, M. M. (1991). *Culture care diversity and universality: A theory of nursing.* New York: National League for Nursing.

Lowe, J. (2002). Cherokee self-reliance. *Journal of Transcultural Nursing, 13,* 287–295.

Mackenzie, E. R., Rajagopal, D. E., Meilbohm, M., & Lavizzo-Mourey, R. (2000). Spiritual support and psychological well-being: Older adults' perceptions of religion and health connection. *Alternative Therapies in Health and Medicine, 6*(6), 37–45.

Malinski, V. M. (1994). Spirituality: A pattern manifestation of human-environment mutual process. *Visions: The Journal of Rogerian Nursing Science, 2,* 12–18.

Malinski, V. M. (2002). Developing a nursing perspective on spirituality and healing. *Nursing Science Quarterly, 15,* 281–287.

Mendelson, C. (2002). Health perceptions of Mexican American women. *Journal of Transcultural Nursing, 13,* 210–217.

Messias, D., Yeager, K., Dibble, S., & Dodd, M. (1997). Patients' perceptions of fatigue while undergoing chemotherapy. *Oncology Nursing Forum, 24,* 43–50.

Neuman, B. (1995). *The Neuman systems model* (3rd ed.). Norwalk, CT: Appleton & Lange.

Newman, M. A. (1994). *Health as expanding consciousness* (2nd ed.). New York: National League for Nursing.

Nightingale, F. (1969). *Notes on nursing: What it is and what it is not.* New York: Dover. (Original work published 1860).

Orem, D. (2001). *Nursing: Concepts of practice* (6th ed.). St. Louis: Mosby.

Paloutzian, R., & Ellison, C. W. (1982). Loneliness, spiritual well-being, and the quality of life. In A. Peplau & D. Perlman (Eds.), *Loneliness: A sourcebook of current theory, research, and therapy* (pp. 224–237). New York: Wiley.

Pargament, K. I., Kennell, J., Hathawary, W., Grevengoed, N., Newman, J., & Jones, W. (1998). Religion and the problem-solving process: Three styles of coping. *Journal for the Scientific Study of Religion, 27,* 90–104.

Parse, R. R. (1981). *Man-living-health: A theory of nursing.* New York: Wiley.

Parse, R. R. (Ed.) (1995). *Illuminations: The human becoming theory in practice and research.* New York: National League for Nursing Press.

Pincharoen, S., & Congdon, J. G. (2003). Spirituality and health in older Thai persons in the United States. *Western Journal of Nursing Research, 25,* 93–108.

Reed, P. G. (1986a). Developmental resources and depression in the elderly. *Nursing Research, 35,* 368–374.

Reed, P. G. (1986b). Religiousness among terminally ill and healthy adults. *Research in Nursing and Health, 9,* 35–41.

Reed, P. G. (1987). Spirituality and well-being in terminally ill and healthy adults. *Research in Nursing and Health, 10,* 335–344.

Reed, P. G. (1989). Mental health of older adults. *Western Journal of Nursing Research, 11,* 143–163.

Reed, P. G. (1991a). Preferences for spiritually related nursing interventions among terminally ill and nonterminally ill hospitalized adults and well adults. *Applied Nursing Research, 4*(3), 122–128.

Reed, P. G. (1991b). Self-transcendence and mental health in oldest-old adults. *Nursing Research, 40,* 5–11.

Reed, P. G. (1991c). Toward a theory of self-transcendence: Deductive reformulation using developmental theories. *Advances in Nursing Science, 13*(4), 64–77.

Reed, P. G. (1992). An emerging paradigm for the investigation of spirituality in nursing. *Research in Nursing and Health, 15,* 349–357.

Rogers, M. E. (1992). Nursing science and the space age. *Nursing Science Quarterly, 5,* 27–34.

Roy, C., & Andrews, H. A. (1999). *The Roy adaptation model* (2nd ed.). Stamford, CT: Appleton & Lange.

Sherman, D. W. (1996). Nurses' willingness to care for AIDS patients and spirituality, social support, and death anxiety. *Image: Journal of Nursing Scholarship, 28,* 205–213.

Smith, D. W. (1994). Toward developing a theory of spirituality. *Visions: The Journal of Rogerian Nursing Science, 2,* 35–43.

Sowell, R. L., Moneyham, L., & Aranda-Naranjo, B. (1999). The care of women with AIDS: Special needs and considerations. *Nursing Clinics of North America, 34*(1), 179–199.

Sowell, R. L., Moneyham, L., Guillory, J., Seals, B., Cohen, L., & Demi, A. (1997). Self-care activities of women infected with human immunodeficiency virus. *Holistic Nursing Practice, 11,* 18–26.

Sowell, R. L., Moneyham, L., Hennessy, M., Guillory, J., Demi, A., & Seals, B. (2000). Spiritual activities as a resistance resource for women with human immunodeficiency virus. *Nursing Research, 49*(2), 73–82.

Swinney, J., Anson-Wonkka, C., Maki, E., & Corneau, J. (2001). Community assessment: A church community and the parish nurse. *Public Health Nursing, 18,* 40–44.

Taylor, E. J. (1993). Factors associated with meaning in life among people with recurrent cancer. *Oncology Nursing Forum, 20,* 1399–1405.

Taylor, E. J. (1995). Whys and wherefores: Adult patient perspectives of the meaning of cancer. *Seminars in Oncology Nursing, 11,* 32–40.

Thorpe, K., & Barsky, J. (2001). Healing through self-reflection. *Journal of Advanced Nursing, 35,* 760–768.

Vance, D. L. (2001). Nurses' attitudes towards spirituality and patient care. *MEDSURG Nursing, 10,* 264–268, 278.

Wallston, K. A., Malcarne, V. L., Flores, L., Hansdottir, I., Smith C. A., & Stein, M. J. (1999). Does God determine your health? The God focus of health control scale. *Cognitive Therapy and Research, 23,* 131–142.

Watson, J. (1999). *Postmodern nursing and beyond.* New York: Churchill Livingstone.

Weaver, A. J., Flannelly, L. T., & Flannelly, K. J. (2001). A review of research on religious and spiritual variables in two primary gerontological nursing journals: 1991–1997. *Journal of Gerontological Nursing, 27*(9), 47–54.

Woodard, E. K., & Sowell, R. (2001). God in control: Women's perspectives on managing HIV infection. *Clinical Nursing Research, 10,* 233–250.

World Health Organization (WHO). (1978). *Alma Ata 1978 primary health care: Report of the International Conference on Primary Health Care, Alma Ata, USSR.* Geneva, Switzerland: Author.

Young, C. A., & Reed, P. G. (1995). Elders' perceptions of the role of group psychotherapy in fostering self-transcendence. *Archives of Psychiatric Nursing, 9,* 338–347.

Recommended Readings

Cooper-Effa, M., Blount, W., Kaslow, N., Rothenberg, R., & Eckman, J. (2001). Role of spirituality in patients with sickle cell disease. *The Journal of the American Board of Family Practice, 14,* 116–122.

Coyle, J. (2002). Spirituality and health: Towards a framework for exploring the relationship between spirituality and health. *Journal of Advanced Nursing, 37,* 589–597.

Dossey, L. (1993). *Healing words: The power of prayer and the practice of medicine.* San Francisco: Harper.

Ellis, M., Campbell, J., Detwiler-Breidenbach, A., & Hubbard, D. K. (2002). What do family physicians think about spirituality in clinical practice? *The Journal of Family Practice, 51,* 249–254.

Hall, B. A. (1997). Spirituality in terminal illness: An alternative view of theory. *Journal of Holistic Nursing, Healthy People 2010.* Available at: http://www.health.gov/healthypeople.

International Center for the Integration of Health and Spirituality, www.icihs.org.

Matthews, D. A., Marlowe, S. M., & Macnutt, F. S. (2000). Effects of intercessory prayer on patients with rheumatoid arthritis. *Southern Medical Journal, 93,* 1177–1186.

Morris, E. L. (2001). The relationship of spirituality to coronary artery disease. *Alternative Therapies, 7,* 96–98.

Newman, J. A., & Reed, B. J. (1998). Mexican-American males with a spinal cord injury. *SCI Psychosocial Process, 11*(1), 14–19.

Pargament, K. I. (1997). *The psychology of religion and coping: Theory, practice, and research.* New York: Guilford.

Pendleton, S. M., Cavalli, K. S., Pargament, K. I, & Nasr, S. Z. (2002). Religious/spiritual coping in childhood cystic fibrosis: A qualitative study. *Pediatrics, 109,* E8.

Plante, T. G., Saucedo, B., & Rice, C. (2001). The association between strength of religious faith and coping with daily stress. *Pastoral Psychology, 49,* 291–300.

Reed, P. G. (1998). A holistic view of nursing concepts and theories in practice. *Journal of Holistic Nursing, 16,* 415–419.

Tanyi, R. A. (2002). Towards a clarification of the meaning of spirituality. *Journal of Advanced Nursing, 39,* 500–509.

Resources

Healthy People 2010
Office of Disease Prevention and Health Promotion, U.S. Department of Health and Human Services, 200 Independence Avenue, S.W., Washington, DC 20201
Phone: (202) 619-0257; Toll Free, (877) 696-6775
http://www.healthypeople.gov

National Institutes of Health
U.S. Department of Health and Human Services, 200 Independence Avenue, S.W., Washington, DC 20201
Phone: (202) 619-0257; Toll Free, (877) 696-6775
http://www.nih.gov

19

The Nurse's Spiritual Health

Susan Weber Buchholz and Karon Schwartz

LEARNING OBJECTIVES

At the end of this chapter, the reader will be able to:
- Identify what constitutes the spiritual self.
- Describe the dynamic interaction of the physical, mental, social, and spiritual dimensions that promotes wellness.
- Recognize the importance of caring for the nurse's spiritual self.
- Discriminate between caregiver fatigue and compassion satisfaction.
- Participate in exercises for physical, mental, social, and spiritual wellness.
- Acknowledge the spiritual energy inherent in nursing.

The **spiritual self** is tied to a person's relationships with self, the divine presence within, and other people. The spiritual self and its experiences vary with the individual. Each person has a path to walk, relationships to develop, and activities in which to engage that are meaningful for his or her own spiritual development.

The spiritual self may be described as a belief or awareness of a presence of a greater power in the realm of a person's spirit. This presence listens to and hears the person's innermost thoughts and prayers. Macrae (2001) wrote of an awareness of a divine presence, noting that for some people this presence may be the Absolute, Allah, Buddha, God, Christ, The Holy Spirit, The Universe, The Great Spirit, or whatever the person understands to be the nature of the higher being or divine presence.

The spirit is inseparable from the body. The spirit also is intangible. It could be compared to breath, which humans often take for granted until they experience shortness of breath. On cool mornings, a person can observe the distillation of his or her breath in the air, heightening awareness of its presence. Likewise, people may experience manifestations of the spirit through miracles or sense divine intervention on behalf of themselves or others. This is especially true in the experiences of birth and death. The spirit also can be compared to the wind. Although the wind cannot be seen, it is felt and its presence is known without doubt. Just as humans know that the wind exists because of its effects on nature, humans know the spirit by its effects on people and the universe.

The essence of the universe is manifest in nature with the growth and beauty of plants and animals. The essence of the spirit within the person, when recognized and honored, allows for spiritual growth and peace with self, others, and the world.

DYNAMIC DIMENSIONS OF WELLNESS MODEL

Wellness means an optimal state of being that generates energy for self and others. In a state of wellness, the person's physical, mental, social, and spiritual dimensions work together toward a meaningful earthly existence. The dimensions are not mutually exclusive; they are intertwined.

Wellness, although often referred to as physical well-being, is not limited to the physical dimension. The wellness of the mind, social interactions, and spirit may take precedence over the condition of the body. Although there are various ways to think about these dimensions, Figure 19-1 suggests one conceptualization, known as the **dy-**

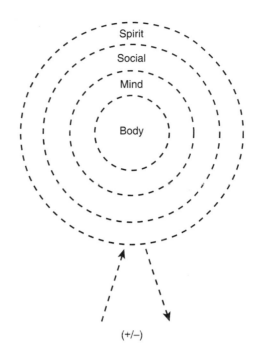

FIGURE 19-1 Dynamic dimensions of wellness model.

(+/−)

namic dimensions of wellness model. The model uses concentric circles to demonstrate the overlapping nature of the four dimensions of wellness: physical, mental, social, and spiritual. The broken lines forming the circles indicate the openness of each dimension, demonstrating a dynamic state that allows energy, as represented by arrows, to flow among the dimensions. Energy can move people in either positive or negative directions. The person constantly exchanges energy with the world.

The body, the center circle, represents the dimension of **physical wellness**. The body is the mechanism by which people live, move, and exist in the physical world. It is the vehicle for meeting and dealing with patients, families, and personal acquaintances. Positive energy in the body means that the body is functioning well and adapting adequately. In other words, the body is healthy. In contrast, people may have chronic physical conditions, such as asthma or arthritis, that move the physical dimension of wellness in a negative direction. Health, illness, or disease may influence energy that flows among the other dimensions.

The next concentric circle depicts **mental wellness**. The mind is the place of mental activity that enables humans to reason, think, know, and understand. Through the mind, people remember, react, and adapt to both internal and external stimuli. It is how people engage in meaningful dialogue with one another. The mind influences, and is influenced by, thinking. People can choose and entertain both negative and positive thoughts in response to internal and external experiences. Mental experiences affect the body, and physical experiences affect the mind. These experiences also intertwine and interact with the social and spiritual dimensions.

The third concentric circle depicts **social wellness**. No man or woman is an island. People spend much time with others, living and interacting with them. Individuals may have different social needs to enhance their well-being. For example, extroverts usually find social interaction easy and stimulating; they may find solitude and lack of socialization to be a physical, mental, and spiritual burden. In contrast, introverts may find social interaction to require greater effort and be less stimulating, leading to physical, mental, and spiritual burdens. Nurses are aware of the necessity for people to balance social interaction with solitude. Both extroverts and introverts will find it beneficial to adjust to various dimensions of social interaction when they consider personal wellness. Extroverts may need to socialize less and take more time to look inward and deal with internal matters. Introverts may need to make the time to socialize and learn from those with whom they live and work.

The outermost circle represents **spiritual wellness**; it encompasses the whole person, permeating the other three dimensions. The spiritual dimension is where people find meaning, draw energy, and gain insights for living meaningful lives in the presence of others. It involves an awareness of a greater power with whom the person communicates in thought or word. The spiritual dimension is not synonymous with a religious dimension. People may find religious rituals, beliefs, and practices beneficial when dealing with the spiritual dimension. This is not to say those who do not express a religious preference are without a spirit (see Chapter 1).

CARING FOR THE NURSE'S SPIRITUAL SELF

To deliver nursing care that is not only safe and effective, but also nourishing and life-giving, nurses must achieve balance in and between their professional and personal lives. Nurses need to take time to reflect on how their personal physical, mental, social, and spiritual health affects their delivery of patient care. Wellness in each dimension is significantly intertwined and interdependent with the other dimensions.

Nursing and Energy

Any dimension of wellness that, for whatever reason, requires special attention or resources can lead to an energy drain on the person. This drain can make a person significantly more vulnerable to professional disappointments and personal health risks. All professions require energy from the people doing the work. The nursing profession requires significant energy at multiple levels from nurses. Thus, for nurses to function at a high level of physical, mental, social, and spiritual health, they must examine each of these dimensions of wellness.

At the physical level, nurses often participate in care delivery that requires significant actual physical labor. Mentally, nurses are aware of the importance that they are taking care of those who may be vulnerable at the moment of care. Often, they put significant energy into being conscious of how to provide care so that patients feel comfortable, protected, and above all trusting that nurses accept them for who they are at that moment. Nurses never view patients in isolation but recognize them as social beings in a larger system, including the family and community. Nurses are also aware that patients address their health and illness needs in the context of personal spiritual beliefs. For nurses to have the energy to address the dimensions of wellness of patients with complex needs, nurses must be aware of the need to make their own wellness, including their spiritual wellness, a priority.

Nursing and Compassion and Caregiving

Nursing is by its nature a caring profession. Nursing combines the science of health care with the art of caring. Health promotion and illness prevention are important components. Likewise, taking care of people who are acutely or chronically ill or injured, disabled, or dying are also important aspects in nursing (International Council of Nursing, n.d.). Taking care of vulnerable people who are in pain and suffering requires significant energy and compassion.

During the past several decades, many terms have been used to describe the frustration, fatigue, and disappointment associated with a professional role. Health care and other service organizations often place the people who choose these professions at significant risk for becoming emotionally depleted and detached from their work. Demands in nursing have increased in recent years because of pressures related to economic changes in health care. As health care organizational budgets tighten, the demands upon the nurse's time and energy often become greater. The increasing complexity of health care related to a rapid expansion of health research and knowledge, people living longer, and paperwork demands can be overwhelming.

Delivering compassionate care involves a desire on the nurse's part to assist patients and their families and to help alleviate their distress. Because nurses and patients are human beings, an intangible human-to-human interaction occurs when they are together. Empathy and sympathy are typical components of compassionate care. In such exchanges, nurses not only give of themselves, but they also receive appreciation, hope, trust, and a sense of worth and purpose in their work.

Although quality nursing is rooted in effective and competent caregiving, it is possible for nurses to deliver care without investing much emotional energy. In a profession that depends on the human-to-human interaction, delivering mechanical care not only cheats the patient, but also the nurse. Thus, nurses need to be able to replenish energy, by delivering compassionate care, restoring personal energy in other ways, or both. If the burden of caregiving becomes overwhelming for whatever reason, nurses are at risk for **caregiver fatigue**.

Different tools in the literature can help people measure any negative impacts associated with their work. The literature also contains an array of definitions associated with negative work experiences leading to dissatisfaction. Interestingly, caregiver fatigue is not a typically used term. However, other terms used actually measure the effects of various levels of caregiver fatigue, including burnout and compassion fatigue, both of which frequently involve the depletion of energy.

Freudenberger (1980) coined the term *burnout*, which is less serious than *compassion fatigue*. Burnout results from stress and psychological strain on the job. Cumulative stressors and hassles can lead to feeling tired and worn down. Typically, nurses at risk for burnout enter their profession with high energy and expectations. As the day-to-day grind of reality sets in, they are at risk for burnout if they cannot adjust their expectations and learn to work successfully within the confines of reality. Nurses at special risk are those who work with difficult patient populations, such as the chronically ill, hospice patients, persons with cognitive deficits, or those with addictions; those expected to produce at a high level with limited resources; those who work long hours, feel their work is not making a difference, or are isolated professionally. Box 19.1 lists symptoms of burnout.

Figley (1995) identified the term *compassion fatigue*, which is all encompassing in that it involves not only physical exhaustion, but also mental, social, and spiritual exhaustion. Nurses with compassion fatigue give a great deal of energy over time; however, they cannot restore their personal energy balance. Compassion fatigue develops gradually, anywhere from several weeks to several years. Unlike burnout, in which nurses withdraw from the situation to recover daily, nurses who experience compassion fatigue continue to try to deliver a high level of care. As nurses use up their compensatory mechanisms, compassion fatigue slowly robs them of their physical, mental, social, and spiritual energy, leaving them with nothing left to give. In addition, nurses also may not be able to receive the respect and appreciation that their patients are trying to return.

The opposite of dissatisfaction is satisfaction. If the experience of being a nurse and delivering compassionate care is positive, nurses experience **compassion satisfaction**. Nursing is an unusual profession in that it has the power to give back so much to those who actually do the job. The human-to-human interaction can be energizing for both patients and nurses. When nurses experience a sense of purpose from being nurses, they can experience compassion satisfaction. As a result, this experience enhances their self-confidence, sense of strength, and spiritual connection.

During their professional careers, nurses may have a wide range of emotional and physical responses to their work. If nurses are concerned that they may be at risk for burnout or compassion fatigue, it may be helpful to take a few minutes to assess the situation. This chapter provides two self-explanatory tests. Figure 19-2 is useful as a quick screening test. Nurses concerned that burnout or compassion fatigue is a serious problem for them can complete a second and more extensive test (Figure 19-3).

B O X 19.1   Symptoms of Burnout and Caregiver Fatigue

SYMPTOMS OF BURNOUT	SYMPTOMS OF CAREGIVER FATIGUE
Loss of compassion	Physical exhaustion
Listlessness	Sleep difficulty
Boredom	Physical symptoms such as
Discouragement	headaches or gastrointestinal
Impatience	symptoms
Alienation	Alcohol, drug, or food abuse
Cynicism	Anger
Negativism	Blaming
Detachment	Hopelessness
Depression	Low self-esteem
	Decreased joy
	Depression
	Workaholism

Answering "yes" or "no" to the following nine statements will help you assess your risk for compassion fatigue:

Personal concerns commonly intrude on my professional role.   Yes No

My colleagues seem to lack understanding.   Yes No

I find even small changes enormously draining.   Yes No

I can't seem to recover quickly after association with trauma.   Yes No

Association with trauma affects me very deeply.   Yes No

My patients' stress affects me deeply.   Yes No

I have lost my sense of hopefulness.   Yes No

I feel vulnerable all the time.   Yes No

I feel overwhelmed by unfinished personal business.   Yes No

Answering "yes" to four or more questions may indicate that you're suffering from compassion fatigue.

FIGURE 19-2 Self-assessment for compassion fatigue. (Pfifferling, J. H., & Gilley, K. [2000]. Overcoming compassion fatigue [Electronic version]. *Family Practice Management, 7*[4], 39. Retrieved June 4, 2003, from http://www.aafp.org/fpm/20000400/39over.html.)

Personal Spiritual Health

Just as it is not possible to totally separate the physical, mental, social, and spiritual dimensions of the individual, it also is not possible for nurses to separate their role as nurse from the rest of their identity. What happens within nurses' professional lives can significantly affect their personal lives, and vice versa. Positive, energizing experiences give nurses more energy and enhance focus within their personal lives.

Professionally, staying healthy has obvious benefits. When nurses experience positive physical, mental, social, and spiritual health, their quality of work is high and everyone benefits. Patients benefit because professionals truly enjoy delivering compassionate nursing care to them. Nurses benefit because they are self-confident and free enough to accept each situation for its potential as well as its limitations, working successfully within those parameters.

Obviously professional energy spills over into one's personal life. When nurses are energized and healthy, they have much to contribute not only professionally but also within their personal lives. As this chapter explores the positive dimensions of wellness, the reader should keep in mind that each dimension affects the other, and

(*text continues on page 336*)

Compassion Satisfaction and Fatigue (CSF) Test

Helping others puts you in direct contact with other people's lives. As you probably have experienced, your compassion for those you help has both positive and negative aspects. This self-test helps you estimate your compassion status: How much at risk you are of burnout and compassion fatigue and also the degree of satisfaction with your helping others. Consider each of the following characteristics about you and your current situation. Write in the number that honestly reflects how frequently you experienced these characteristics in the last week. Then follow the scoring directions at the end of the self-test.

0 = Never 1 = Rarely 2 = A few times 3 = Somewhat often 4 = Often 5 = Very often

Items About You

_____ 1. I am happy.

_____ 2. I find my life satisfying.

_____ 3. I have beliefs that sustain me.

_____ 4. I feel estranged from others.

_____ 5. I find that I learn new things from those I care for.

_____ 6. I force myself to avoid certain thoughts or feelings that remind me of a frightening experience.

_____ 7. I find myself avoiding certain activities or situations because they remind me of a frightening experience.

_____ 8. I have gaps in my memory about frightening events.

_____ 9. I feel connected to others.

_____ 10. I feel calm.

_____ 11. I believe that I have a good balance between my work and my free time.

_____ 12. I have difficulty falling or staying asleep.

_____ 13. I have outbursts of anger or irritability with little provocation.

_____ 14. I am the person I always wanted to be.

_____ 15. I startle easily.

_____ 16. While working with a victim, I thought about violence against the perpetrator.

_____ 17. I am a sensitive person.

_____ 18. I have flashbacks connected to those I help.

_____ 19. I have good peer support when I need to work through a highly stressful experience.

_____ 20. I have had first-hand experience with traumatic events in my adult life.

_____ 21. I have had first-hand experience with traumatic events in my childhood.

_____ 22. I think that I need to "work through" a traumatic experience in my life.

_____ 23. I think that I need more close friends.

_____ 24. I think that there is no one to talk with about highly stressful experiences.

_____ 25. I have concluded that I work too hard for my own good.

_____ 26. Working with those I help brings me a great deal of satisfaction.

_____ 27. I feel invigorated after working with those I help.

FIGURE 19-3 Compassion Satisfaction and Fatigue (CSF) test. (© B. Hudnall Stamm, 2003. Professional quality of life: Compassion fatigue and satisfaction subscales, R-III [Pro-QOL]. Retrieved August 6, 2003, from http://www.isu.edu/~bhstamm/tests/satfat_english.htm.)

_____ 28. I am frightened of things a person I helped has said or done to me.

_____ 29. I experience troubling dreams similar to those I help.

_____ 30. I have happy thoughts about those I help and how I could help them.

_____ 31. I have experienced intrusive thoughts of times with especially difficult people I helped.

_____ 32. I have suddenly and involuntarily recalled a frightening experience while working with a person I helped.

_____ 33. I am pre-occupied with more than one person I help.

_____ 34. I am losing sleep over a person I help's traumatic experiences.

_____ 35. I have joyful feelings about how I can help the victims I work with.

_____ 36. I think that I might have been "infected" by the traumatic stress of those I help.

_____ 37. I think that I might be positively "inoculated" by the traumatic stress of those I help.

_____ 38. I remind myself to be less concerned about the well being of those I help.

_____ 39. I have felt trapped by my work as a helper.

_____ 40. I have a sense of hopelessness associated with working with those I help.

_____ 41. I have felt "on edge" about various things and I attribute this to working with certain people I help.

_____ 42. I wish that I could avoid working with some people I help.

_____ 43. Some people I help are particularly enjoyable to work with.

_____ 44. I have been in danger working with people I help.

_____ 45. I feel that some people I help dislike me personally.

Items About Being a Helper and Your Helping Environment

_____ 46. I like my work as a helper.

_____ 47. I feel like I have the tools and resources that I need to do my work as a helper.

_____ 48. I have felt weak, tired, run down as a result of my work as helper.

_____ 49. I have felt depressed as a result of my work as a helper.

_____ 50. I have thoughts that I am a "success" as a helper.

_____ 51. I am unsuccessful at separating helping from personal life.

_____ 52. I enjoy my co-workers.

_____ 53. I depend on my co-workers to help me when I need it.

_____ 54. My co-workers can depend on me for help when they need it.

_____ 55. I trust my co-workers.

_____ 56. I feel little compassion toward most of my co-workers.

_____ 57. I am pleased with how I am able to keep up with helping technology.

_____ 58. I feel I am working more for the money/prestige than for personal fulfillment.

_____ 59. Although I have to do paperwork that I don't like, I still have time to work with those I help.

_____ 60. I find it difficult separating my personal life from my helper life.

FIGURE 19-3 (Continued)

_____ 61. I am pleased with how I am able to keep up with helping techniques and protocols.

_____ 62. I have a sense of worthlessness/disillusionment/resentment associated with my role as a helper.

_____ 63. I have thoughts that I am a "failure" as a helper.

_____ 64. I have thoughts that I am not succeeding at achieving my life goals.

_____ 65. I have to deal with bureaucratic, unimportant tasks in my work as a helper.

_____ 66. I plan to be a helper for a long time.

Scoring Instructions

Please note that research is ongoing on this scale and the following scores should be used as a guide, not confirmatory information.

1. Be certain you respond to all items.
2. Mark the items for scoring:
    a. Put an x by the following 26 items: 1–3, 5, 9–11, 14, 19, 26–27, 30, 35, 37, 43, 46–47, 50, 52–55, 57, 59, 61, 66.
    b. Put a check by the following 16 items: 17, 23–25, 41, 42, 45, 48, 49, 51, 56, 58, 60, 62–65.
    c. Circle the following 23 items: 4, 6–8, 12, 13, 15, 16, 18, 20–22, 28, 29, 31–34, 36, 38–40, 44.
3. Add the numbers you wrote next to the items for each set of items and note:
    a. *Your potential for Compassion Satisfaction (x):* 118 and above = extremely high potential; 100–117 = high potential; 82–99 = good potential; 64–81 = modest potential; below 63 = low potential.
    b. *Your risk for Burnout (check):* 36 or less = extremely low risk; 37–50 = moderate risk; 51–75 = high risk; 76–85 = extremely high risk.
    c. *Your risk for Compassion Fatigue (circle):* 26 or less = extremely low risk, 27–30 = low risk; 31–35 = moderate risk; 36–40 = high risk; 41 or more = extremely high risk.

FIGURE 19-3 (Continued)

that having spiritual wellness means that our physical, mental, and social dimensions are energy producing. Nurses dedicate themselves to the care of other people. It is equally important that the nurses make their own health a priority. For nurses who have been ignoring their own needs, the moment will arrive when it is time to reorganize priorities, taking notice of physical, mental, social, and spiritual health. To have the energy needed to be a compassionate caregiver, nurses must intentionally examine each dimension of wellness in their own lives and make personal plans to obtain optimal wellness.

MOVING TOWARD POSITIVE DIMENSIONS OF WELLNESS

Each dimension of wellness is important. If one dimension of wellness is stagnant or moving in a negative direction, it drains energy, which could begin to negatively affect the other dimensions. Thus, nurses should take a personal inventory of all aspects of their lives. It is likely they will find some dimensions moving in a positive direction, whereas other dimensions could be enhanced to achieve higher wellness. The next section addresses each dimension of wellness from the inside of the circle outward (see Figure 19-1).

Exercises for Physical Wellness

At the center of well-being is the physical self. According to Maslow's (1954) hierarchy of needs, people must address the most basic physical needs before they can fulfill the next levels of needs, such as safety, love, and self-actualization. To have the energy and focus needed to examine personal mental, social, and spiritual dimensions, nurses need to provide themselves with a strong physical core.

Peaceful Sleep

Foundational to the maintenance of physical energy is the ability to obtain not only sufficient, but also restorative, rest. Sleep is restorative in that it re-energizes and heals the body. It is necessary for our bodies to function properly.

The amount of sleep a person needs depends on several factors. Age is one of the most significant factors. Children require more sleep than adults. Elderly people typically experience fragmented nighttime sleep; they may sleep less during the night but nap more during the day. In general, adults need 7 to 8 hours of sleep each night to prevent a sleep debt; some people need 9 hours, whereas others can sleep 6 or fewer hours and not experience daytime drowsiness. Short naps also help prevent daytime sleepiness and are an effective strategy for preventing a sleep debt.

Sleep is often one of the first activities compromised when demands become heavy. Many people simply do not sleep because they need to spend the time just getting through the normal tasks of the day. In addition, the modern fast-paced world often rewards being a high achiever. However, striving toward achievement often comes with a price. Emotional, intellectual, and physical challenges can affect not only the amount, but also the quality, of sleep. The National Sleep Foundation has found that more than 50% of U.S. adults have a sleep problem that affects them at least once a week. Daytime sleepiness that compromises the ability to engage in daily activities affects more than 40% of adults at least several days a month. Nurses are at particular risk for fatigue because of the significant amount of shift work that around-the-clock nursing care involves. In addition, some nurses work overtime hours, back-to-back shifts, or rest only a few hours between shifts.

Several sleep disorders affect the amount of sleep a person can obtain. *Insomnia*, or the inability to initiate sleep, occasionally happens to most people. Nurses experiencing frequent schedule changes or significant stress may suffer insomnia. A person regularly experiencing insomnia that affects quality of life should seek medical treatment. More serious disorders, such as *sleep apnea* (which causes interruption of breathing during sleep) and *narcolepsy* (which causes a person to fall asleep without warning during the day), are serious medical problems in need of treatment by a health care provider.

Fortunately, nurses can use various strategies to obtain a good night's rest and to prevent daytime drowsiness:

- *Set a schedule and stick with it.* Go to bed at the same time each night and rise at the same time each morning.

- *If you are tired during the day, a short nap may be energizing.* Avoid long naps and naps later in the day because they may delay your readiness for usual sleep. If tired during the day, especially when driving, try to take a rest break—even 10 minutes can be energizing.
- *Exercise daily.* Moderately intense exercise (e.g., brisk walking for 30 minutes 4 or more days a week) promotes restful sleep. If this is not possible, shorter and more frequent exercise during the day can help. Plan exercise early in the day if possible. It is important not to exercise within several hours of the time that you plan to go to sleep.
- *Monitor use of caffeine, nicotine, and alcohol.* Avoid excessive consumption of caffeine during the day or too close to bedtime. Also avoid smoking before bedtime. Alcohol consumed too close to nighttime hours can cause a sleep disruption.
- *Use your bed for sleeping and lovemaking only.* If you can not get to sleep, go to another place in your home and relax. Do not watch television or do paperwork in bed.
- *Establish an environment that promotes sleeping.* A comfortable mattress and pillow and a cool room temperature all enhance sleep.
- *If you are a shift worker, set an intentional schedule for sleeping and stick with it.* Experiment with different sleep schedules. Some shift workers find that sleeping in two segments works best. Others can get one block of sleep during the day. Either way, ensure that the bedroom is quiet and that sunlight (a natural trigger for alertness) is adequately blocked from the sleep area. Find a way to manage typical daytime interruptions with tools such as answering machines. Do not let other demands take priority over your need for sleep. Do not be afraid to set limits with those working daytime hours. After all, you would likely not call them at 3 a.m. to chat! It is up to you to carefully guard your sleeping time.
- *Make an appointment with your health care provider if you experience ongoing insomnia or other sleep disorders.* Multiple health conditions can affect the quality and quantity of sleep. Your health care provider can determine the need for medication as well as an appropriate diagnostic work-up.

Physical Activity

Adequate exercise and physical activity are important to care of the physical self. In a society that has become increasingly sedentary, lack of exercise and obesity are now significant contributors to disease and premature death.

Regular physical activity provides multiple benefits. It decreases risks of obesity, heart disease, diabetes, hypertension, and certain types of cancer. It also promotes strong muscles and joint and bone health. In addition, regular physical activity enhances mental well-being and lessens feelings of depression and anxiety (U.S. Department of Health and Human Services, 1996).

There are four components of physical activity (Figure 19-4), each of which is important. Aerobic training is moderate intensity exercise that promotes cardiovascular health. Examples include brisk walking, jogging, running, bicycling, Tae Bo, and lap swimming. A person should engage in aerobic exercise at least three to four times a week for 30 minutes or more. Activities that increase heart rate to a target of 50% to 70% above normal for at least 10 minutes will improve cardiovascular and general health.

Flexibility is achieved primarily through stretching, which can be part of the warm-up for aerobic exercise or done separately. Stretching involves gentle and

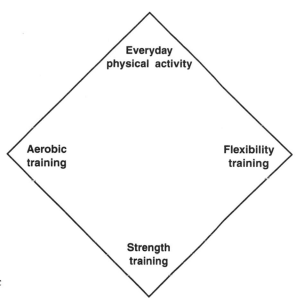

FIGURE 19-4 Quadratic components of physical activity.

repetitive movement of the various aspects of our body. A person should stretch regularly at least three to four times a week, preferably daily. A simple plan is to begin with gentle head rolls, moving to stretching the shoulders and upper arms, followed by gentle stretches of the chest and back, and ending with stretches of the upper and lower leg muscles. Incorporating daily stretching not only improves flexibility but also decreases general body aches and discomfort.

Strength training involves the use of weights three to four times a week. Some people prefer to use actual weight-training equipment; others prefer to use their own body weight (e.g., push-ups). Either way, strength training is an essential component of weekly physical activity. Increasing upper and lower body strength also increases muscle mass. This not only boosts body metabolism, but it also decreases risks for lower back injury. Research also has shown strength training to reduce the risk of osteoporosis (loss of bone density) (Allen, 1994).

In addition to planned aerobic exercise, flexibility, and strength training, increasing everyday activity can significantly improve overall physical well-being. Such things as taking a walk instead of driving, moving quickly when doing household chores, planting a garden, or getting out and playing ball with neighborhood children are small ways to increase activity levels. To examine overall physical activity, nurses should consider taking an inventory of daily activity. To maximize physical wellness, it is important to be intentional and schedule regular aerobic, flexibility, and strength training as well as just simply moving more.

Sound Nutrition

Making wise food choices is one way for nurses to easily and quickly influence their health positively. The Food Pyramid provides a guide as to what and how much to eat each day (United States Department of Agriculture, 1996). It illustrates a suggested daily intake: many servings of bread, cereal, rice, and pasta; several servings of fruits and vegetables; two to three servings of dairy products as well as meat or beans; and only a few fats and sweets.

The following steps provide a guide for enhancing nutritional health:

• Eat a diet low in refined sugars and fats. The more processed the food is, the less of it you should eat.
• Monitor fat intake. Choose lean meats (e.g., broiled, baked, or grilled fish or chicken).
• Eat a diet high in natural grains. Eat meat substitutes high in protein (e.g., tofu, beans).
• Increase daily fruits and vegetables. Eat at least 5 servings, preferably fresh or lightly steamed, each day.
• Eat breakfast (even just a morning snack) every day.
• Smaller, more frequent meals are preferable to one or two larger meals.
• Monitor caffeine intake. Limit caffeine to 1 to 2 cups of coffee, tea, or soda pop daily.
• Drink adequate fresh water every day, preferably 4 to 6 cups.

In addition to sound eating, monitoring the quantity of food intake is important. Obesity is a growing problem in the United States. Figure 19-5 provides a tool for calculating Body Mass Index (BMI), which indicates healthy and unhealthy weights. Nurses with a BMI that indicates obesity are placing themselves at significant risk for several chronic medical problems. There is no magic and quick answer to losing weight and maintaining a healthy weight. The general formula is to consume fewer calories than expended. When healthy food choices are a consistent part of a nurse's lifestyle, it becomes easier to travel the pathway to a healthy weight.

Avoiding Hurtful Habits

Tobacco use continues to be a leading contributor to U.S. morbidity and mortality (American Lung Association, 2002). It contributes significantly to the development of lung cancer, chronic obstructive pulmonary disease, and coronary artery disease.

Body Mass Index (BMI)

English Formula
BMI = [weight in pounds ÷ height in inches ÷ height in inches] × 703

Metric Formula
BMI = weight in kilograms ÷ [height in meters]^2

The BMI value for adults is one fixed number, regardless of age or sex, using the following guidelines:

Underweight	BMI less than 18.5
Overweight	BMI of 25.0 to 29.9
Obese	BMI of 30.0 or more

FIGURE 19-5 Body mass index (BMI) formula. (U.S. Department of Health and Human Services. [n.d.]. *BMI for adults: Body mass index formula.* Retrieved August 12, 2003, from http://www.cdc.gov/nccdphp/dnpa/bmi/bmi-adult-formula.htm.)

Cigarette smoking is among the most difficult habits to break. Two things must happen to stop smoking. First, smokers have to break their actual physical addiction to nicotine. Second, they must break the habit of smoking. Box 19.2 lists tips on quitting smoking.

Moderate alcohol use typically is not a problem for most people. When alcohol consumption begins to interfere with physical health, employment, and family activities, or when a person drives while intoxicated, alcohol use has become a hurtful habit. Nurses who are concerned about alcohol use and consumption should visit the Alcoholics Anonymous Web site (see Recommended Readings and Resources). The site provides a short self-assessment for problems with alcohol.

Illicit drug use can be seen in several forms. Use of marijuana, cocaine, heroin, and other substances continues to be a significant problem in the United States. Nurses have the additional risk of access to controlled substances (e.g., narcotics). The use of illicit drugs and narcotics without prescriptions is not only dangerous physically, but also has considerable legal and professional implications. State boards of nursing spend significant time addressing the practice and licensing of impaired nurses.

If nurses are engaging in illicit drug use and desire to quit, it is important for them to follow-up with a drug rehabilitation center. They also can contact Narcotics Anonymous (NA), an association of recovering drug addicts who help fellow members stay clean.

Vitamin and Herbal Therapy

Although a sound diet typically provides adequate vitamin and mineral intake, there are times when nurses may need to enhance their physical health. A general multivitamin/mineral supplement with 100% daily requirements for most nutrients is sufficient (Fletcher & Fairfield, 2002). If a woman has a history of heavy menstruation, anemia, or both, her health care provider may recommend a multivitamin/mineral with iron. In addition to a regular multipurpose vitamin, certain vitamins work particularly well as antistress agents (Baer & Williams, 1996; Shealy, 1998):

- Vitamin B6 (pyridoxine), 50 mg three times daily
- Vitamin B5 (pantothenic acid), 500 mg daily

BOX 19.2   Tips on Quitting Smoking

- Use the American Lung Association (ALA) as a resource. The ALA has a Web site with information on how to quit.
- Pick a time to quit that is not particularly stressful. It is important to pick an actual quit date.
- Everyone experiences nicotine withdrawal differently. You may experience a wide variety of symptoms from sleepiness to irritability.
- Balance your health with adequate rest, exercise, and good nutrition.
- Find family and friends who are willing to be supportive.
- Talk to your health care provider about nicotine replacement agents and medications available to assist with smoking cessation. If you have quit before and are trying again, keep believing in yourself that you can kick the habit once and for all.

- Vitamin C, 500 mg every day
- Vitamin E, 400 IU every day
- Vitamin A, 5000 IU every day

If a vitamin has the label of a stress tablet (or uses a similar label), it typically contains these particular vitamin components and is easier to take than using several different vitamins every day.

In addition to vitamins, certain herbs seem to facilitate energy. Ginkgo and ginseng are both important mental enhancers. Herbs that help enhance relaxation include motherwort, valerian, and chamomile (Shealy, 1998; Springhouse, 2001). Because of the lack of regulation on the processing of vitamins and minerals, and the lack of sufficient rigorous studies, nurses who use vitamins/mineral supplements and herbs should proceed with caution. Normal kidney and liver function are essential before taking any of these substances. In addition, several herbs have the potential to interfere with prescription medications (Cupp, 1999) or are not recommended for use during pregnancy or lactation (Mattison, n.d.). A consultation with a health care provider who is knowledgeable about vitamins, minerals, and herbal therapy is advised before taking any of these substances. Natural food energy boosters such as apples, orange juice, beans, oatmeal, and water are also effective and probably safer.

Aromatherapy

Aromatherapy involves the use of essential oils to enhance psychological and physical well-being. Essential oils are concentrated and combined with a carrier oil before they are applied to the skin; they can be used not only in creams, gels, compresses, and salves, but also in bath therapy and with steam inhalation. More than 70 essential oils are available. Some people use rosemary and peppermint to help combat fatigue. Others use chamomile, lavender, and geranium to help decrease anxiety and encourage relaxation (Shealy, 1998).

Separate from aromatherapy is the use of various scents in everyday life. Smell is an extremely strong sense that can easily evoke memories. For many, bayberry candles evoke a time of long ago, as do clove-studded oranges hung on pine trees at Christmas. The use of incense is ancient, and incense is still a part of many religions today. Lemon and oranges evoke a sense of freshness. The wafting smell of vanilla and cinnamon instills an expectation for many people of something good coming out of the oven. Intentionally using scents that evoke peaceful and happy times for you is one way of helping to re-energize yourself (Shealy, 1998).

Yoga

Many people use the ancient art of yoga to bring the body and mind together in harmony. The word *yoga* actually means to "join or yoke together." Three main structures to yoga work together synergistically: exercise, breathing, and meditation. Through appropriate exercise and breathing, the body and mind become quiet and have a chance to heal and recover from daily stressors.

There are many different types of yoga. One of the best known is Hatha Yoga, which combines specific postures and physical movements with breathing techniques. Yoga can be self-taught with books or videotapes; however, novice yoga students may find it useful to enroll in a class with a teacher who has had significant experience and training, is willing to work closely with students, and implements a holistic approach. Although yoga is commonly misperceived to have developed from

Hinduism, yoga is not a religion. People of all religions can practice yoga without any conflicts with their beliefs.

Massage Therapy

From infancy onward, the act of touching and being touched by other human beings is important and necessary. Giving a loved one a hug expresses trust and comfort. Nurses often touch other people. They take great care to be gentle and respectful.

Massage therapy takes touch a step further. *Massage therapy* is the application of manual soft tissue manipulation. It uses multiple movements, including applying pressure, holding, and causing movement of the body. Massage therapy is widely accepted and is used to treat multiple health problems as well as to simply enhance general health (Field, 1998; Field et al., 1999; Hernandez-Reif, Field, & Hart, 1999; Hernandez-Reif, Field, Krasnegor, et al., 1999)

Nurses looking for a qualified massage therapist should consider several things. In the United States, more than 25 states now regulate massage therapists. Thus, the nurse would want to find out if a massage therapist is licensed (or certified or registered). The nurse should learn where a massage therapist trained, how long it took to acquire training, and if the therapist has any advanced training. It is also important to know if the massage therapist is a graduate of a program approved by the Commission on Massage Therapy Accreditation or certified by the National Certification Board of Therapeutic Massage and Bodywork.

Once satisfied with a massage therapist's credentials, the nurse can concentrate on finding one he or she likes. It is important to be comfortable with the massage therapist. It is also important to find the type of massage therapy most useful to the nurse.

Achieving Overall Physical Wellness

In the end, all these suggestions mean little if a nurse cannot incorporate them into life. Developing and adhering to a realistic plan is essential. Changing health habits is not always easy, but is well worth it in the long run. People who tend to succeed are motivated by the knowledge that what they are doing will truly improve the quality of their life. In addition, those most likely to stick with changes make progressive small changes and incorporate them into everyday life. Figure 19-6 is a personal exercise form for recording a physical wellness plan.

Another important aspect of wellness is establishing a relationship with a health care provider. Nurses must remember that they are not always supposed to be on the giving side of health care delivery. As individuals, they also have unique health care needs to fully care for and address. Making their own health care needs a priority is vital. Doing so will enhance a nurse's wellness, allowing him or her to bring more energy to the all-important human-to-human interactions that occur daily in nursing.

Exercises for Mental Wellness

The ability to think at a highly cognitive level gives people the freedom to make many choices. They can use this freedom in a positive or negative way. This discussion provides a list of tools to enhance mental wellness.

Journaling

Journaling is a nonverbal method of capturing personal thoughts and later taking time to reflect upon what was written. There is no right or wrong way to use a jour-

Date	Area of Physical Wellness	Is it satisfactory?	If not, what changes can I make?
	Peaceful rest		
	Physical activity		
	Sound nutrition		
	Avoiding hurtful habits		
	Appropriate health care follow-up		
	Other applicable areas		

FIGURE 19-6   Exercise for developing a physical wellness plan.

nal. A person keeps a journal simply to use pen and paper (or perhaps a computer) as an outlet for thinking. How often a person writes in a journal depends on the purpose. Some people prefer to write every day, perhaps early in the morning or before they go to bed. Others use the journal only once a week or when they have difficult decisions.

Journaling fosters sorting through ideas and expressing both negative and positive thoughts without interference from anyone else. Nurses can use a journal to write down random thoughts or specific ideas about how to handle situations. For many people, journals are private affairs. A journal represents who that person is—from the cover housing the journal to the thoughts expressed on the pages. Some people prefer to share their journals with close family members or friends. By doing so, others can understand aspects that the writer may be unable to share verbally.

Reading

Even in an age of media frenzy, nothing replaces a book's ability to transport a person for a short time. Books are a great escape from daily hassles. Nurses can use books for several different reasons, depending on their needs:

- *Inspirational books.* Multiple inspirational books are available today. Inspirational books discuss specific topics such as rest and reflection. Some books facilitate increased motivation and help provide readers with reassurance and encouragement. The type preferred depends on a person's needs.
- *Instructional books.* People have long used books as a primary mode of teaching. If a person is seeking to learn, a book is a tangible way to increase knowledge.
- *Books for relaxation.* This category separates into two sections: fiction and nonfiction. Fiction provides an opportunity to go to a totally different place. A myriad of books also are available on travel, romance, mystery, and other topics. Nurses should take time to decide what they want to read because some books may not

be beneficial if their stories induce fear, negative thoughts, and skepticism. The second type is nonfiction. Books about other people and civilizations often enhance the ability to view one's own life with more depth and breadth and to think more creatively.

- *Spiritual books.* People may find that these books assist them to deepen their own spirituality. The Bible, Torah, Koran, and other spiritual writings provide age-old guidance. Memorizing significant phases often allows a nurse to draw on comfort in times of stress and when actual reading would not be feasible.

Visualization

Visualization is the art of placing oneself in a specific setting without actually being there and using the process to promote relaxation and positive thinking. Nurses also can use visualization to help see themselves as having already achieved a desired goal. When using visualization for relaxation, nurses should employ the following steps:

- Sit or lie down in a comfortable and quiet place.
- Close your eyes.
- Tighten then relax your face and neck muscles.
- Tighten, then relax, your arms, chest, and back muscles.
- Tighten, then relax, your abdomen, hip, and leg muscles.
- Think about a place that brings you joy or comfort.
- Hear the sounds of that place; see the sights of that place.
- Feel the warmth of being in that place.
- The healing nature of your chosen place will allow your mind to rest.

When using visualization toward a specific goal, nurses can use the following steps, which help to reorganize thoughts and focus on priorities:

- Find a relaxing place.
- Close your eyes and sit comfortably.
- Picture yourself as the person that you would like to become.
- Remember that you are a unique creation. There is no one else like you. You have unique gifts and capabilities. You have a unique contribution to make. You are a unique and wonderful creation.

If time is very limited, nurses can do brief deep-breathing exercises:

- Sit in a relaxed posture with your feet squarely on the floor, arms at your side.
- Bend head forward, backward, to left, to right. Do not roll your head.
- Rotate your shoulders slowly and relax your arms, chest, back, abdomen, and legs. Slowly take a deep breath. Exhale intentionally and slowly through your mouth. As you breathe in, think about inhaling life-giving oxygen. As you exhale, let go of negative thoughts and feelings. Repeat this several times.
- Although this takes only a few minutes, it will leave you feeling refreshed.

Music

Hearing cues people in about things that they may not be able to see at that moment. Music affects mood within a very short time. Selection of music is a very personal choice, reflecting one's culture, current physical and mental state, and age.

Nurses can use music to enhance well-being. Music can set the tone for relaxation and restoration within the setting of one's vehicle and home. Upbeat music can provide motivation to get things done. Soft music can help people unwind. Because music has ancient roots in church and religious history, it sets the tone for worship. Many religious groups today use the foundational elements of old chants or liturgies.

Silence
Although music is a wonderful way to help improve mood and setting, there are times when silence is equally powerful. In the busyness of life, it is easy to miss out on the importance of solitude and silence. By taking a few moments each day to be alone in thoughts and to reflect quietly from deep within, a person has the chance to reflect upon where he or she is that day and where her or she hopes to go. Turning off the television, computer, and radio and not answering the telephone can provide precious time for reorganizing and thinking about what is important.

Counseling
Sometimes, life simply becomes overwhelming. When a person finds that he or she cannot handle a difficult situation alone or within the context of his or her family, he or she should seek counseling. Counseling helps to solve personal and interpersonal crises, resolve past issues, and deal with ongoing psychological problems. Counseling allows people to rebuild their lives based on identified strengths, such as support systems and values.

Seeking the right counselor is important. Insurance resources may limit available choices. Many workplaces provide confidential counseling through employee assistance programs. Typically, these programs provide limited counseling to help employees formulate a plan for appropriate follow-up psychological care if needed. Many insurance companies also now have telephone numbers dedicated to mental health questions. Another accessible resource is local community mental health services.

People dealing with anxiety, depression, unreal thoughts, or suspicious thinking may need both psychological counseling and a psychiatric evaluation, including short-term or long-term medication use. People with suicidal thoughts or thoughts of harming others require immediate assistance from a physician, nurse practitioner, or local hospital emergency room, crisis center, or psychiatric center.

Humor
Laughter is, by nature, healing. A strong and hearty laugh causes most people to smile and feel good inside. Healthy humor is never at the expense of another person but is uplifting for those privileged to hear or participate in it. Many humorous books, calendars, pictures, and movies make people laugh.

If nurses find their attitudes about situations becoming overly intense, they should ask themselves if they are taking the situation too seriously. Life is far from perfect, and humor is one way to cope with life's daily imperfections. Your optimism or lack thereof and your belief in what you can or cannot accomplish go a long way to either giving or taking away additional mental power and energy.

Additional Education
For nurses who have mastered their clinical area, going to school may provide the intellectual challenges missing from the work environment. Attaining an advanced degree or taking a class in an area of interest can help nurses to gain new perspectives

as they consider new ideas. Earning a degree also can have the added benefit of preparation for alternative jobs should opportunities arise.

Exercises for Social Wellness

Healthy Relationships with Family and Friends

Relationships with family and friends are often complex. One of the most important aspects of any relationship is communication. If communication in not adequate and honest, it is very difficult to have healthy relationships with family and friends. When disagreements arise, certain rules foster healthy relationships:

- Accept family and friends for who they are, not who you wish they were. One of the greatest gifts we can give one another is unconditional acceptance.
- Set ground rules for handling disagreements. Demeaning and belittling language is never useful. Respect helps facilitate communication.
- Communicate honestly and openly. Hiding feelings only leads to frustration. Use "I" language, not "You" language. For instance: "I feel disappointed that this didn't occur," rather than "You really disappointed me." Using "you" is accusatory and puts the other person on the defensive.
- Try to respond, not react, to the situation.
- Attempt to achieve a compromise that works for both parties.
- Remember that no one, including you, is perfect. Forgiveness goes a long way.

Nurses experiencing physical, mental, or sexual abuse need to seek help from a religious counselor, therapist, or someone they trust. These people can help nurses design a safety plan. Important contingencies to address are found in Boxes 19.3 and 19.4. A nurse who is truly at serious physical risk must leave his or her home immediately and seek help from the police or a shelter.

People have limited choices regarding many relationships in their lives. For example, we cannot choose our birth or adoptive families. However, we can choose life partners and friends. Wise choices are especially important when decisions affect one's entire life. Seeking guidance to make wise decisions can be very useful. Meditation, prayer, and religious rituals are also helpful. Nurses who find themselves in difficult situations based on poor choices (or no choice) also should look for guidance to improve their relationships.

Healthy Relationships with Other Nurses

Nurses face many job-related stressors. Taking care of ill and needy patients requires special gifts and abilities. Co-workers can significantly influence the energy nurses have to complete the work that needs to be done. All nurses sometimes get frustrated, tired, and angry. However, nurses must be careful not to take out their frustrations on patients or to focus their negative energy on the nurses around them. When that happens, no one wins.

Nurses need to foster honesty and communication in their relationships with colleagues. When communication breaks down, typical pitfalls include withdrawal, passive-aggressive behavior, and gossiping, all of which can erode teamwork. These behaviors are not helpful and ultimately will affect not only nurses but also the patients they serve. Nurses already face many challenges delivering patient care; they do not need the additional challenge of dealing with negative attitudes from colleagues.

When nurses face difficult communication situations, it is important for them to talk openly and respectfully with the others involved. If this is not effective, it may be necessary to share the problems with a manager who will plan a strategy for improving relationships to resolve communication issues. If nurses find themselves in a situation they cannot change, they may need to practice in a different setting.

BOX 19.3   Personal Safety Plan for Nurses in Abusive Relationships

IN THE RELATIONSHIP
- Have important telephone numbers available for self and children.
- Tell two people about the violence; ask them to call the police if they hear suspicious noises from the home.
- Know four places to go if leaving home.
- Leave extra money, car keys, clothes, and copies of documents with one person.
- Obtain a protective order; keep it with you at all times and give a copy to another person.
- Ensure safety and independence by:
  - Always having change for phone calls.
  - Opening a personal savings account.
  - Rehearsing your escape route with your support person.
  - Reviewing safety plan regularly.
- If leaving, bring items on the checklist (see Box 19.4).

WHEN THE RELATIONSHIP IS OVER
- Change locks; install a security system, smoke detector, and outside lighting.
- Inform two people that the partner no longer lives there and they should call the police if they observe him or her.
- Tell people who take care of the children who is allowed to visit or collect them.
- Avoid stores, banks, and other places you frequented when you were living with the abusive partner.
- Save threatening e-mails and voice messages.
- Identify a support person to call if you are feeling depressed and ready to return to an abusive situation.
- Notify people at work:
  - Have calls screened.
  - Provide photograph of abuser to security.
  - Change your work schedule.
  - Identify an emergency contact person for your employer to telephone if you are absent from work.
  - Find an escort to transportation.
  - Maintain copies of the restraining order.

> **BOX 19.4 Checklist for Items Needed When Leaving an Abusive Relationship**
>
> ☐ Identification
> ☐ Birth certificates
> ☐ Social security cards
> ☐ School/medical records
> ☐ Keys: car, home, office
> ☐ Driver's license
> ☐ Medications
> ☐ Change of clothes
> ☐ Address book
> ☐ Children's favorite toys/ blankets
>
> ☐ Welfare identification
> ☐ Passport/green card/work permits
> ☐ Divorce/court papers
> ☐ Lease/rental agreement, house deed
> ☐ Mortgage payment book/ unpaid bills
> ☐ Insurance papers
> ☐ Pictures/jewelry/items of sentimental value

Mentoring

Mentoring is when a person in a senior position guides and supports a person in a junior position to ensure the success of the person being mentored. Nurses have been mentoring other nurses since Florence Nightingale, although the process may not have been labeled as such until recently.

Mentoring fits well within the concept of nursing. Much knowledge of nursing is gained through experience. The level of knowledge and ability of nurses to comprehend human-to-human interactions evolves with time, making them experts in their specialty. Because of the way in which nurses become experts, experienced nurses must be generous in sharing their knowledge with newer nurses. More experienced nurses also can guide junior nurses in their career trajectory. In addition, they can help facilitate the relationships of junior nurses with other experts in their field. These measures help the nursing profession to thrive.

Support Groups

Support groups have been discussed in relationship to personal health habits. A multitude of support groups also is available for different types of problems. For some people, support groups work very well. Others view such groups as an invasion of privacy and not necessarily helpful. People must decide for themselves if a support group would be useful. For many, it is significant relief to know that others are dealing with similar problems.

Nurses involved in particularly difficult crises may be given the opportunity to participate in a support group. In addition, nurses experiencing personal illness or loss may find a support group useful. Support groups offer a method of replenishing personal energy by letting others who have walked similar paths offer help and guidance in difficult situations.

Recreational Activities

Recreational restoration comes in many different forms. Not to be overlooked are smaller recreational activities that can be used on a daily and weekly basis to restore energy. Recreational activities allow you to give something back to yourself and are as varied as people are. Box 19.5 offers some suggestions about things you can do to restore your energy.

Retreats

A retreat is a time set aside to reflect, reorganize priorities, and re-energize. A retreat can be with other people who share a joint purpose (e.g., nurse colleagues in a work setting), a group of people from a place of worship, or simply by oneself. Retreats vary in length. It may be possible to accomplish what is needed in one morning. Longer and more complicated issues may take several days. Depending on resources, a person may want to go to a quiet and reflective setting to think without the interruptions of typical daily demands.

A retreat requires personal preparation. Although the direction may change somewhat once reflection begins, it is important to have at least a few basic ideas of what is to be accomplished. Groups should consider appointing a leader for the retreat. If a nurse is conducting a self-retreat, he or she should consider asking a neutral party to discuss thoughts and ideas. When a person leaves a retreat, he or she should feel more focused and ready to address the tasks at hand.

Vacations

Most people look forward to taking time away from their daily grind of home and work responsibilities. The problem with vacations is that people often come back from them exhausted. If at all possible, vacations should provide time for rest before and after engaging in strenuous or emotionally demanding activities. The type of vacation varies according to need. Vacations can range from rugged and sports based, to taking in tourist sites, to simply being pampered. It is useful for the nurse to choose a vacation that would bring personal joy and enhance his or her energy.

Vacations provide an excellent diversion from life. Often 1 or 2 weeks away from a situation helps people feel refreshed and offers them a new perspective on their current setting. However, sometimes a vacation is not enough. Nurses who are truly exhausted or frustrated may need a more substantial break. The duration depends on the financial resources available to the nurse who would be away from work for an extended time. In some cases, nurses may opt to change their job setting. Sometimes a change of pace helps a nurse escape a career rut. Whether a vacation from a work setting is short or long, such a break typically gives a nurse space and perspective and leaves him or her renewed and ready to tackle the many demands of the job.

Volunteering

Nurses are not strangers to the idea of helping others. Just as nurses can derive energy from professional encounters, volunteering also can energize nurses. On mission trips, many nurses, along with other health care providers, share their professional expertise with those who lack basic or specialized health care. But not all volunteering must be professional. Sharing one's expertise in a hobby or interest with youth or older adults can move the social dimension in a positive direction.

B O X 1 9 . 5   Suggestions for Recreational Activities

- Take a leisurely walk.
- Color a picture.
- Engage in a sport such as bowling, golfing, fishing, or playing tennis.
- Eat a cold ice cream cone on a hot summer day.
- Sit on a bench and watch the sunset.
- Pet a dog or cat.
- Sing a song.
- Fly a kite.
- Drink a cup of hot chocolate on a cold winter day.
- Appreciate the rain as you sit in your home listening to it.
- Reflect on all the good things in your life.

Exercises for Spiritual Wellness

Worship in a Community of Faith

Participating in a faith community enriches the spirit. Many people find solace in the company of others with similar beliefs. The ritual of worship can be a reassuring source of comfort; it is not surprising that churches and temples are considered places of sanctuary. As with volunteering, people who use their talents and gifts to honor God find that doing so moves the spiritual dimension of wellness in a positive direction. Chapter 15 provides more information about various therapeutic modalities that energize the spirit.

Prayer and Devotion

Praying, spending time alone reading, meditating, reflecting on blessings, and committing those things over which we do not have control to a higher power are useful exercises. A person can pray in a moment—a prayer can be as simple as a thought for help or a blessing.

Songs, Hymns, and Poetry

Listening to or reading songs, hymns, and poetry are excellent ways to renew strength and faith. Often the words of a verse or a hymn can encourage and uplift the nurse as he or she ministers to others or finds self in need of solace.

Meditation

Meditation can take different forms. Although some people use exercises such as yoga, meditation also can include focusing on a hymn or verse of scripture and thinking about the words to discover their significance and meaning.

Positive Affirmations

Positive affirmations are helpful in stressful situations. One form of positive affirmation is to dwell on a verse of scripture or song. The blessing at the end of this chapter is a positive affirmation that can be used aloud or silently in ministering to self and to others.

Spiritual Journaling

Spiritual journaling can be done with other journaling. It is beneficial to write down any spiritual inspirations and thoughts that come to mind; one can then return to these inspirations and renew oneself when going through difficult situations.

Spiritual Support

Spiritual support comes in various forms. One can seek support in a community of believers in regularly scheduled meetings at churches, mosques, synagogues, or temples. Other ways to seek spiritual support are to share with others of like mind and to seek a mentor who will offer spiritual support and guidance. Counselors, known as spiritual directors, have specialized training and often mentor others on their spiritual journey.

Spiritual Energy Derived from Nursing

Nursing is not just a job or a profession. It is a calling that includes arts and talents. It is intuitive and spiritual. The ability to be with another person, ministering without forethought of being ministered to in return is a unique gift to both patient and self. As Mother Teresa (1995) said: "It is not how much we do—it is how much love we put into the doing." It is not the "doing" but the "being" that shares and regenerates energy.

ENERGY DERIVED FROM GIVING TO OTHERS

In nursing, the spiritual dimension is where spirits blend and nurses are truly present with patients. Nurses know that they have ministered to others, which encompasses all dimensions of wellness. Ministering to others is like a boomerang—the energy nurses give comes back quickly, generating more energy for nurses. In turn, nurses can keep passing that energy along to others.

PERSONAL REFLECTIONS

- How much importance do you place on caring for your own spiritual self?
- What do you see as the relationship between the spiritual self and nursing?
- What do you understand to be the "Dynamic Dimensions of Wellness" as presented in this chapter?
- Are you comfortable with body, mind, social, and spiritual connectedness?
- Would you be able to personally integrate the various aspects of physical, mental, social, and spiritual wellness discussed in this chapter?
- Do you get energy from delivering nursing care?
- Are you comfortable with the human-to-human interaction in the nursing arena?
- Would you feel comfortable relating one or more experiences in which you felt truly connected with a patient?

Nurses must truly listen and know their cues. They must use compassionate touch when communicating and performing tasks (O'Brien, 2001). True presence is being with patients, looking into their eyes, allowing personal woundedness to be present in an effort to bring about healing in others. Trina Paulus (1972), in her book *Hope for the Flowers,* says that when we communicate with another, stopping to listen, fear subsides and we can make sense of our world and what we are to become. We no longer just barely touch in passing but are connected in the process of becoming what we are truly meant to be.

The challenge for nurses as caregivers is to give without thought of "what's in it for me." When nurses approach each patient with "How can I make a positive difference in this patient's life today?" and then wait for intuitive cues and respond with true compassion, nurses will experience high personal returns of spiritual, social, mental, and physical wellness. Helping others with only the intellect and not from the heart may be the cause of "compassion fatigue." True compassion knows no fatigue of spirit. The caregiver who is afraid of pain may, in subtle and sometimes not so subtle ways, distance his or her heart from the ill or dying person with whom he or she is working (Dass & Bush, 1992). A nurse may experience fatigue of body, mind, and social interaction; however, fatigue of the spirit, which is the source of compassion, is nonexistent.

CASE STUDY 19.1

Sam is a full-time school nurse for three grade schools, one junior high school, and one high school. Sam is expressing his frustrations to colleagues at a conference. Sam took the job 2 years ago, planning to implement health promotion programs for students, faculty, and staff throughout the school district. Sam tells how the number of acute illnesses in children who report to the office allows him enough time to complete only mandatory screenings and paperwork. Sam feels disconnected from the school faculty and staff because of the unique role of the school nurse. He wonders if the nursing care "is really making a difference in the health of the children," noting that "so much more could be done." Comparing being a school nurse to volunteering at a church youth summer camp, Sam states that "school nursing is so draining compared to how energizing summer camp is. I wonder if it's time to change jobs."

Critical Thinking
- If you were Sam's colleague, how would you respond?
- From the information given, which dimensions of wellness can you identify quickly as needing to move in a positive direction?
- To find out about the other dimensions of wellness, what questions would you ask Sam?
- Would you use any screening tools presented in this chapter?
- Could you recommend any exercises to Sam based on the information provided in the brief discussion?

May you be filled with loving-kindness
May you be well
May you be peaceful and at ease
May you be happy
May I be filled with loving kindness
May I be well,
May I be peaceful and at ease
May I be happy.

Author unknown

Key Points

- The spiritual self of the nurse affects the nurse's personal and professional life.
- The nurse's spiritual self is multidimensional; it incorporates the integration of the physical, mental, social, and spiritual dimensions of wellness.
- The body, mind, social, and spiritual dimensions are dynamic, open systems in which each dimension affects the other.
- The nurse can experience symptoms that indicate burnout or caregiver fatigue.
- The nurse may experience compassion satisfaction in caregiving.
- There are various exercises that can be used to enhance physical, mental, social, and spiritual wellness.
- The human-to-human interaction is an integral part of nursing that can be beneficial to both the nurse and the patient.
- The nurse receives spiritual energy from participating in patient care.

References

Allen, S. H. (1994). Exercise considerations for postmenopausal women with osteoporosis. *Arthritis Care and Research, 7*(4), 205–212.

American Lung Association. (2002, June). *Quitting smoking.* Available at: http://www.lungusa.org/tobacco/quitting_smoke.html.

American Nurses Association. (2002). Available at: http://www.nursingworld.org.

Baer, C. L., & Williams, B. R. (1996). *Clinical pharmacology and nursing* (3rd ed.). Springhouse, PA: Springhouse.

Cupp, M. J. (1999). Herbal remedies: Adverse effects and drug interactions. *American Family Physician, 59*(5), 1239–1245.

Dass, R., & Bush, M. (1992). *Compassion in action: Setting out on the path of service.* New York: Belltower.

Field, T. (1998). Massage therapy effects. *The American Psychologist, 53,* 1270–1281.

Field, T., Hernandez-Reif, M., Hart, S., Theakston, H., Schanberg, S., & Kuhn, C. (1999). Pregnant women benefit from massage therapy. *Journal of Psychosomatic Obstetrics and Gynaecology, 20*(1), 31–38.

Figley, C. R. (Ed.). (1995). *Compassion fatigue: Coping with secondary traumatic stress disorder in those who treat the traumatized.* New York: Brunner/Mazel.

Fletcher, R. H., & Fairfield, K. M. (2002). Vitamins for chronic disease prevention in adults: Clinical applications. *Journal of the American Medical Association, 287*(23), 3127–3129.

Freudenberger, H. J. (1980). *Burn-out: The high cost of high achievement.* Garden City, NY: Doubleday and Company, Inc.

Hernandez-Reif, M., Field, T., & Hart, S. (1999). Smoke cravings are reduced by self-massage. *Preventive Medicine, 28,* 28–32.

Hernandez-Reif, M., Field, T., Krasnegor, J., Martinez, E., Schwartzman, M., & Mavunda, K. (1999). Children with cystic fibrosis benefit from massage therapy. *Journal of Pediatric Psychology, 24,* 175–181.

International Council of Nursing. (n.d.). *The ICN definition of nursing*. Retrieved August 12, 2003, from http://www.icn.ch/definition.htm.

Macrae, J. A. (2001). *Nursing as a spiritual practice: A contemporary application of Florence Nightingale's views*. New York: Springer Publishing.

Maslow, A. H. (1954). *Motivation and personality*. New York: Harper and Row Publishers.

Mattison, D. (n.d.). *Herbal supplements: Their safety, a concern for health care providers*. Retrieved August 12, 2003, from http://www.marchofdimes.com.

Mother Teresa. (1995). *A simple path*. New York: Ballantine Books.

O'Brien, M. E. (2001). *The nurse's calling: A Christian spirituality of caring for the sick*. New York: Paulist Press.

Paulus, T. (1972). *Hope for the flowers*. New York: Paulist Press.

Shealy, C. N. (1998). *The illustrated encyclopedia of healing remedies*. New York: Barnes & Noble.

Springhouse. (2001). *Nursing herbal medicine handbook*. Springhouse, PA: Author.

U.S. Department of Agriculture. (1996). *The food guide pyramid*. Available at: http://www.pueblo.gsa.gov/cic_text/food/food-pyramid/main.htm.

U.S. Department of Health and Human Services. (1996). *Physical activity and health: A report of the Surgeon General*. Washington, DC: Author.

Recommended Readings

Barnum, B. (1996). *Spirituality in nursing: From traditional to new age*. New York: Springer Publishing Co.

Breathnach, S. (1995). *Simple abundance: A daybook of comfort and joy*. New York: Warner Books.

Callanan, M., & Kelly, P. (1992). *Final gifts: Understanding the special awareness, needs, and communications of the dying*. New York: Bantam Books.

Canfield, J., Hansen, M., Mitchell-Autio, N., & Theiman, L. (2001). *Chicken soup for the nurse's soul: 101 stories to celebrate, honor and inspire the nursing profession*. Deerfield Beach, FL: Health Communications Inc.

Chopra, D. (1997). *The path of love: Renewing the power of spirit in your life*. New York: Harmony Books.

Dass, R., & Gorman, P. (1991). *How can I help?: Stories and reflections on service*. New York: Alfred Knopf.

Davis, M., Eschelman, E. R., & McKay, M. (2000). *The relaxation and stress reduction workbook* (5th ed.). Oakland, CA: New Harbinger.

Dement, W. C. (1999). *The promise of sleep*. New York: Random House.

Dyer, W. (2001). *There is a spiritual solution to every problem*. New York: HarperCollins Publishing.

Fish, S., & Shelly, J. (1978). *Spiritual care: The nurse's role*. Downer's Grove, IL: InterVarsity Press.

Jones, W. B., & Levin, J. S. (Eds.). (1999). *Essentials of complimentary and alternative medicine*. Philadelphia: Lippincott Williams & Wilkins.

Kelsey, M. T. (1981). *Caring: How can we love one another?* New York: Paulist Press.

Kelsey, M. T. (1981). *Transcend: A guide to the spiritual quest*. New York: Crossroad.

Knaack, T. (1981). *Special friends who reflect the fruit of the spirit*. Waco, TX: Word Books.

Mann, S. T. (1949). *Change your life through love*. New York: Dodd Mead & Co.

Mayeroff, M. (1971). *On caring*. New York: HarperCollins Publishers.

McNamara, J. (1983). *The power of compassion: Innocence and powerlessness as adversaries of the spiritual life*. New York: Paulist Press.

Micozzi, M. S. (Ed.). (2001). *Fundamentals of complimentary and alternative medicine* (2nd ed.). New York: Churchill Livingstone.

Moffat, M., & Vickery, S. (1999). *Book of body maintenance and repair*. New York: Henry Holt and Company.

Norcross, J. C., Santrock, J. W., Campbell, L. F., Smith, T. P., Sommer, R., & Zuckerman, E. L. (2000). *Authoritative guide to self-help resources in mental health*. New York: The Guilford Press.

Remen, R. N. (1996). *Kitchen table wisdom: Stories that heal*. New York: Riverhead Books.

Remen, R. N. (2000). *My grandfather's blessings: Stories of strength, refuge, and belonging*. New York: Riverhead Books.

Rowe, L. (1958). *On call: Devotionals for nurses.* Grand Rapids, MI: Baker Publishing.

Santorelli, S. (1999). *Heal thy self: Lessons on mindfulness in medicine.* New York: Belltower.

Simoton, O. C., Henson, R., & Hampton, B. (1992). *The healing journey: Restoring health and harmony to body, mind, and spirit.* New York: Bantam Books.

Smith, D. C. (1997). *Caregiving: Hospice-proven techniques for healing body and soul.* New York: Macmillan.

U.S. Department of Health and Human Services. (2002). *BMI for adults: Body mass index formula.* Retrieved August 12, 2003, from http://www.cdc.gov/nccdphp/dnpa/bmi/bmi-adult-formula.htm.

Vaughn, F., & Walsh, R. (Eds.). (1983). *Accept this gift: Selections from 'A course in miracles.'* Los Angeles: Jeremy P. Thatcher, Inc.

Watson, J. (1999). *Postmodern nursing and beyond.* New York: Churchill Livingstone.

Wiancek, D. A. (2000). *The natural healing companion: Using alternative medicines.* Emmaus, PA: Rodale.

Willett, W. C., & Stampfer, M. J. (2001). What vitamins should I be taking, Doctor? *New England Journal of Medicine, 345,* 1819–1823.

Resources

Alcoholics Anonymous
Grand Central Station, P.O. Box 459, New York, NY 10163
http://www.alcoholics-anonymous.org

American Botanical Council
6200 Manor Road, Austin, TX 78723
Phone: (512) 926-4900
Fax: (512) 926-2345
http://www.herbalgram.org

American Lung Association
61 Broadway, 6th Floor, New York, NY 10006
Phone: (212) 315-8700
http://www.lungusa.org

American Massage Therapy Association
820 Davis Street, Suite 100, Evanston, IL 60201-4444
Phone: (847) 864-0123
Fax: (847) 864-1178
http://www.amtamassage.org
Maintains referral information.

American Yoga Association
P.O. Box 19986, Sarasota, FL 34276
Phone: (941) 927-4977
Fax: (941) 921-9844
http://www.americanyogaassociation.org

Cybergrrl Safety Net
http://www.cybergrrl.com/views/dv//book/safe.html
Personalized Safety Plan: information on creating a safety plan for domestic violence.

Division of Nutrition and Physical Activity
National Center for Chronic Disease Prevention and Health Promotion
Centers for Disease Control and Prevention
4770 Buford Highway, NE, MS/K-24, Atlanta, GA 30341-3717
Phone: (770) 488-5820
Fax: (770) 488-5473
http://www.cdc.gov/nccdphp/dnpa/physical/index.htm
Provides information about physical activity.

Family Violence Prevention Fund
383 Rhode Island Street, Suite 304, San Francisco, CA 94103
http://www.silcom.com/~paladin/madv/safetyplan.html
What Is a Safety Plan? *Information for creating a safety plan for domestic violence.*

Fetzer Institute
9292 West KL Avenue, Kalamazoo, MI 49009
Phone: (269) 375-2000
Fax: (269) 372-2163
http://www.fetzer.org
The Fetzer Institute is a nonprofit, private operating foundation that supports research, education, and service programs exploring the integral relationships among body, mind, and spirit. "The key to humanity's future lies in the productive linkage of the mind, body, and spirit."—John E. Fetzer

The March of Dimes
1275 Mamaroneck Avenue, White Plains, NY 10605
Phone: (800) MODIMES
http://www.marchofdimes.com
Information about contraindicated herbs during pregnancy and lactation.

Narcotics Anonymous
World Service Office
P.O. Box 9999, Van Nuys, CA 91409
Phone: (818) 773-9999
Fax: (818) 700-0700
http://www.na.org

The National Association for Holistic Aromatherapy
4509 Interlake Avenue N., #233, Seattle, WA 98103-6773
Phone: (888) ASK-NAHA; (206) 547-2164
Fax: (206) 547-2680
http://www.naha.org

National Center for Post Traumatic Stress Disorder
Phone: (802) 296-6300
http://www.ncptsd.org

The National Sleep Foundation
1522 K Street, NW, Suite 500, Washington, DC 20005
Phone: (202) 347-3471
Fax: (202) 347-3472
http://www.sleepfoundation.org

Nutrition.gov
http://www.nutrition.gov
Information on nutrition.

Office of Dietary Supplements
National Institutes of Health
6100 Executive Boulevard, Room 3B01, MSC 7517, Bethesda, MD 20892-7517
http://www.cc.nih.gov/ccc/supplements
Information on vitamin supplements.

Index

Page numbers followed by f indicate figures; those followed by t indicate tables; and those followed by b indicate boxed material.